Smart Biomimetic Coatings

Woodhead Publishing Series in Biomaterials

Smart Biomimetic Coatings

Design, Properties, and Biomedical Applications

Edited by

JEENAT ASLAM

SAMAN ZEHRA

RUBY ASLAM

CHAUDHERY MUSTANSAR HUSSAIN

ELSEVIER

WP
WOODHEAD
PUBLISHING
An imprint of Elsevier

Woodhead Publishing is an imprint of Elsevier
50 Hampshire Street, 5th Floor, Cambridge, MA 02139, United States
125 London Wall, London EC2Y 5AS, United Kingdom

ISBN: 978-0-443-21738-8 (print)
ISBN: 978-0-443-21739-5 (online)

For information on all Woodhead Publishing publications
visit our website at https://www.elsevier.com/books-and-journals

Publisher: Matthew Deans
Acquisitions Editor: Sabrina Webber
Editorial Project Manager: Fernanda A. Oliveira
Production Project Manager: Prasanna Kalyanaraman
Cover Designer: Mark Rogers

Typeset by MPS Limited, Chennai, India

Contents

List of contributors

Tejas Girish Agnihotri
Department of Pharmaceutics, National Institute of Pharmaceutical Education and Research (NIPER)-Ahmedabad, Gandhinagar, Gujarat, India

Faiza Amin
Department of Science of Dental Materials, Dow University of Health Sciences, Karachi, Pakistan

Afroz Aslam
Department of Chemistry, Constituent Government College, M.J.P. Rohilkhand University, Bareilly, Uttar Pradesh, India

Jeenat Aslam
Department of Chemistry, College of Science, Taibah University, Yanbu, Al-Madina, Saudi Arabia

Ruby Aslam
School of Civil Engineering and Architecture, Chongqing University of Science and Technology, Chongqing, P.R. China

Muhammad Awais
Department of Industrial Engineering, Faculty of Engineering, Taibah University, Madinah, Saudi Arabia

Safee Ullah Chaudhary
Biomedical Informatics & Engineering Research Laboratory, Department of Life Sciences, Lahore University of Management Sciences, Lahore, Pakistan

H. Eivaz Mohammadloo
Color, Resin and Surface Coatings Department, Iran Polymer and Petrochemical Institute, Tehran, Iran

Muhammad Amber Fareed
Clinical Sciences Department, College of Dentistry, Ajman University, Ajman, United Arab Emirates; Center of Medical and Bio-allied Health Sciences Research, Ajman University, Ajman, United Arab Emirates

Shyam Sudhakar Gomte
Department of Pharmaceutics, National Institute of Pharmaceutical Education and Research (NIPER)-Ahmedabad, Gandhinagar, Gujarat, India

Aakanchha Jain
Department of Pharmaceutics, National Institute of Pharmaceutical Education and Research (NIPER)-Ahmedabad, Gandhinagar, Gujarat, India

Naresh Kumar
Department of Science of Dental Materials, Dow University of Health Sciences, Karachi, Pakistan

Nasreena Lone
School of Allied Healthcare & Sciences, JAIN (Deemed-to-be University), Bangalore, Karnataka, India

Nazrah Maher
Department of Science of Dental Materials, Dow University of Health Sciences, Karachi, Pakistan

N. Mehranshad
Department of Polymer Engineering and Color Technology, Amirkabir University of Technology, Tehran, Iran

Mohammad Mobin
Corrosion Research Laboratory, Department of Applied Chemistry, Faculty of Engineering and Technology, Aligarh Muslim University, Aligarh, Uttar Pradesh, India

Hilal Ahmad Parray
Department of Pathology, University of Texas, Dallas, TX, United States

Vasu Peddinti
Department of Pharmaceutics, National Institute of Pharmaceutical Education and Research (NIPER)-Ahmedabad, Gandhinagar, Gujarat, India

B. Ramezanzadeh
Department of Surface Coating and Corrosion, Institute for Color Science and Technology, Tehran, Iran

Andreas Rosenkranz
Department of Chemical Engineering, Biotechnology and Materials, Universidad de Chile, Santiago, Chile

Sh. Roshan
Department of Polymer Engineering and Color Technology, Amirkabir University of Technology, Tehran, Iran

Biswajit Rout
Department of Pharmaceutics, National Institute of Pharmaceutical Education and Research (NIPER)-Ahmedabad, Gandhinagar, Gujarat, India

Qihui Wang
School of Civil Engineering and Architecture, Chongqing University of Science and Technology, Chongqing, P.R. China

Zhitao Yan
School of Civil Engineering and Architecture, Chongqing University of Science and Technology, Chongqing, P.R. China

Muhammad Sohail Zafar
Center of Medical and Bio-allied Health Sciences Research, Ajman University, Ajman, United Arab Emirates; Department of Restorative Dentistry, College of Dentistry, Taibah University, Madinah, Saudi Arabia; Department of Dental Materials, Islamic International Dental College, Riphah International University, Islamabad, Pakistan

Saman Zehra
Corrosion Research Laboratory, Department of Applied Chemistry, Faculty of Engineering and Technology, Aligarh Muslim University, Aligarh, Uttar Pradesh, India

Qi Zhang
School of Civil Engineering and Architecture, Chongqing University of Science and Technology, Chongqing, P.R. China

Chongkang Zhao
School of Civil Engineering and Architecture, Chongqing University of Science and Technology, Chongqing, P.R. China

About the editors

Dr. Jeenat Aslam

Department of Chemistry, College of Science, Taibah University, Yanbu, Al-Madina, Saudi Arabia

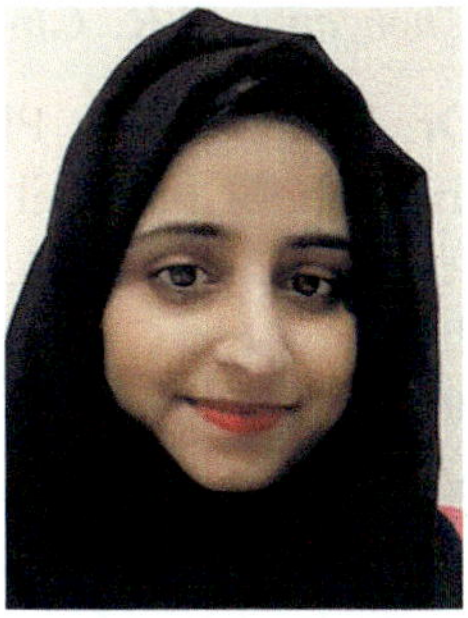

Dr. Jeenat Aslam, PhD, currently serves as an associate professor in the Department of Chemistry at the College of Science, Taibah University, Yanbu, Al-Madina, Saudi Arabia. She has earned her MSc and PhD degrees in surface science/chemistry from Aligarh Muslim University, Aligarh, India. Her research primarily focuses on materials and corrosion, nanotechnology, and surface chemistry. Dr. Jeenat has contributed significantly to her field, publishing numerous research and review articles in esteemed peer-reviewed international journals, including ACS, Wiley, Elsevier, Springer, Taylor & Francis, and Bentham Science. In addition, she has authored more than 40 book chapters and edited more than 30 books for prestigious publishers such as the American Chemical Society, Elsevier, Royal Society of Chemistry, Springer, Wiley, De Gruyter, and Taylor & Francis.

Dr. Saman Zehra

Corrosion Research Laboratory, Department of Applied Chemistry, Faculty of Engineering and Technology, Aligarh Muslim University, Aligarh, India

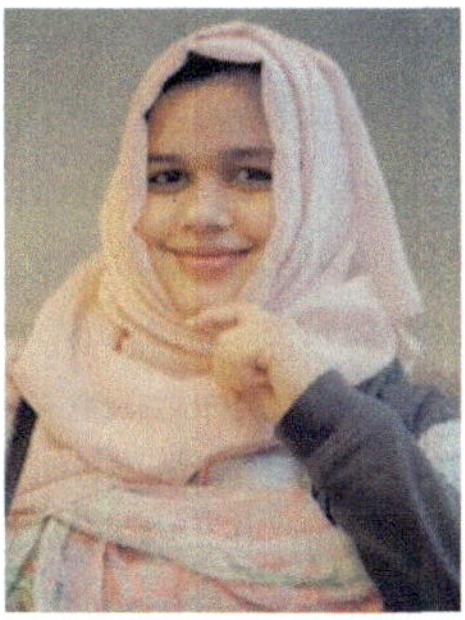

Dr. Saman Zehra, PhD, works at the Women Scientist Program (WOS-A) of DST, New Delhi, in the Department of Applied Chemistry of Aligarh Muslim University, Aligarh, India. Her area of research broadly covers stimuli-responsive smart functional anticorrosion coatings and corrosion inhibitors. She received her PhD and MSc degrees from the same university. She has published 51 articles in international peer-reviewed journals, including reviews, book chapters, and 3 books. With active participation in conferences, her work significantly advances the field of corrosion research.

Dr. Ruby Aslam
School of Civil Engineering and Architecture, Chongqing University of Science and Technology, Chongqing, P.R. China

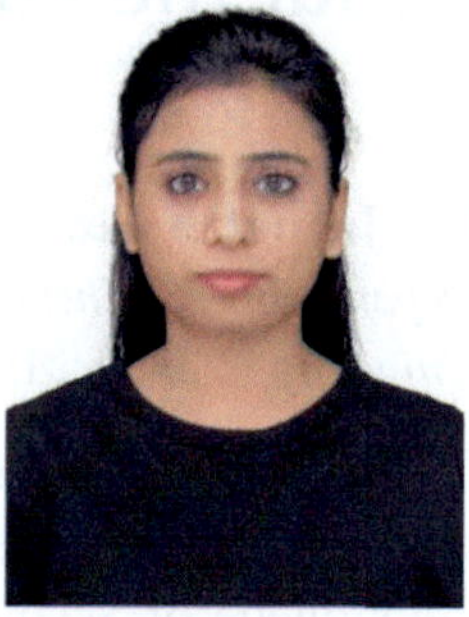

Dr. Ruby Aslam, PhD, is a postdoctoral fellow in the School of Civil Engineering and Architecture at Chongqing University of Science and Technology, Chongqing, China. She received her MSc, MPhil, and PhD degrees from Aligarh Muslim University, India. She has authored/coauthored more than 80 research articles in international peer-reviewed journals of wide readership, including critical reviews and book chapters. She has edited more than 10 books.

Dr. Chaudhery Mustansar Hussain
Department of Chemistry and Environmental Science, New Jersey Institute of Technology, Newark, NJ, United States

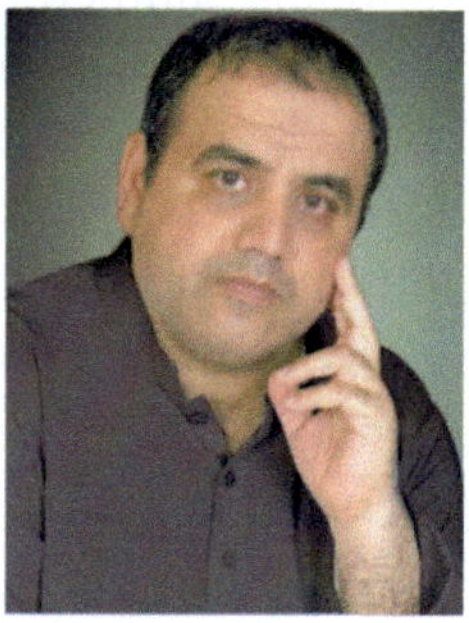

Dr. Chaudhery Mustansar Hussain, PhD, is an adjunct professor and director of laboratories in the Department of Chemistry and Environmental Sciences at the New Jersey Institute of Technology (NJIT), Newark, New Jersey, United States. His research is focused on the applications of nanotechnology and advanced materials, environmental management, analytical chemistry, and other various industries. Dr. Hussain is the author of numerous papers in peer-reviewed journals as well as a prolific author and editor of around 150 books, including scientific monographs and handbooks in his research areas. He has published with Elsevier, American Chemical Society, Royal Society of Chemistry, John Wiley & Sons, CRC Press, and Springer.

Preface

The biomimetic surface coating process stands out as a highly versatile technique, demonstrating its efficacy in coating diverse surfaces for various applications. Coatings, whether applied for decorative, protective, or functional purposes, often serve a combination of these roles. Bioinspired materials present a sustainable solution, mitigating catastrophic failure and extending service life. Despite their potential, the intricate fabrication process poses scalability challenges. Nature, with its millions of years of evolution, offers a wealth of ingeniously engineered materials. The complex and spontaneous multifunctionality observed in natural systems serves as a wellspring of inspiration for materials scientists developing multifunctional surface coating formulations. The book highlights the importance of understanding the intricate architecture of natural composites, derived from extensive evolutionary changes, to create composite materials with exceptional performance. Drawing inspiration from plants, arthropods, mammals, and marine organisms such as nacre, bone, and lotus leaf, the biomimetic approach extends beyond mimicking biological structures to include replicating biological functions.

This comprehensive book, structured into 12 chapters, consolidates essential research on multifunctional surface coatings. The focus spans diverse applications such as orthopedic and dental implants, tissue engineering, marine systems, and sensors. Aimed at scholars in academia and industry, corrosion engineers, and materials science students, the book serves as a valuable resource for applied and engineering chemistry. The structured format provides readers with a systematic and up-to-date reference, offering a concentrated exploration of fundamental aspects, applications, and implementation studies related to biomimetic coatings.

Chapter 1 sets the stage by providing a comprehensive overview of biomimetic coatings. Delving into the foundational concepts, it aims to establish a solid understanding of this innovative field. Following this introduction, Chapter 2 delves into the intricacies of the synthesis processes and key properties associated with biomimetic coatings. Moving forward, Chapter 3 focuses on the application of the biomimetic technique in coating various surfaces of orthopedic implants, offering insights into advancements in medical technology. Chapters 4–9 explore diverse applications, including dental implants, marine antifouling coatings, self-cleaning technologies, bone regeneration, drug delivery, and anticorrosion measures. Chapter 10 specifically investigates the impact of biomimetic coatings on tribocorrosion. Chapter 11 delves into their effectiveness in antimicrobial applications. Finally, Chapter 12 provides a forward-looking perspective on the future of biomimicry in smart coatings, projecting potential advancements and applications across various fields. This comprehensive journey through biomimetic coatings underscores their multifaceted contributions to science and technology.

The principal aim of this book is to present the most recent advancements in the application of biomimetic coatings across various industrial and medical contexts. Tailored for a diverse audience in materials chemistry, chemical engineering, and related fields, it stands as a valuable resource for professionals, researchers, and students within academic, government, and nonprofit sectors. Designed to address contemporary research needs, this book serves as a comprehensive guide for those seeking profound insights into the utilization of biomimetic coatings.

Each chapter has undergone meticulous editing by esteemed academic and professional researchers, scientists, and subject matter specialists. The book expresses gratitude to the chapter authors for their exceptional and sincere contributions to this work. Special acknowledgment is extended to Dr. Sabrina Webber (Acquisitions Editor), Ms. Fernanda A. Oliveira (Editorial Project Manager), and the Editorial Team at Elsevier for their unwavering support and assistance throughout the project. The commendable release of the book by Elsevier is an achievement deserving of praise.

Jeenat Aslam
Saman Zehra
Ruby Aslam
Chaudhery Mustansar Hussain

CHAPTER 1

Biomimetic coatings: an introduction

Saman Zehra and Mohammad Mobin
Corrosion Research Laboratory, Department of Applied Chemistry, Faculty of Engineering and Technology, Aligarh Muslim University, Aligarh, Uttar Pradesh, India

1.1 Introduction

The natural world harbors a plethora of remarkable structures, offering sustainable solutions to human challenges through time-tested patterns. The interdisciplinary pursuit of drawing inspiration, adapting, or deriving designs from nature is known as biomimetics (Xia, 2016). This evolving field has witnessed a surge in research interest, with no signs of regression (Vijayan & Puglia, 2019; Zhan et al., 2018). Harnessing the secrets of nature has been a historical endeavor to enhance the quality of life, especially as we navigate the current millennium heralded as the "age of materials."

Biomimetics entails understanding the functions, structures, and principles of biological entities, and the term itself emerged in 1974, denoting the study of biologically produced substances and materials for the synthesis of similar products through artificial mechanisms (Zhan et al., 2018).

Nature's materials exhibit exceptional properties—biodegradability, self-generation, antireflection, self-cleaning, protective qualities, and self-healing mechanisms (Jiang et al., 2022). Consequently, scientists and engineers have increasingly turned to nature for inspiration in developing bioinspired or biomimetic materials, forming a bridge between biology and engineering (Bar-Cohen, 2006, 2011; Perera & Coppens, 2019). Biomimicry is one type of bioinspired design, but not all bioinspired designs are Biomimicry. The difference between the nature-inspired materials can be understood with the help of the illustration in Fig. 1.1.

As a burgeoning scientific discipline, bioinspired engineering extends its applications to medicine, industries, the environment, and beyond. Precisely, bioinspired coatings mimic the structures, properties, or functions of natural materials, necessitating a deep exploration into how living entities adapt to their environments (Chen et al., 2021; Harun-Ur-Rashid et al., 2023).

Smart Biomimetic Coatings
DOI: https://doi.org/10.1016/B978-0-443-21738-8.00001-1

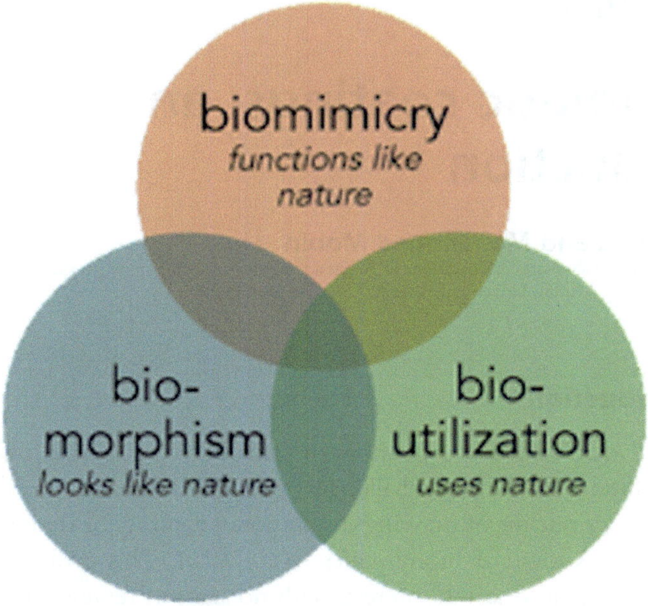

Figure 1.1 Classification of bioinspired materials.

This chapter explores the profound impact of Biomimicry on coatings, delving into how biological principles are employed to create innovative solutions, and examines Biomimicry in the context of its applications in coatings, offering an in-depth analysis of the basics of biomimetic coatings. This interdisciplinary approach aims to transform biological insights into engineering solutions, tools, and mechanisms by uncovering the potential inherent in nature's capabilities. The collaborative efforts of experts from biology and engineering are essential in bridging these fields and categorizing biological capabilities into technological advancements.

1.2 Historical overview of the biomimetic coatings

Biomimetic coatings are coatings that mimic the properties or functions of natural materials or systems. They are inspired by the shapes, structures, or principles of nature to achieve desired biological responses or improve the performance of the coated materials or surfaces. The idea of biomimetics, involving the study and emulation of nature, has roots in ancient times. During those early periods, humans observed and replicated behaviors or characteristics of animals and plants for diverse purposes like hunting, fishing, or achieving flight (Antony et al., n.d.).

Otto Schmitt, an American biophysicist and polymath, introduced the term biomimetics in the 1950s. During this period, he devised the Schmitt trigger, a device that mimicked the biological nerve propagation system. This innovation was inspired by Schmitt's study of nerves in squid (Harkness, 2002). The first evidence of crude dental implants, which can be considered as a form of biomimetic coating, was found in Roman and pre-Columbian cultures of Central and South America in the first and second centuries. Dental amalgam, a blend of metals designed to replicate the characteristics of natural teeth, made its inaugural appearance in Chinese literature in the year BCE 659 (Singer et al., 2023).

During the 1960s, Janine Benyus, an American natural sciences writer, played a pivotal role in advancing and promoting the concept of biomimetics. Her book, *Biomimicry: Innovation Inspired by Nature*, became a seminal work, introducing numerous instances of biomimetic technologies and their applications across various fields (Singer et al., 2023). In the 1970s, the progress of biomimetic coatings received a significant boost with the identification of hydroxyapatite. Larry Hench, an American materials scientist, discovered this mineral, which constitutes the primary component of natural bone. Hench then synthesized it into a biocompatible and bioactive ceramic material specifically for the purpose of bone repair and regeneration (Mozafari et al., 2018).

During the 1980s, the exploration of biomimetic coatings broadened to encompass a range of other natural materials or systems. This expansion included investigations into insect eyes, butterfly wings, sharkskin, lotus leaves, and seaweed, each exhibiting diverse functions such as optical, mechanical, chemical, or antifouling properties (Wang et al., 2016). In the 1990s, the progress in nanotechnology and microfabrication facilitated the development of biomimetic coatings, allowing for meticulous control of surface morphology and processes. This advancement spanned from the macroscale to the nanoscale, accompanied by a high degree of fault tolerance (Wang et al., 2016).

Throughout the 2000s, the realm of biomimetic coatings reached a stage of maturity and diversification. Novel and enhanced technologies surfaced across various stages of development, spanning from laboratory experimentation to commercialization. These innovations found extensive applications in diverse domains, including engineering, medicine, energy, and biotechnology (Wang et al., 2016). The literature from 2000 to 2023 has immensely increased as can be seen in Fig. 1.2.

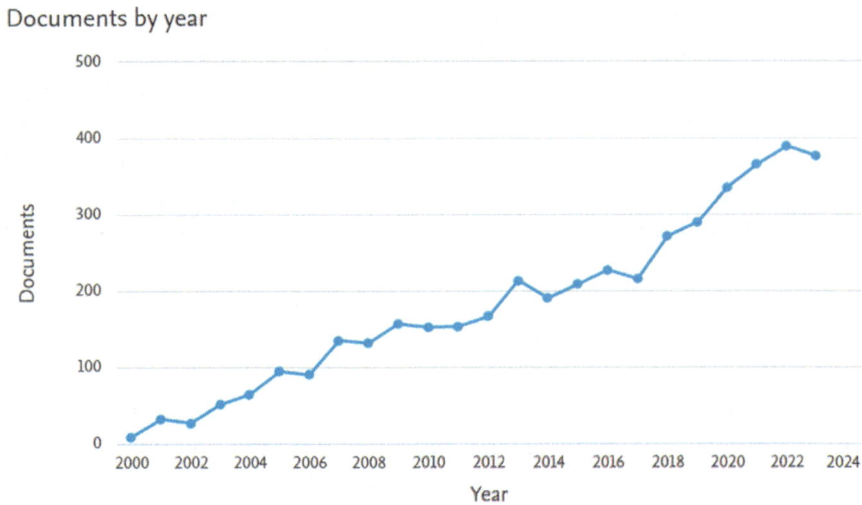

Figure 1.2 Literature from 2000 to 2023 as per the Scopus database by searching the keywords biomimetic coatings and biomimicry.

1.3 Key concept of biomimetic coatings

Through careful observation and comprehension of natural processes, humans can create products, processes, and systems that align more harmoniously with the environment and the interconnected web of life on Earth. As scientists and engineers delve deeper into understanding biological principles, new possibilities for biomimetic applications continue to emerge, paving the way for advancements in materials science and technology. Some of the key concepts involved in the field of biomimetic coatings are discussed in the following sections.

1.3.1 Nature-inspired design

Biomimetic coatings draw inspiration from nature's diverse forms, structures, and mechanisms. By emulating natural strategies, these coatings aim to replicate and harness the efficiency and functionality inherent in biological systems.

1.3.2 Functional mimicry

The primary goal of biomimetic coatings is to mimic specific functions or properties observed in nature. This includes replicating features such as self-cleaning, antifouling, superwettability, and other unique attributes found in biological organisms and materials.

1.3.3 Interdisciplinary approach

The development of biomimetic coatings involves collaboration across multiple disciplines, including biology, chemistry, physics, and engineering. This interdisciplinary approach is essential for understanding the underlying biological principles and translating them into practical coating applications.

1.3.4 Biocompatibility

Biomimetic coatings are designed to be biocompatible, ensuring that they can interact harmoniously with biological systems without causing harm. This feature makes them suitable for applications in medicine, such as orthopedic implants or drug delivery systems.

1.3.5 Environmental friendliness

One of the key advantages of biomimetic coatings is their environment-friendly nature. Often derived from natural materials or inspired by sustainable processes, these coatings offer a greener alternative to traditional coatings that may rely on synthetic and potentially harmful chemicals.

1.3.6 Versatility in applications

Biomimetic coatings find applications across various industries, including engineering, medicine, energy, and biotechnology. Their adaptability allows for a wide range of uses, from enhancing the performance of medical implants to improving the efficiency of solar cells.

1.3.7 Innovative material synthesis

The development of biomimetic coatings often involves innovative material synthesis methods. This may include creating bioinspired materials or replicating intricate surface topographies to achieve the desired functional properties.

1.3.8 Responsive mechanisms

Biomimetic coatings can incorporate responsive mechanisms inspired by biological systems. This adaptability allows the coatings to respond to environmental stimuli, contributing to their self-healing, self-cleaning, or other dynamic functionalities.

1.4 Inspiration of the biomimetic coatings

Biomimetic coatings are used in various fields such as aerospace, automotive, solar energy, marine technology, electronics, architecture, and medical. Many fields use nature for inspiration because it has worked for thousands of years.

The fundamentals involved in the design of the biomimetic coatings are represented in Fig. 1.3. Several coatings have multipurposes and can be used in many fields. There are a variety of bioinspired coatings, and naming them all could take a while. The brief outlines of various inspirations used in the biomimetic coatings are discussed in the following sections.

1.4.1 Shark skin

Inspiration: The unique dermal denticles of sharks reduce drag and inhibit the attachment of marine organisms. Biomimetic engineering of shark skin surfaces to study antibiofouling properties has attracted considerable interest in recent years (Liu & Li, 2012; Munther et al., 2018). Sharkskin exhibits a highly complex surface structure, consisting of micro-arrays named placoid scales or dermal denticles. Denticles exhibit a riblet-like morphology; the surface of concave grooves was found to exhibit nanostructured protuberances (Feld et al., 2019; Xia et al., 2018). The unique structure of the denticles allows sharks to reduce drag and move more efficiently through water (Wen et al., 2015) as well as prevents the attachment and growth of microorganisms (Zhang et al., 2017). The structure of shark skin and biomimetic shark skin is shown in Fig. 1.4.

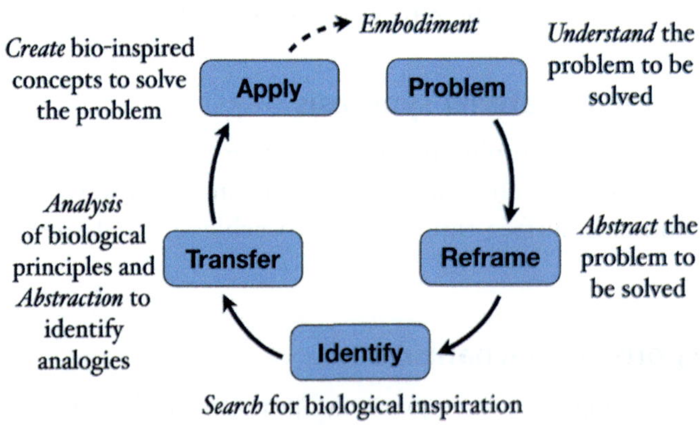

Figure 1.3 Scanning electron Micrographs of shark skin and biomimetic shark skin: (A) the riblet structures of shark surface; (B) the surface of biomimetic shark skin prepared.

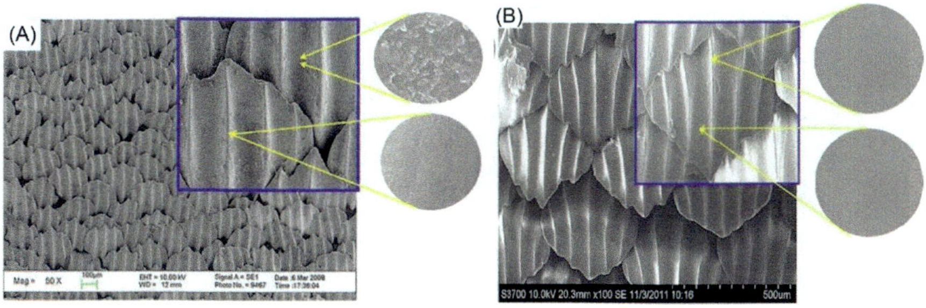

Figure 1.4 Two-level hierarchical structure of the water strider's leg, which exhibits microstructures with fine nanoscale grooves under the field emission scanning electron mircographs of eye: (A) a G. remigis insect, which is floating in a pond, (B) the water strider's frontal leg, which is covered by numerous oriented needle-shaped microsetae, (C) the nanogrooves of a microseta, which is composed of several papillae (D). *From Pu, X., Li, G., & Huang, H. (2016).* Biology Open. *5. (Original work published 2016.)*

Application: Antifouling coatings for ship hulls and underwater structures.

1.4.2 Lotus leaf

Inspiration: The lotus leaf's self-cleaning ability is due to its micro- and nanostructured surface. Lotus leaf, specifically the *Nelumbo nucifera*, has the natural ability to repel water droplets at a high contact angle (>150 degrees), thus being superhydrophobic (Latthe et al., 2014; Mozumder et al., 2011). In addition the lotus leaf utilizes its high contact angle to cause the water droplets to roll off the leaf at a low sliding angle (<5 degrees)—the rolling droplets collect any debris that the leaf contains, thus providing a naturally occurring self-cleaning property (Zorba et al., 2008). This is referred to as the "Lotus Effect." This can be best demonstrated by Fig. 1.5A.

The unique nature of the lotus leaf appears more obvious when examined by a scanning electron microscope, as viewed in Fig. 1.5B, which resembles a natural terrain consisting of hills and valleys. The valleys exist between and around the hills, which can be alluded to form the earlier discussed microscale structure. The water droplets cannot reach the valley areas due to their larger size. In addition the debris never enters deep enough into the valleys due to the repelling nature of the nanoscale hair-like structure, which pushes the debris up so it can be collected by the rolling water droplets (Cheng et al., 2006). Fig. 1.5C provides a simple diagram of the hydrophobic structure of a lotus leaf that governs the lotus

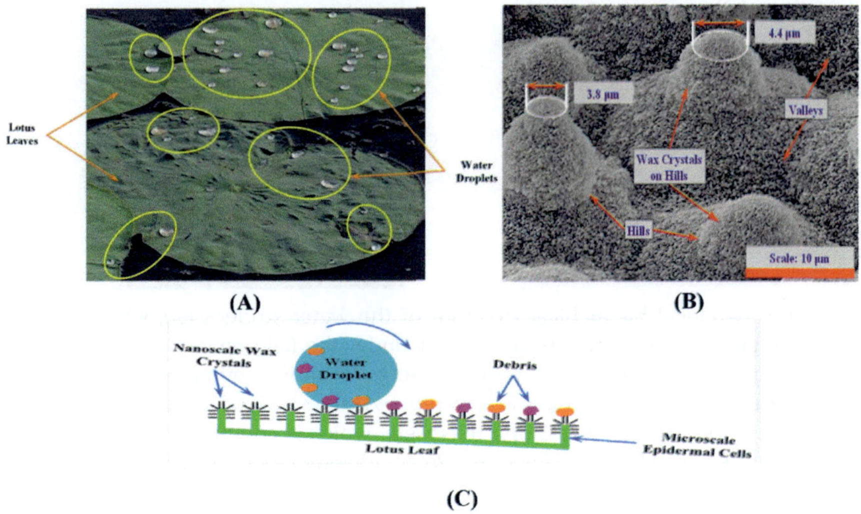

Figure 1.5 (A) Lotus leaves with "lotus effect," (B) an scanning electron mircographs image of the lotus leaf, and (C) A simple schematic for understanding of the lotus effect. *From Poole, B. (2007). (Original work published 2007.)*

effect. The high contact angle creates a rolling effect of the water droplets supported by the micro-protrusions (microscale epidermal cells). The nanoscale wax crystals facilitate the water droplets to remain buoyant, roll down, and collect the debris before descending from the leaf.

Application: Coatings with self-cleaning properties for surfaces like glass and solar panels.

1.4.3 Butterfly wings

Inspiration: Nanostructures on butterfly wings that create vibrant colors and superhydrophobicity. The various optical properties are one of the most outstanding features of the butterfly wings (Pantelić et al., 2011; Vukusic et al., 2000). The Morpho butterflies are known for the brilliant color of their wings (Niu et al., 2015), while the Greta oto butterfly exhibits omnidirectional antireflection property (Siddique et al., 2015). Besides the optical properties, the surface wettability of the butterfly wings has also been studied in recent researches. These researches have demonstrated the extremely hydrophobicity and directional adhesion properties of the wing scales, which indicate that the butterfly wings may be applied in directional coatings and novel microfluidic systems.

Application: Coatings for optical devices, lenses, and solar cells with enhanced properties.

1.4.4 Water striders

Inspiration: The hydrophobic legs of water striders (*Gerris remigis*) that enable them to walk on water. The water strider is a wonderful case that we can learn from nature to understand how to stride on the water surface (Fig. 1.6). It possesses an impressive capability to effortlessly stand, walk, and even leap on the surface of water (Dickinson, 2003). Original investigations into the physical mechanism have unveiled that the force supporting the water strider comprises three primary components: buoyancy force, curvature force, and deformation force (Hu et al., 2003). The water strider's movement is rooted in the momentum generated by swirling vortices beneath the water surface, resembling the action of an oar. Additionally,

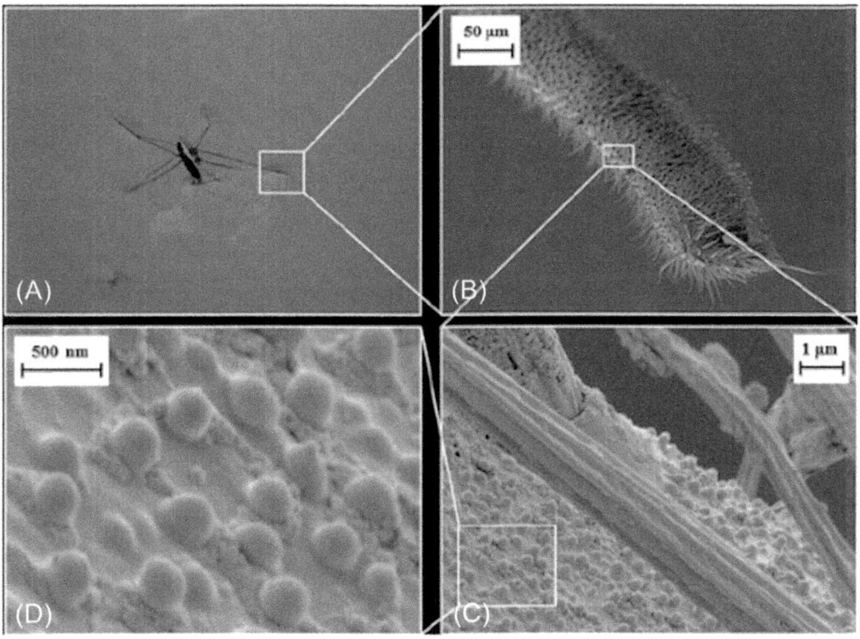

Figure 1.6 Two-level hierarchical structure of the water strider's leg, which exhibits microstructures with fine nanoscale grooves under the field emission scanning electron mircographs eye: (A) a *Gerris remigis* insect, which is floating in a pond, (B) the water strider's frontal leg, which is covered by numerous oriented needle-shaped microsetae, (C) the nanogrooves of a microseta, which is composed of several papillae (D) (Lepore et al., 2013).

chemical studies have delved deeper into the water strider, revealing that its exceptional water-walking ability arises from the remarkable water repellency of its legs (Gao & Jiang, 2004). These legs feature thousands of tiny setae with intricate nanogroove structures. These setae and nanogrooves effectively trap numerous air bubbles under the water, providing robust support for the water strider to traverse and move effortlessly on the water surface.

Application: Superhydrophobic coatings for water-resistant surfaces.

1.4.5 Chameleons

Inspiration: Chameleons' ability to change color for communication and camouflage. The radiative control by a chameleon, which controls visible (VIS) light and reflects near-infrared (NIR) light, is ideal in many cases. A chameleon controls light by dispersion (or aggregation) of pigment-containing organelles within its dermal chromatophores. It organizes iridophores into two superposed layers to create efficient camouflage with spectacular display while potentially providing a passive thermal protection. Within the superficial thick layer of the dermal iridophores, chameleons change color (VIS light) by active tuning a lattice of guanine nanocrystals. A denser population of iridophores with large crystals reflects a substantial proportion of sunlight, especially in the NIR range (Fig. 1.7A). For example, products such as cars and buildings are usually exposed to too much sunlight. In many cases, dark-color coatings are preferably used in these products for appearance purposes. However, these dark coatings absorb a large amount of solar irradiation in the VIS and NIR regions. Therefore the interior temperature becomes high and creates a large cooling load in air-conditioning systems. The resultant energy consumption contributes to environmental problems such as the greenhouse effect (Seneviratne et al., 2016) and urban heat islands. In a situation where a surface must be kept cool when exposed to sunlight, the surface should have maximum solar-energy reflectance. The biomimetic coatings inspired by the chameleons can be used (Fig. 1.7B and C).

Application: Developments in adaptive coatings for textiles or materials with color-changing capabilities.

1.4.6 Gecko feet

Inspiration: Gecko feet's adhesive properties due to microscopic hairs (Fig. 1.8).

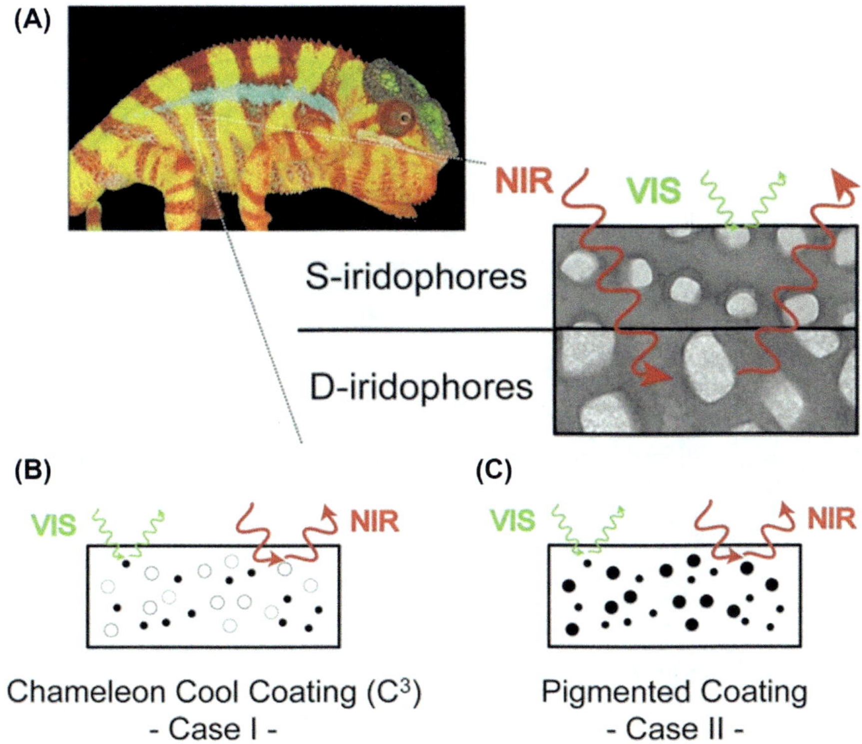

Figure 1.7 C3 concept. (A) Schematic of the thermal barrier in a chameleon. Picture of chameleon and transmission electron microscope image of guanine nanocrystals in superficial (S-) and deep (D-) iridophores obtained from a paper written by Teyssier et al. (B) Schematic of C3. The black particle controls the VIS light, and the white particle reflects the NIR light. (C) Schematic of a usual coating pigmented by a single particle. *NIR*, Near-infrared; *VIS*, visible. *From Gonome, H., Nakamura, M., Okajima, J., & Maruyama, S. (2018).* Scientific Reports. *8. (Original work published 2018.)*

Application: Adhesive coatings for temporary attachment or climbing applications.

1.4.7 Spider silk

Inspiration: The strength and flexibility of spider silk. Spider silks produced by spiders are unique protein-based biofibres possessing extraordinary properties, such as high tensile strength and toughness as well as super contraction (Bell et al., 2002; Omenetto & Kaplan, 2010). Meanwhile, spider silks are biocompatible and biodegradable (Chung et al., 2012).

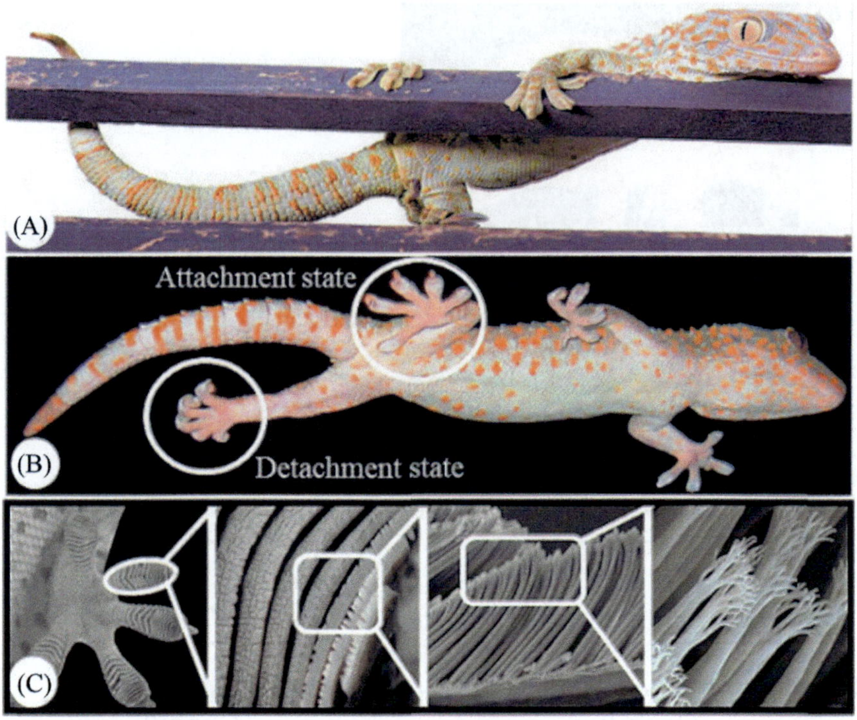

Figure 1.8 Morphological features of a gecko: (A) the climbing state of a gecko on a wooden pole; (B) the attachment state and detachment state of gecko feet; (C) The microscopic structure of gecko feet. *From Autumn, K., & Gravish, N. (2008).* Philosophical Transactions of the Royal Society A: Mathematical, Physical and Engineering Sciences. *366. (Original work published 2008.)*

Application: Creating durable and flexible coatings for various applications, such as medicine, textiles, and engineering.

1.4.8 Mussel adhesion

Inspiration: The adhesive properties of mussel proteins for strong and resilient underwater adhesion.

Application: Developing coatings for underwater structures and medical adhesives.

1.4.9 Moth eyes

Inspiration: Nanostructures on moth eyes that minimize reflection and enhance light absorption (Fig. 1.9). The surfaces of their eyes are covered with a layer of a subwavelength structure that eliminates reflections of

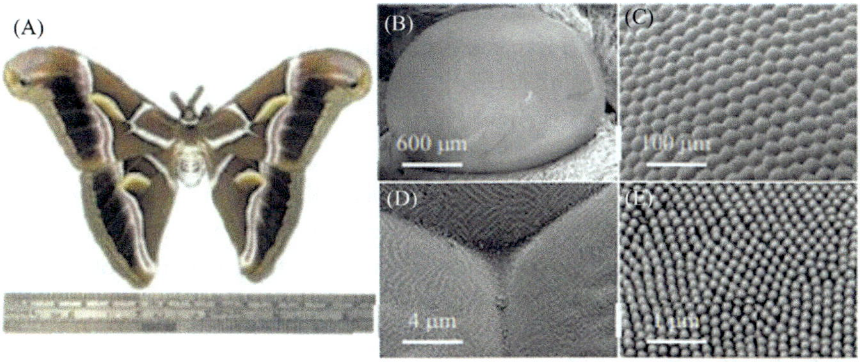

Figure 1.9 (A) The photograph of the adult Philosamia cynthia ricini was obtained from the Miaoli District Agricultural Research and Extension Station, Council of Agricultural, Taiwan. Scanning electron micrographs images of the Philosamia cynthia ricini moth-eye structure at different magnifications: (B) the complete compound eyes, (C) the hexagonal arrangement of ommatidia, (D) the details of the ommatidia, and (E) the corneal nipple arrays in one ommatidium. *From Kuo, W. -K., Hsu, J. -J., Nien, C.-K., & Yu, H. H. (2016).* ACS Applied Materials & Interfaces. *8. (Original work published 2016.)*

VIS light. This layer allows the eyes of moths to escape detection in darkness, without reflections that could reveal the position of the moths to potential predators.

Application: Coatings for reducing glare in optical devices.

These diverse inspirations from the natural world serve as blueprints for developing biomimetic coatings with unique and beneficial properties, showcasing the versatility of nature-inspired design in materials science and technology.

1.5 Application of biomimetic coatings in various fields

Biomimetic coatings serve the purpose of enhancing the performance, durability, and functionality of coated surfaces or materials. Biomimetic coatings draw inspiration from nature but can surpass natural capabilities by combining different features or incorporating synthetic materials to achieve novel or improved functions. Notably, these coatings are recognized for their environment-friendly, biocompatible, and cost-effective characteristics, providing sustainable alternatives to conventional coatings reliant on synthetic chemicals or additives. With their versatility, biomimetic coatings are anticipated to find widespread applications across various fields, spanning engineering, medicine, energy, and biotechnology.

Their applications are diverse, aiming to address specific challenges and improve various aspects. Here are some notable areas where biomimetic coatings are applied (Li et al., 2023).

1.5.1 Medical devices

Biomimetic coatings can be used on medical implants and devices to improve biocompatibility, reduce rejection rates, and promote tissue integration. Examples include coatings mimicking the structure of natural bone or enhancing the blood compatibility of surfaces.

1.5.2 Antifouling surfaces

Coatings inspired by marine organisms, such as the lotus leaf or shark skin, can be applied to ship hulls to reduce biofouling and increase hydrodynamics, leading to improved fuel efficiency.

1.5.3 Self-cleaning surfaces

Mimicking the self-cleaning properties of certain plants and insects, biomimetic coatings can be used on surfaces exposed to environmental elements, such as building exteriors and car windshields, to repel dirt and maintain cleanliness.

1.5.4 Optics and sensors

Biomimetic coatings can enhance the performance of optical devices by mimicking the nanostructures found in butterfly wings or moth eyes, improving light absorption or reflection for various applications, including sensors and imaging systems.

1.5.5 Energy harvesting

Coatings inspired by photosynthetic processes in plants can be applied to capture and convert solar energy efficiently. These biomimetic coatings have potential applications in solar panels and other energy-harvesting devices.

1.5.6 Aerospace materials

Biomimetic coatings with lightweight and strong structures, inspired by natural materials like bird feathers or insect cuticles, can be utilized in the aerospace industry to improve the strength-to-weight ratio of components.

1.5.7 Water harvesting

Coatings inspired by desert beetles or cacti can be used to collect water from the atmosphere, offering a potential solution for water scarcity in arid regions.

1.5.8 Textiles and fabrics

Biomimetic coatings can be applied to textiles to impart water-repellent, stain-resistant, or antibacterial properties, mimicking the characteristics of certain plant surfaces or animal fur.

The versatility of biomimetic coatings across these diverse applications highlights the potential for nature-inspired solutions to address challenges in various industries.

1.6 Conclusion

In this chapter, it becomes evident that nature stands as an unparalleled source of inspiration and innovation for materials science and engineering. The exploration of biomimicry, a concept rooted in learning from nature's time-tested solutions, has paved the way for the development of coatings that emulate the remarkable properties found in diverse biological systems. From the antifouling abilities inspired by shark skin to the self-cleaning attributes borrowed from lotus leaves, biomimetic coatings exhibit a remarkable capacity to enhance the performance, durability, and functionality of diverse surfaces. The mimicry of structures, chemical compositions, and functional mechanisms found in nature has led to coatings with self-healing capabilities, superwettability, and responsiveness to environmental stimuli.

The interdisciplinary nature of biomimetic coatings, bridging biology, chemistry, physics, and engineering, underscores the importance of collaboration and knowledge integration across these domains. This collaborative effort has enabled the translation of biological principles into practical solutions, opening avenues for sustainable and environment-friendly alternatives to conventional coatings.

As biomimetic coatings continue to evolve, they hold great promise in addressing global challenges across various industries. Their applications in engineering, medicine, energy, and biotechnology showcase the versatility and adaptability of these coatings in providing innovative solutions. Moreover, the ethical and philosophical underpinnings of biomimicry urge us to respect and appreciate nature not only as a resource but as a source of wisdom, fostering a deeper connection between scientific advancement and ecological harmony.

In essence, this chapter has provided a comprehensive introduction to the world of biomimetic coatings, offering insights into the fundamental concepts, applications, and future directions of this exciting and rapidly advancing field. As researchers and practitioners delve further into nature's intricacies, the potential for biomimetic coatings to shape a more sustainable and resilient future remains both promising and inspiring.

Acknowledgment

One of the authors gratefully acknowledges funding from the Department of Science and Technology (DST), New Delhi, India, for the funding under the Women Scientist (WOS-A) program [File number: SR-WOS-A-ET-54-2019].

References

Antony, S., Anju, T.R., & Thomas, B. (n.d.). *Handbook of biopolymers* (pp. 1–31). Springer Nature Singapore.

Bar-Cohen, Y. (2006). *Bioinspiration & Biomimetics, 1*, P1–P12.

Bar-Cohen, Y. (2011). *Biomimetics: Nature-based innovation*. CRC press.

Bell, F. I., McEwen, I. J., & Viney, C. (2002). *Nature, 416*.

Chen, L., Duan, Y., Cui, M., Huang, R., Su, R., Qi, W., & He, Z. (2021). *Science of the Total Environment, 766*.

Cheng, Y. T., Rodak, D. E., Wong, C. A., & Hayden, C. A. (2006). *Nanotechnology, 17*.

Chung, H., Kim, T. Y., & Lee, S. Y. (2012). *Current Opinion in Biotechnology, 23*.

Dickinson, M. (2003). *Nature, 424*.

Feld, K., Kolborg, A. N., Nyborg, C. M., Salewski, M., Steffensen, J. F., & Berg-Sørensen, K. (2019). *Biomimetics, 4*.

Gao, X., & Jiang, L. (2004). *Nature, 432*.

Harkness, J. M. (2002). *Physics in Perspective, 4*.

Harun-Ur-Rashid, M., Jahan, I., Foyez, T., & Imran, A. B. (2023). *Micromachines, 14*.

Hu, D. L., Chan, B., & Bush, J. W. (2003). *Nature, 424*.

Jiang, S., Diao, Y., & Yang, H. (2022). *Advances in Colloid and Interface Science*.

Latthe, S. S., Terashima, C., Nakata, K., & Fujishima, A. (2014). *Molecules, 19*.

Lepore, E., Giorcelli, M., Saggese, C., Tagliaferro, A., & Pugno, N. (2013). *Journal of Materials Research, 28*.

Li, K., Liu, X., & Zhang, Y. (2023). *Biogeotechnics, 1*.

Liu, Y., & Li, G. (2012). *Journal of Colloid and Interface Science, 388*.

Mozafari, M., Rajadas, J., & Kaplan, D. L. (2018). *Nanoengineered biomaterials for regenerative medicine* (pp. 1–488). Elsevier. Available from http://www.sciencedirect.com/science/book/9780128133552, 10.1016/C2016-0-03951-7.

Mozumder, M. S., Zhang, H., & Zhu, J. (2011). *Macromolecular Materials and Engineering, 296*.

Munther, M., Palma, T., Angeron, I. A., Salari, S., Ghassemi, H., Vasefi, M., Beheshti, A., & Davami, K. (2018). *Applied Surface Science, 453*.

Niu, S., Li, B., Mu, Z., Yang, M., Zhang, J., Han, Z., & Ren, L. (2015). *Journal of Bionic Engineering, 12.*

Omenetto, F. G., & Kaplan, D. L. (2010). *Science, 329.*

Pantelić, D., Ćurčić, S., Savić-Šević, S., Korać, A., Kovačević, A., Ćurčić, B., & Bokić, B. (2011). *Optics Express, 19.*

Perera, A. S., & Coppens, M.-O. (2019). *Philosophical Transactions of the Royal Society A, 377.*

Poole, B. (2007). *Biomimetics: Borrowing from Biology. Science Features.* The Naked Scientists, 2007. Available online: https://www.thenakedscientists.com/articles/science-features/biomimetics-borrowing-biology (accessed on 29 December 2020).

Seneviratne, S. I., Donat, M. G., Pitman, A. J., Knutti, R., & Wilby, R. L. (2016). *Nature, 529.*

Siddique, R. H., Gomard, G., & Hölscher, H. (2015). *Nature Communications, 6.*

Singer, L., Fouda, A., & Bourauel, C. (2023). *BMC Oral Health, 23.*

Vijayan, P. P., & Puglia, D. (2019). *Emergent Materials, 2.*

Vukusic, P., Sambles, J., & Lawrence, C. (2000). *Nature, 404.*

Wang, Z., Elimelech, M., & Lin, S. (2016). *Environmental Science & Technology, 50.*

Wen, L., Weaver, J. C., Thornycroft, P. J., & Lauder, G. V. (2015). *Bioinspiration & Biomimetics, 10.*

Xia, P., Guangji, L., Hanlu, H., Yunhong, L., & Ashraf, M. A. (2018). *Brazilian Archives of Biology and Technology, 60.*

Xia, Z. (2016). *Biomimetic principles and design of advanced engineering materials.* Wiley. Available from 10.1002/9781118926253.

Zhan, Y., Zhang, J., Wan, X., Long, Z., He, S., & He, Y. (2018). *Applied Surface Science, 436.*

Zhang, Y., Zhao, W., Chen, Z., Liu, Z., Cao, H., Zhou, C., & Cui, P. (2017). *Colloids and Surfaces A: Physicochemical and Engineering Aspects, 528.*

Zorba, V., Stratakis, E., Barberoglou, M., Spanakis, E., Tzanetakis, P., Anastasiadis, S. H., & Fotakis, C. (2008). *Advanced Materials, 20.*

CHAPTER 2

Synthesis and properties of biomimetic coatings

Saman Zehra
Corrosion Research Laboratory, Department of Applied Chemistry, Faculty of Engineering and Technology, Aligarh Muslim University, Aligarh, Uttar Pradesh, India

2.1 Introduction

In the pursuit of fabricating advanced materials with unprecedented properties, scientists and engineers have increasingly turned to nature as a source of inspiration (Wang, Hu et al., 2020). The remarkable adaptability, efficiency, and multifunctionality found in biological systems have sparked a burgeoning field at the intersection of biology and materials science: biomimicry (Gebeshuber, 2023). One particularly captivating facet of this interdisciplinary exploration is the synthesis and properties of biomimetic coatings.

Biomimetic coatings seek to emulate the structural intricacies and functional prowess observed in nature's diverse array of organisms. From the self cleaning surfaces inspired by the lotus leaf to the gecko's remarkable ability to cling effortlessly to vertical surfaces, researchers are harnessing the design principles refined by evolution for millions of years (Lin et al., 2011; Xu, Zhang et al., 2016). The pursuit of these coatings is driven by the desire to mimic nature's elegance and the practical implications they hold across a spectrum of applications. From enhancing the durability of everyday materials to revolutionizing medical devices and advancing technology, biomimetic coatings offer a glimpse into a future where materials are functional and dynamically responsive to their environment (Liu et al., 2023).

In this chapter, the main aim is to explore how biomimetic coatings draw inspiration from the lotus leaf's hydrophobicity, the gecko's adhesive prowess, and the photonic brilliance of butterfly wings (Collins & Safiuddin, 2022). Additionally, the mechanical, thermal, and chemical properties that make these coatings not only intriguing but also immensely practical for a

Smart Biomimetic Coatings
DOI: https://doi.org/10.1016/B978-0-443-21738-8.00002-3

myriad of applications are also scrutinized. On the exploration, it becomes clear that the synthesis and properties of biomimetic coatings represent a scientific endeavor and a bridge between the natural world and human ingenuity. The knowledge gained from this synthesis propels the field forward and opens doors to novel possibilities, pushing the boundaries of what materials can achieve.

This chapter serves as a comprehensive guide, navigating through the various synthesis methods employed in creating biomimetic coatings and unraveling the multifaceted properties exhibited by these marvels of biomimicry. This chapter embarks on a journey into the heart of biomimetic coatings, unraveling the synthesis techniques that enable the replication of nature's ingenuity and exploring the diverse properties that emerge.

2.2 Background on biomimicry in materials science

In the realm of materials science, the quest for innovation often takes inspiration from the extraordinary designs perfected by nature over millions of years. This approach, known as biomimicry, represents a paradigm shift where scientists and engineers look to the inherent wisdom embedded in the biological world for solutions to complex challenges (Ali Hussein Mohamed et al., 2022).

The background on biomimicry in materials science is rooted in the realization that living organisms have evolved efficient and optimized structures that outperform many human-made materials. The lotus leaf's ability to repel water, the spider's silk strength, and the gecko's adhesive capabilities are just a few examples of nature's unparalleled craftsmanship (Barhoum et al., 2022). In the pursuit of sustainability, efficiency, and enhanced performance, researchers have turned their attention to understanding and replicating these remarkable biological designs (Moshood et al., 2022).

Biomimicry in materials science is not a recent phenomenon but a continuum of discoveries and breakthroughs. As technological advancements allow for deeper exploration of biological structures at the microscopic and nanoscopic levels, scientists are uncovering novel insights that guide the development of materials with superior properties (Hwang et al., 2015). The biomimetic approach extends beyond mere imitation; it involves deciphering the underlying principles governing biological systems and adapting them to create synthetic materials with similar functionalities (Gerola et al., 2023).

This shift towards biomimicry signifies a departure from traditional trial and error methods in materials science. Instead, it heralds an era where researchers study nature's blueprints, unlocking secrets that can be harnessed to revolutionize the properties of materials. The background on biomimicry in materials science is a rich tapestry woven with discoveries from various disciplines, converging to redefine how to conceptualize, design, and fabricate materials for a spectrum of applications. It stands as a testament to the transformative power of learning from the natural world, where each biological marvel serves as a guidepost for the next generation of innovative materials.

2.3 Biomimetic coating synthesis techniques

2.3.1 Self-assembly method

Self-assembly techniques in biomimetic coatings represent a sophisticated approach inspired by nature's ability to organize and structure materials at the molecular and nanoscale levels (Chai et al., 2022; Lombardo et al., 2020; Sola et al., 2023). Mimicking the inherent order found in biological systems, researchers harness self-assembly to create coatings with tailored properties and functionalities. In the "top-down" approach, biomaterials are generated by stripping down a complex entity into its component parts (e.g., paring a virus particle down to its capsid to form a viral cage) whereas, in the "bottom-up" approach, materials are assembled molecule by molecule (and in some cases even atom by atom) to produce novel supramolecular architectures. The latter approach is likely to become an integral part of nanomaterials manufacture and requires a deep understanding of individual molecular building blocks and their structures, assembly properties, and dynamic behaviors. This section explores key self-assembly techniques employed in biomimetic coatings, shedding light on their principles and applications:

2.3.2 Molecular self assembly

The process of molecular self assembly is dependent on noncovalent interactions, including hydrogen bonding, van der Waals forces, and pi—pi stacking, which cause molecules to spontaneously arrange into well defined patterns (Swiegers, 2004).

Weak, noncovalent links, such as hydrogen bonds, ionic bonds (electrostatic interactions), hydrophobic contacts, van der Waals interactions, and water-mediated hydrogen bonds, are the main mediators of molecular self-assembly (Ugwu & Conradie, 2023). While individually these bonds may not seem like much, collectively they control the structural shape of all biological macromolecules and affect how they interact with other molecules. Since water is a component of every biological substance, the water-mediated hydrogen bond is particularly significant for living systems (Schiebel et al., 2018). Every biomolecule, including proteins and peptides, interacts with one another and organizes itself to create distinct structures linked to specific functions. Through an examination of the mechanisms involved in the construction of supramolecular structures in nature, self assembly may be used to create totally new synthetic materials. Proteins and peptides make excellent building blocks when creating new materials (Shen et al., 2021). They have previously been utilized by nature as scaffolds to create an astounding variety of materials, such as collagen, keratin, pearl, shell, microlenses, made of coral and calcite, and optical waveguides.

Applications: Producing biomimetic coverings with particular molecular architectures, such as those that imitate lipid membranes or proteins' organized structures.

2.3.3 Colloidal self assembly

Colloidal self assembly is the process by which colloidal particles are arranged into ordered structures by use of factors such as capillary forces or electrostatic interactions. Direct self assembly of microspheres, which has been developed since the early 1950s, is the tight packing or systematic arrangement of microspheres driven by an external force (Xu, Wang et al., 2016). More specifically, the capillary action, charge compensation effect, hydrophilic and hydrophobic effect, electrostatic contact, hydrogen bonding interaction, and charge compensation effect can all operate as driving forces between microspheres. Because of its low cost, ease of processing, high throughput, and superior controllability, direct self-assembly of colloidal particles has been widely used in recent decades to build a variety of hierarchical and periodic micro-/nanostructure arrays on a large scale (Tian et al., 2010; Ye & Qi, 2011; Zhang et al., 2010).

2.3.4 Template-assisted methods

Hard or soft templates guide the arrangement of building blocks during coating formation, providing a scaffold for organized growth. In terms of geometry, templates are substrates (in 1D, 2D, or 3D) that have active spots on their surface that have been changed and can cause nanoparticles deposition to occur selectively. These templates may now be separated into soft and hard categories (Nie et al., 2010). Soft templates in polymer science include single molecules, microstructures (like carbon nanotubes), block copolymers, and microstructures. These templates have a spatial distribution of specific reactive sites and are frequently used as scaffolds to arrange different particles into targeted structures (like DNA) that have complementary morphologies to the templates. Physical hard templates can be produced more accurately than soft templates by the use of photolithography, reactive ion etching, electronic etching, focused ion beam (FIB) etching, and other etching techniques. Template approaches are frequently used with other techniques, such as evaporation, convection capillary force, and spin coating process, to get the colloidal self-assembly (Dai et al., 2013; Xia et al., 2007). Recently, Kim et al. used nanoporous templates to develop high-resolution light-emitting diodes based on well-defined nanoarrays of colloidal quantum dots of various sizes over a wide area (Kim et al., 2019). Gupta and colleagues have created a stretchable periodic square lattice of gold nanoparticles on macroscopic areas using a combination of soft lithography and template-assisted colloidal self-assembly. This has allowed them to create low-loss, mechanically tunable plasmonic nanostructures that exhibit strong optical anisotropy upon mechanical deformation. The process is economical and efficient (Gupta et al., 2019). Simultaneously, as Fig. 2.1 illustrates, Xu and colleagues have created nanohole arrays using FIB as templates for PS microsphere self-assembly (Hu et al., 2015). In addition, Yin and colleagues conducted a number of investigations to enhance the physical template self-assembly technique for assembling monodispersed spherical colloids on intricately patterned templates, such as circular rings, polygonal or polyhedral clusters, linear or zigzag chains, and photolithographically produced polygonal or polyhedral clusters, as illustrated in Fig. 2.2 (Lu et al., 2001; Yin & Xia, 2001; Yin et al., 2001; Zhang et al., 2020). It has been discovered that there is sufficient capillary force to cause a preferred orientation in the solid substrate's plane.

2.3.5 Layer by layer assembly

Alternating layers of positively and negatively charged materials are sequentially deposited, allowing precise control over coating thickness and

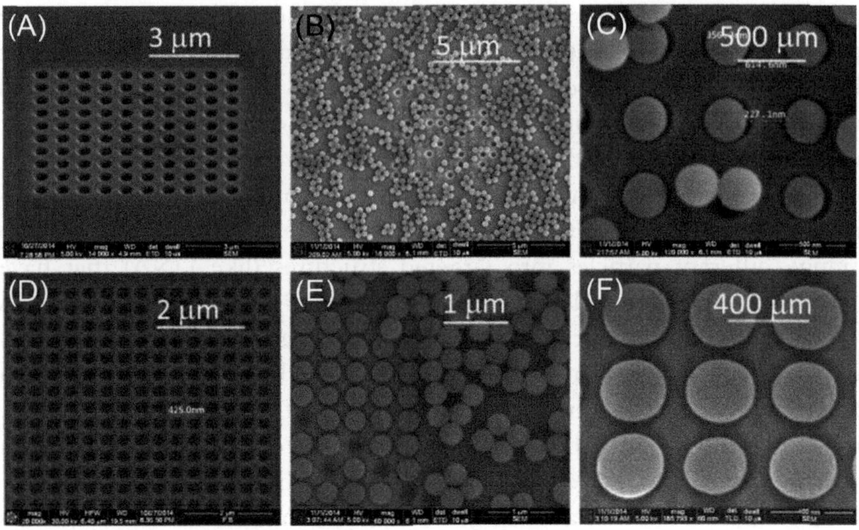

Figure 2.1 (A–F) Scanning electron mircrographs of surface-enhanced Raman scattering substrates with different sizes by FIB nanopatterning regulation and subsequent PS microspheres self-assembling, respectively. *FIB*, Focused ion beam. *Reproduced with permission from Hu X., Xu, Z., Li, K., Fang, F., Wang, L. (2015).* Applied Surface Science, 355; *Zhang, H., Bu, X., Yip, S., Liang, X., & Ho, J. C. (2020).* Advanced Intelligent Systems, 2. *(Original work published 2020).*

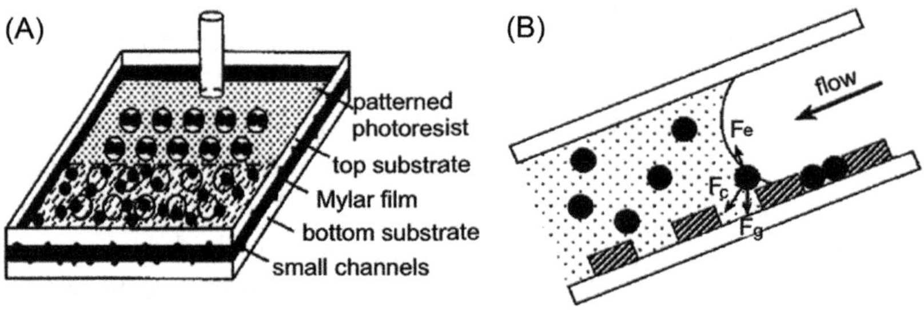

Figure 2.2 (A) Schematic diagram of template colloidal self-assembly combined with convection capillary force. (B) The stress diagram of particles when they are on the rear edge of the liquid slug. *Fc*, capillary force, *Fg*, gravitational force, *Fe*, electrostatic force. *Reproduced with permission from Zhang, H., Bu, X., Yip, S., Liang, X., & Ho, J. C. (2020).* Advanced Intelligent Systems, 2. *(Original work published 2020).*

composition. Layer by layer (LbL) assembly is an alternative to self-assembled monolayer assembly and Langmuir Blodgett deposition, which are two dominant techniques for obtaining solid films at the molecular level. LbL assembly was first proposed by Iler in 1966 and achieved substantial development after the pioneering work of Decher et al. in the 1990s (Borges & Mano, 2014; Decher, 1997; Tang et al., 2006). Since then, LbL assembly technique has become an efficient, facile, flexible, and versatile strategy to coat substrates with multilayers of controlled structures, properties, and functions for various applications (Decher, 1997). The process of LbL assembly is simple and can be accurately controlled to create finely tailored structures (Li et al., 2005; Zhong et al., 2006). Typically, the LbL assembly process includes the sequential adsorption of complementary molecules on a substrate surface, driven by multiple interactions involving electrostatic and/or nonelectrostatic interactions. Washing and drying steps are typically added in between the adsorption stages for each layer deposition to elute loose molecules and stabilize them in the formed layers, as well as to prevent contamination of the subsequent solution from liquid adhering on substrates from the previous solution. To get the required number of deposition layers, repeat these deposition and wash stages. Furthermore, by modifying the assembly parameters, including solution characteristics like concentration, ionic strength, and pH, as well as process factors like temperature, duration, and drying conditions, precise control of composition, thickness, and topography may be accomplished (Chang et al., 2008; Zou & Kim, 2014). Natural polymers, synthetic polymers, peptides, clays, metal oxides, polymer gels, and complexes of these materials are some of the building blocks that are utilized for LbL assembly (Li & Haynie, 2004; Li et al., 2006). The LbL assembly technique has three main advantages over other methods of fabricating nanofilms: it allows for precise control over the composition and structure of the nanofilms, large-scale fabrication on a variety of substrates regardless of size and shape, and mild and confined formation environments.

Numerous deposition technologies, such as dipping, centrifugation, roll to roll, calculated saturation, creaming, immobilization, atomization, spinning, spraying, magnetic assembly, high gravity, electrodeposition, electrocoupling, filtration, fluidics, and fluidized beds, have been designed and developed as a result of the widespread use of LbL assembly for a variety of applications with different processing requirements and tools (Grigoriev et al., 2008; Ma et al., 2012; Shim et al., 2007). As seen in Fig. 2.3, these methods may be broadly classified into five categories: immersion, spin, spray, electromagnetic driven, and fluidic assembly. Typically, it produces enormous nanofilms with a brief assembly process; yet, it can only coat tiny planar substrates, as seen in Fig. 2.3.

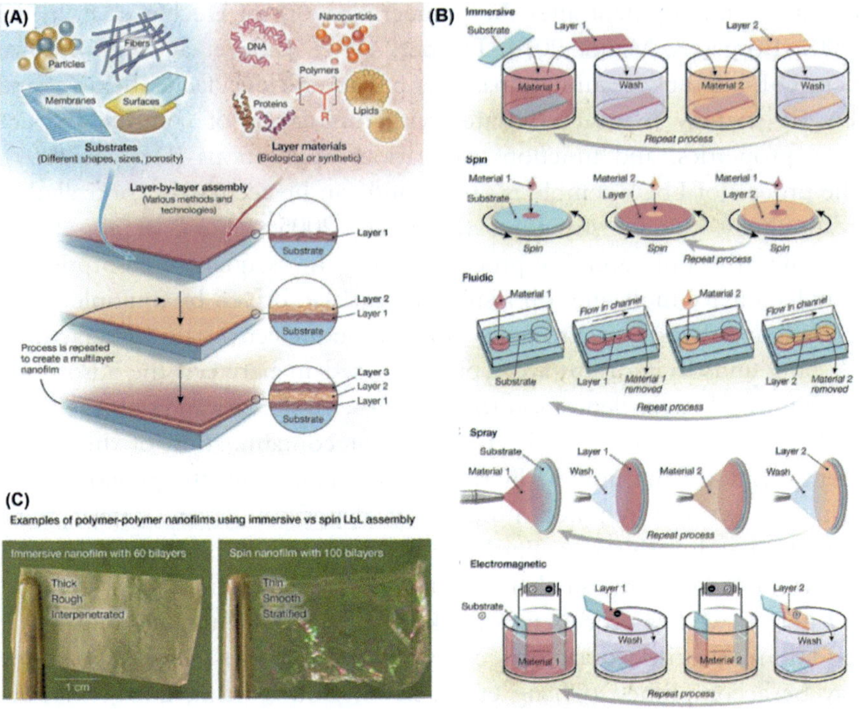

Figure 2.3 (A) Schematic overview of LbL assembly technique with fabrication capacity on any type of substrates and from an extensive choice of materials; (B) schematics showing the five main technology categories for LbL assembly; (C) a typical comparison of different films using immersive and spin assembly (Richardson et al., 2015). *LbL*, Layer-by-layer *From Richardson, J. J., Björnmalm, M., & Caruso, F. (2015).* Science, *348. (Original work published 2015).*

Applications: Mimicking the layered structures found in certain natural surfaces, like fish scales or bird feathers, to achieve enhanced mechanical properties and multifunctionality.

2.3.6 Sol gel methods

In the process of sol gel fabrication, a liquid precursor undergoes a chemical transformation to produce a solid gel, facilitating the development of coatings with controlled porosity and composition. From a purely physical standpoint, sol gel techniques are valuable because they enable the direct creation of multicomponent materials in various configurations (such as monoliths, coatings, foams, and fibers) without the need for powder intermediates (Rosenholm et al., 2010; Yang et al., 2012) or the utilization of costly processing methods like vacuum techniques. The versatility of materials achievable through the sol–gel method has established it as a crucial synthesis pathway in multiple research domains, including optics, electronics, semi/superconductors, and biomaterials. In this context, the methods employed do not impact the final chemical composition of the material; rather, the manner in which the material is obtained provides the advantage. The roots of sol–gel science trace back over 150 years, with the term "sol gel" first coined by Graham in 1864 during his research on silica sols (Barhoum et al., 2022). Even though van Helmont had discovered "water glass" in 1640 by dissolving silicate materials in alkali and precipitating silica gel upon acidification (Moshood et al., 2022), true sol gel experiments commenced in 1846 when Ebelmen observed the formation of transparent glass after exposing a silane obtained from SiCl4 and ethanol to the atmosphere (Gerola et al., 2023; Hwang et al., 2015). Patrick's efforts during his doctoral studies in 1912–15 led to the development of an economically viable and rapid sol gel method for producing silica gel from sodium silicate (Na_2SiO_3) in large quantities (Lombardo et al., 2020). Additionally, Kistler and Caldwell (1934) described the initial synthesis of a highly porous silica (SiO_2) form, termed "aerogel," by supercritically drying the gel obtained through the hydrolytic polycondensation of silicic acid [Si(OH)4]. Each of these endeavors serves as a starting point for the modern sol gel approach, culminating in its widespread application in biomedical contexts.

Sol gel thin film processing presents several advantages, including low-temperature processing, ease of fabrication, and precise control over microstructure and chemical composition. Various synthesis routes are currently available for producing such materials, and sol gel stands out as one of these pathways. In essence, all sol gel methods involve two distinct phases: solution and gelation. A sol, as the name suggests, is a colloidal suspension of solid particles, while a gel constitutes an interconnected network of solid-phase particles forming a continuous entity within a secondary, typically liquid, phase. In sol gel technology, these phases are preserved through chemical reactions during gel evolution and can be manipulated in numerous ways, such as altering initial precursors, gelation time, catalysts, degree of solvation, gelation conditions, or the physical processing of the gel itself. Sol gel processes enable the formation of solid materials through solution gelation, offering the flexibility to produce a wide array of beneficial morphologies (see Fig. 2.4).

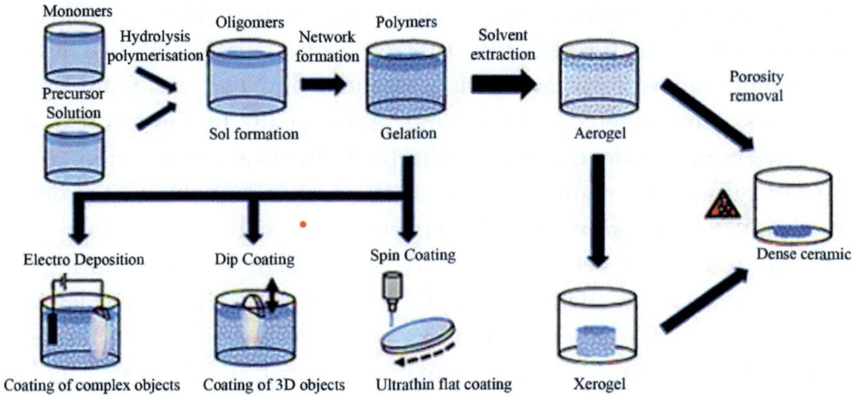

Figure 2.4 Sol gel synthesis routes. Processes are defined as sol gel by the transition of colloidal solution to an interconnected gel network (gelation). The further processing stages illustrated are nonredundant and may be combined depending on the specific needs of the application. *From Owens, G. J., Singh, R. K., Foroutan, F., Alqaysi, M., Han, C. M., Mahapatra, C., Kim, H. W., & Knowles, J. C. (2016). Sol-gel based materials for biomedical applications.* Progress in Materials Science, *77, 1–79. https://doi.org/10.1016/j.pmatsci.2015.12.001.*

Applications: Developing coatings that emulate the porous structures seen in bones or shells for improved mechanical strength and lightweight properties.

2.4 Properties of biomimetic coatings

2.4.1 Mechanical properties

2.4.1.1 Toughness and flexibility

Biomimetic coatings, inspired by the structural resilience of natural materials, have emerged as pioneers in the quest for toughness and flexibility in engineered surfaces. The ability to mimic nature's ingenious designs enables the creation of coatings that not only withstand external forces but also adapt to dynamic environments (Bhushan, 2009). In the realm of biomimetic coatings, achieving toughness and flexibility involves a delicate balance of structural design, material composition, and innovative engineering. By understanding and replicating nature's solutions, researchers are paving the way for coatings that not only resist mechanical stress but also adapt to the ever-changing demands of real-world applications (Arzt et al., 2021). The integration of these principles holds the promise of ushering in a new era of resilient and adaptable biomimetic materials.

This section delves into the key considerations and breakthroughs in achieving toughness and flexibility within biomimetic coatings.

1. Hierarchical structural designs:

   Inspiration from nature: Natural materials often exhibit hierarchical structures that dissipate stress and enhance toughness. Biomimetic coatings leverage this concept by integrating hierarchical architectures at different length scales (Wei et al., 2023).

   Applications: Creating coatings with enhanced toughness for applications in impact-resistant surfaces, such as those found in shells or bones.

2. Adaptive layering and composition:

   Inspiration from nature: Mimicking the layered structures found in certain biological tissues, biomimetic coatings utilize adaptive layering and composition to distribute stress and improve flexibility (Wang et al., 2013).

   Applications: Developing coatings for flexible electronics or wearable devices, where mechanical adaptability is crucial for performance and comfort.

3. Molecular mimicry for enhanced toughness:

   Inspiration from nature: Natural materials often derive their toughness from specific molecular arrangements. Biomimetic coatings employ molecular mimicry to replicate these arrangements, enhancing toughness at the molecular level (Wang, Naleway et al., 2020).

   Applications: Designing coatings with improved resistance to cracking and abrasion in high-stress environments.

4. Dynamic bonding and self healing capabilities:

   Inspiration from nature: Biomimetic coatings incorporate dynamic bonding mechanisms inspired by biological systems, allowing for self healing capabilities. These coatings can repair damage autonomously, restoring their toughness and flexibility (Speck & Speck, 2019).

   Applications: Enhancing the durability of coatings in applications where maintenance is challenging, such as in aerospace or marine environments.

5. Mimicking natural fibrous structures:

   Inspiration from nature: Natural fibers, such as collagen or silk, exhibit exceptional toughness and flexibility. Biomimetic coatings replicate fibrous structures to impart similar mechanical properties (Eadie & Ghosh, 2011).

Applications: Developing coatings for textiles, medical implants, or structural materials where flexibility and strength are critical.

6. Environmental responsiveness:

Inspiration from nature: Some biomimetic coatings can adjust their mechanical properties in response to environmental stimuli, such as temperature or humidity changes, allowing for tailored performance in varying conditions (Sommese et al., 2023).

Applications: Creating coatings for outdoor structures or transportation systems that need to adapt to fluctuating environmental conditions.

7. Lessons from biological joints and tissues:

Inspiration from nature: Biomimetic coatings draw inspiration from the mechanical properties of biological joints and tissues, incorporating flexibility and toughness into synthetic materials (Vincent, 2014).

Applications: Designing coatings for prosthetics or implants that require both strength and flexibility to mimic natural movement.

2.4.2 Fatigue resistance in biomimetic coatings

Biomimetic coatings, inspired by the endurance observed in natural materials, are pushing the boundaries of fatigue resistance in engineered surfaces. Mimicking the strategies employed by biological systems to withstand repeated stress and strain, these coatings are designed to exhibit prolonged durability under cyclic loading conditions (Tu et al., 2021). The pursuit of fatigue resistance in biomimetic coatings involves a holistic approach, considering not only material composition and structural design but also dynamic adaptability and self-repair mechanisms. By emulating the resilience found in the natural world, biomimetic coatings are poised to redefine the standards for durability under cyclic loading, offering solutions for industries where extended operational life is paramount (Assadi-Langroudi et al., 2021). This section explores the key principles and advancements in achieving fatigue resistance within biomimetic coatings.

1. Hierarchical architecture for enhanced endurance:

Inspiration from nature: Natural materials often feature hierarchical architectures that contribute to their fatigue resistance. Biomimetic coatings incorporate similar structures to enhance endurance and mitigate the effects of cyclic loading.

Applications: Developing coatings for components in machinery or infrastructure subjected to repetitive stress, where extended service life is critical.

2. Dynamic adaptability and stress redistribution:

   Inspiration from nature: Biomimetic coatings integrate dynamic adaptability, allowing them to redistribute stress during cyclic loading. This adaptability minimizes localized damage, contributing to increased fatigue resistance.

   Applications: Creating coatings for components in transportation systems or industrial machinery, where cyclic loading is a common operational condition.
3. Self-repair mechanisms to counter fatigue damage:

   Inspiration from nature: Some biomimetic coatings incorporate self repair mechanisms inspired by natural systems. These mechanisms enable the coating to autonomously repair damage incurred during cyclic loading, maintaining fatigue resistance over time.

   Applications: Enhancing the longevity of coatings in applications where manual maintenance is challenging, such as in offshore structures or aerospace components.
4. Mimicking fibrous reinforcement for strength:

   Inspiration from nature: Natural materials often employ fibrous reinforcements to enhance their strength and fatigue resistance. Biomimetic coatings replicate these fibrous structures to improve overall endurance.

   Applications: Designing coatings for components in automotive or marine applications that experience repetitive stress and require high fatigue resistance.
5. Adaptive damping for reduced vibrations:

   Inspiration from nature: Biomimetic coatings can incorporate adaptive damping mechanisms to reduce vibrations induced by cyclic loading. This damping capability helps in minimizing the fatigue damage caused by oscillations.

   Applications: Developing coatings for structural elements in buildings or bridges to reduce the impact of cyclic loads and vibrations.
6. Environmental stability and resistance:

   Inspiration from nature: Biomimetic coatings designed for fatigue resistance also consider environmental factors. Resistance to environmental degradation, such as corrosion or chemical exposure, contributes to prolonged fatigue life.

   Applications: Coatings for outdoor structures or components in aggressive environments where fatigue resistance is coupled with protection against external factors.

7. Lessons from biological motion:

Inspiration from nature: Biomimetic coatings draw insights from the fatigue-resistant structures observed in biological systems that undergo repetitive motion. Lessons from joints and tissues guide the design for improved endurance.

Applications: Developing coatings for flexible electronics or wearable devices that experience frequent bending or flexing.

2.4.3 Thermal properties of biomimetic coatings

Biomimetic coatings, inspired by nature's thermal adaptations, exhibit a diverse range of thermal properties that make them invaluable in various applications. This section delves into two crucial aspects of the thermal performance of these coatings: heat resistance and thermal insulation.

2.4.3.1 Heat resistance

Heat resistance in biomimetic coatings is a testament to their ability to withstand elevated temperatures and thermal stresses. Drawing inspiration from natural materials that thrive in extreme environments, biomimetic coatings are engineered to maintain structural integrity and functionality under high temperature conditions (Jamei & Vrcelj, 2021).

1. Heat-resistant biological structures:

   Inspiration from nature: Biomimetic coatings often take cues from organisms inhabiting extreme environments, such as thermophilic bacteria or heat resistant plant structures.

   Applications: Designing coatings for aerospace components, automotive parts, or industrial machinery exposed to high temperature conditions.

2. Structural optimization for thermal stability:

   Inspiration from nature: Biomimetic coatings optimize their structures at various scales to enhance heat resistance. This may involve the use of heat-resistant materials or the incorporation of heat dissipating features.

   Applications: Creating coatings for electronic devices, where heat dissipation is crucial for optimal performance and longevity.

3. Adaptive thermal response:

Inspiration from nature: Some biomimetic coatings exhibit adaptive thermal responses, altering their properties in the presence of heat to maintain functionality.

Applications: Developing coatings for components in close proximity to heat sources, where adaptive thermal behavior can enhance overall system performance.

2.4.3.2 Thermal insulation

Thermal insulation is a critical property in biomimetic coatings, allowing them to regulate heat flow and provide protection against temperature variations. Borrowing strategies from natural insulating materials, these coatings are designed to minimize heat transfer.

1. Inspiration from natural insulators:

   Inspiration from nature: Biomimetic coatings often take inspiration from the insulating properties of natural materials like fur, feathers, or the insulating layer in the skin of certain animals.

   Applications: Creating coatings for buildings, pipelines, or electronic devices where thermal insulation is essential for energy efficiency and performance.

2. Nanostructure design for insulation:

   Inspiration from nature: Biomimetic coatings leverage nanostructure design to incorporate insulating air pockets or layers, reducing heat transfer.

   Applications: Developing coatings for energy efficient windows or electronic devices, where thermal insulation enhances overall efficiency.

3. Multifunctional insulation with other properties:

   Inspiration from nature: Biomimetic coatings often combine thermal insulation with other functionalities, such as mechanical strength or flexibility, to create multifunctional materials.

   Applications: Designing coatings for wearable technologies or outdoor equipment, where a combination of thermal insulation and other properties is advantageous.

4. Environmentally responsive thermal insulation:

Inspiration from nature: Some biomimetic coatings can adapt their thermal insulation properties in response to environmental conditions, providing dynamic heat regulation.

Applications: Coatings for energy efficient building materials that adjust insulation based on external temperature changes.

In the realm of thermal properties, biomimetic coatings offer a versatile toolbox for engineers and researchers, enabling the creation of materials that not only resist high temperatures but also regulate heat flow for enhanced efficiency and performance in diverse applications.

2.4.4 Chemical resistance of biomimetic coatings

Biomimetic coatings, drawing inspiration from the chemical adaptations observed in nature, exhibit remarkable resistance to corrosive environments and chemical challenges. This section explores two crucial aspects of the chemical resistance of these coatings: corrosion resistance and chemical stability.

2.4.4.1 Corrosion resistance

Corrosion resistance in biomimetic coatings is a vital property that protects underlying materials from degradation caused by chemical reactions with the surrounding environment. Borrowing strategies from nature, these coatings are designed to withstand corrosive agents and extend the lifespan of coated surfaces.

1. Inspiration from corrosion-resistant biological structures:

   Inspiration from nature: Biomimetic coatings often take inspiration from organisms exposed to corrosive environments, such as marine organisms with protective coatings or extremophiles thriving in acidic or alkaline conditions.

   Applications: Designing coatings for marine structures, pipelines, or metallic components in industrial settings where corrosion resistance is critical.

2. Barrier layer formation:

   Inspiration from nature: Biomimetic coatings may form dense and protective barrier layers that prevent corrosive agents from reaching the substrate material.

   Applications: Developing coatings for automotive components, infrastructure, or offshore structures where exposure to harsh environmental conditions requires robust corrosion protection.

3. Self-healing corrosion protection:

Inspiration from nature: Some biomimetic coatings incorporate self-healing mechanisms to repair any damage or breaches in the coating, maintaining continuous corrosion protection.

Applications: Enhancing the longevity of coatings in applications where manual maintenance for corrosion protection is challenging, such as in marine environments.

2.4.4.2 Chemical stability

Chemical stability in biomimetic coatings ensures that the coating's structure remains intact when exposed to various chemical substances. By emulating the chemical resilience found in biological systems, these coatings offer stability in the face of diverse chemical challenges. In the realm of chemical resistance, biomimetic coatings offer a robust defense against degradation, providing a shield that enables materials to endure corrosive environments and maintain stability in the face of diverse chemical challenges.

1. Molecular design for chemical inertness:

   Inspiration from nature: Biomimetic coatings may employ molecular design strategies to enhance chemical inertness, minimizing reactivity with different substances.

   Applications: Creating coatings for chemical processing equipment, laboratory surfaces, or medical devices where resistance to chemical reactions is crucial.

2. Adaptive chemical response:

   Inspiration from nature: Some biomimetic coatings exhibit adaptive chemical responses, altering their properties in the presence of specific chemicals to maintain stability.

   Applications: Designing coatings for components in chemical manufacturing or storage facilities where exposure to a variety of chemicals is inevitable.

3. Resistance to harsh environmental conditions:

   Inspiration from nature: Biomimetic coatings are designed to withstand exposure to harsh environmental conditions, including exposure to acids, bases, and other aggressive chemicals.

   Applications: Coatings for architectural structures, transportation infrastructure, or electronic components where resilience to diverse environmental challenges is essential.

4. Hydrophobicity and oleophobicity:

Inspiration from nature: Biomimetic coatings may incorporate hydrophobic and oleophobic properties, preventing the absorption of liquids and oils that could lead to chemical degradation.

Applications: Developing coatings for surfaces in kitchens, laboratories, or industrial settings where resistance to liquid chemicals and oils is crucial.

2.5 Challenges and future directions in biomimetic coatings

2.5.1 Challenges associated with the biomimetic coatings

Biomimetic coatings hold immense promise in revolutionizing material science, but as with any emerging field, they face challenges that require innovative solutions. The future directions of biomimetic coatings involve addressing these challenges while exploring new frontiers for enhanced performance and broader applications.

- **Reproducibility and scalability:** Achieving consistent and reproducible results in the synthesis of biomimetic coatings remains a significant challenge. The intricate structures inspired by nature often require precise control, making it difficult to replicate these coatings on a large scale.
- **Durability and long-term stability**: Ensuring the long-term stability and durability of biomimetic coatings, particularly in real-world conditions, poses a challenge. Environmental factors, wear and tear, and the dynamic nature of many applications require coatings to withstand prolonged exposure.
- **Integration into existing manufacturing processes**: The seamless integration of biomimetic coatings into existing manufacturing processes is essential for their practical implementation across industries. Adapting these coatings to conventional production methods and ensuring compatibility with existing materials can be challenging.
- **Emerging trends and cutting-edge research in biomimetic coatings**: Keeping abreast of the latest trends and cutting-edge research is crucial for the continued advancement of biomimetic coatings. The field is dynamic, with new discoveries and innovations emerging rapidly.

2.5.2 Future directions

- Develop standardized protocols: Establishing standardized procedures for the synthesis of biomimetic coatings can enhance reproducibility across different laboratories.
- Automation and robotics: Leveraging automation and robotics in the fabrication process can improve precision and scalability, reducing variability in coating properties.
- Collaboration and knowledge-sharing: Encouraging collaboration among researchers and fostering open sharing of knowledge can accelerate progress in achieving reproducibility.
- Materials engineering: Investigate and develop new materials with enhanced durability, weather resistance, and mechanical strength, drawing inspiration from nature's most resilient structures.
- Long-term testing protocols: Establish comprehensive and standardized long-term testing protocols to assess the durability and stability of biomimetic coatings under varying conditions.

- Continuous monitoring and maintenance strategies: Implementing systems for continuous monitoring of coating performance and developing maintenance strategies can extend the lifespan of biomimetic coatings.
- Process optimization: Investigate methods for optimizing existing manufacturing processes to accommodate the unique requirements of biomimetic coatings.
- Customization for industry-specific needs: Develop biomimetic coatings tailored to specific industries, considering their manufacturing processes and material compatibility.
- Industry collaboration: Foster collaboration between biomimetic researchers and industry experts to bridge the gap between academic advancements and industrial applications.
- Multidisciplinary research: Encourage collaboration among researchers from diverse disciplines, including materials science, biology, and engineering, to explore new avenues for biomimetic coatings.
- Investment in research and development: Allocate resources for continued research and development in biomimetic coatings to explore novel concepts and push the boundaries of what is currently achievable.
- Stay informed about emerging technologies: Actively engage with emerging technologies, such as nanotechnology and 3D printing, to explore their potential applications in advancing biomimetic coatings.

As biomimetic coatings transition from innovative concepts to practical applications, addressing these challenges and pursuing these future directions will play a pivotal role in unlocking their full potential across various industries. The collaborative efforts of researchers, industry partners, and policymakers will be instrumental in shaping the trajectory of biomimetic coatings in the coming years.

2.6 Conclusion

In conclusion, biomimetic coatings stand at the forefront of materials science, offering a glimpse into a future where materials draw inspiration from the elegance of the natural world, pushing the boundaries of what is achievable and opening new frontiers in innovation.

2.6.1 Recap of key findings

In the exploration of biomimetic coatings, a realm has been uncovered where the brilliance of nature converges with human ingenuity to create materials with unprecedented properties. The synthesis methods, properties, and applications of these coatings reveal a tapestry woven with inspiration drawn from the intricate designs found in the natural world.

From self-assembly techniques mimicking molecular precision to coatings exhibiting remarkable toughness, flexibility, and resistance to thermal and chemical challenges, biomimetic coatings stand as a testament to the remarkable progress made in materials science. The journey through hierarchical structures, adaptive responses, and innovative fabrication methods has provided insights into the versatility and potential of these coatings.

2.6.2 Significance of biomimetic coatings in advancing materials science

Biomimetic coatings represent a paradigm shift in materials science, offering solutions that transcend the limitations of conventional materials. The significance of biomimetic coatings lies not only in their ability to replicate nature's efficiency but also in their potential to redefine the performance and functionality of materials across diverse applications.

These coatings hold promise in enhancing the durability and resilience of materials, making them indispensable in industries ranging from aerospace and automotive to healthcare and electronics. By unlocking the secrets embedded in natural structures, biomimetic coatings pave the way for materials that are not only high-performing but also environmentally responsive and adaptable.

2.7 Prospects and potential breakthroughs

Peering into the future of biomimetic coatings, exciting prospects and potential breakthroughs beckon, as the challenges of reproducibility, scalability, durability, and integration into existing manufacturing processes offer opportunities for innovation. Researchers are poised to discover novel materials, fabrication techniques, and applications that will propel biomimetic coatings into mainstream use.

The continuous evolution of biomimetic coatings holds the promise of groundbreaking advancements. From self-healing coatings and dynamically adaptive materials to coatings tailored for specific industries, the future is ripe with possibilities. The collaboration between academia, industry, and policymakers will be pivotal in unlocking the full potential of biomimetic coatings, ushering in an era where materials are not just inspired by nature but intricately woven into the fabric of sustainable and resilient technological solutions.

Acknowledgments

One of the authors gratefully acknowledges funding from the Department of Science and Technology (DST), New Delhi, India, for the funding under the Women Scientist (WOS-A) program [File number: SR-WOS-A-ET-54-2019].

References

Ali Hussein Mohamed, N., Mandour, M., & Marey, S. (2022). *Engineering Research Journal, 176*, 90–109.

Arzt, E., Quan, H., McMeeking, R. M., & Hensel, R. (2021). *Progress in Materials Science, 120*, 100823.

Assadi-Langroudi, A., Kelly, B. C., Barreto, D., Cotecchia, F., Dicks, H., Ekinci, A., Garcia, F. E., Harbottle, M., Tagarelli, V., Jefferson, I., Maghoul, P., Masoero, E., El Mountassir, G., Muhunthan, B., Geng, X., Ghadr, S., Mirzababaei, M., Mitrani, H., & van Paassen, L. (2021). *International Journal of Geosynthetics and Ground Engineering, 8*, 3.

Barhoum, A., García-Betancourt, M. L., Jeevanandam, J., Hussien, E. A., Mekkawy, S. A., Mostafa, M., Omran, M. M., Abdalla, M. S., & Bechelany, M. (2022). *Nanomaterials*, 177.

Bhushan, B. (2009). *Philosophical Transactions of the Royal Society A: Mathematical, Physical and Engineering Sciences, 367*, 1445.

Borges, J., & Mano, J. F. (2014). *Chemical Reviews, 114*, 8883.

Chai, Z., Childress, A., & Busnaina, A. A. (2022). *ACS Nano, 16*, 17641.

Chang, L., Kong, X., Wang, F., Wang, L., & Shen, J. (2008). *Thin Solid Films, 516*, 2125.

Collins, C. M., & Safiuddin, M. (2022). *Infrastructures*, 46.

Dai, Q., Frommer, J., Berman, D., Virwani, K., Davis, B., Cheng, J. Y., & Nelson, A. (2013). *Langmuir: the ACS Journal of Surfaces and Colloids, 29*, 7472.

Decher, G. (1997). *Science (New York, N.Y.), 277*, 1232.

Eadie, L., & Ghosh, T. K. (2011). *Journal of the Royal Society, Interface/the Royal Society, 8*, 761.

Gebeshuber, I. C. (2023). *Biomimetics*.

Gerola, A., Robaey, Z., & Blok, V. (2023). *Philosophy & Technology, 36*, 65.

Grigoriev, D., Bukreeva, T., Möhwald, H., & Shchukin, D. (2008). *Langmuir: the ACS Journal of Surfaces and Colloids, 24*, 999.

Gupta, V., Probst, P. T., Goßler, F. R., Steiner, A. M., Schubert, J., Brasse, Y., König, T. A., & Fery, A. (2019). *ACS applied materials & interfaces, 11*, 28189.

Hu, X., Xu, Z., Li, K., Fang, F., & Wang, L. (2015). *Applied Surface Science, 355*, 1168.

Hwang, J., Jeong, Y., Park, J. M., Lee, K. H., Hong, J. W., & Choi, J. (2015). *International Journal of Nanomedicine, 10*, 5701.

Jamei, E., & Vrcelj, Z. (2021). *Applied Sciences*, 7514.

Kim, J., Hwang, G. S., Lee, D.-E., Ahn, J., Hwang, C.-S., Chin, B. D., & Lee, D. H. (2019). *ACS Applied Electronic Materials, 1*, 1626.

Kistler, S., & Caldwell, A. G. (1934). *Industrial Engineering and Chemistry, 26*(6), 658–662.

Li, B., & Haynie, D. T. (2004). *Biomacromolecules, 5*, 1667.

Li, B., Haynie, D. T., Palath, N., & Janisch, D. (2005). *Journal of Nanoscience and Nanotechnology, 5*, 2042.

Li, B., Rozas, J., & Haynie, D. T. (2006). *Biotechnology Progress, 22*, 111.

Lin, J., Cai, Y., Wang, X., Ding, B., Yu, J., & Wang, M. (2011). *Nanoscale, 3*.

Liu, S., Yu, J.-M., Gan, Y.-C., Qiu, X.-Z., Gao, Z.-C., Wang, H., Chen, S.-X., Xiong, Y., Liu, G.-H., Lin, S.-E., McCarthy, A., John, J. V., Wei, D.-X., & Hou, H.-H. (2023). *Military Medical Research, 10*.

Lombardo, D., Calandra, P., Pasqua, L., & Magazù, S. (2020). *Materials, 13*, 1048.
Lu, Y., Yin, Y., & Xia, Y. (2001). *Advanced Materials, 13*, 34.
Ma, L., Cheng, M., Jia, G., Wang, Y., An, Q., Zeng, X., Shen, Z., Zhang, Y., & Shi, F. (2012). *Langmuir: the ACS Journal of Surfaces and Colloids, 28*, 9849.
Moshood, T. D., Nawanir, G., Mahmud, F., Mohamad, F., Ahmad, M. H., & AbdulGhani, A. (2022). *Cleaner Engineering and Technology, 6*, 100404.
Nie, Z., Petukhova, A., & Kumacheva, E. (2010). *Nature nanotechnology, 5*, 15.
Richardson, J. J., Björnmalm, M., & Caruso, F. (2015). *Science (New York, N.Y.), 348*, 2491.
Rosenholm, J. M., Sahlgren, C., & Lindén, M. (2010). *Nanoscale, 2*, 1870.
Schiebel, J., Gaspari, R., Wulsdorf, T., Ngo, K., Sohn, C., Schrader, T. E., Cavalli, A., Ostermann, A., Heine, A., & Klebe, G. (2018). *Nature Communications, 9*, 3559.
Shen, Y., Levin, A., Kamada, A., Toprakcioglu, Z., Rodriguez-Garcia, M., Xu, Y., & Knowles, T. P. J. (2021). *ACS Nano, 15*, 5819.
Shim, B. S., Podsiadlo, P., Lilly, D. G., Agarwal, A., Lee, J., Tang, Z., Ho, S., Ingle, P., Paterson, D., & Lu, W. (2007). *Nano Letters*, 7, 3266.
Sola, A., Trinchi, A., & Hill, A. J. (2023). *Smart Materials in Manufacturing, 1*, 100013.
Sommese, F., Badarnah, L., & Ausiello, G. (2023). *Renewable and Sustainable Energy Reviews, 188*, 113847.
Speck, O., & Speck, T. (2019). *Biomimetics (Basel).*
Swiegers, G. F. (2004). *Assemblies and self-assembly, Comprehensive Coordination Chemistry II* (1, pp. 747–759). Australia: Elsevier Ltd Available from. Available from http://www.sciencedirect.com/science/referenceworks/9780080437484 Available from.
Tang, Z., Wang, Y., Podsiadlo, P., & Kotov, N. A. (2006). *Advanced Materials, 18*, 3203.
Tian, J., Jin, J., Zheng, F., & Zhao, H. (2010). *Langmuir: the ACS Journal of Surfaces and Colloids, 26*, 8762.
Tu, Z., Liu, W., Wang, J., Qiu, X., Huang, J., Li, J., & Lou, H. (2021). *Nature Communications, 12*, 2916.
Ugwu, D. I., & Conradie, J. (2023). *Journal of Molecular Structure, 1293*, 136275.
Vincent, J. F. V. (2014). *Materials experience* (pp. 235–246). Butterworth-Heinemann.
Wang, P., Hu, M., Wang, H., Chen, Z., Feng, Y., Wang, J., Ling, W., & Huang, Y. (2020). *Advanced Science*, 7, 2001116.
Wang, X., Ding, B., & Li, B. (2013). *Materials Today, 16*, 229.
Wang, Y., Naleway, S. E., & Wang, B. (2020). *Bioactive Materials, 5*, 745.
Wei, J., Pan, F., Ping, H., Yang, K., Wang, Y., Wang, Q., & Fu, Z. (2023). *Research. A Journal of Science and its Applications, 6*, 0164.
Xia, D., Li, D., Ku, Z., Luo, Y., & Brueck, S. (2007). *Langmuir: The ACS Journal of Surfaces and Colloids, 23*, 5377.
Xu, Q., Zhang, W., Dong, C., Sreeprasad, T. S., & Xia, Z. (2016). *Journal of the Royal Society, Interface/the Royal Society, 13.*
Xu, Z., Wang, L., Fang, F., Fu, Y., & Yin, Z. (2016). *Current Nanoscience, 12*, 725.
Yang, P., Gai, S., & Lin, J. (2012). *Chemical Society Reviews, 41*, 3679.
Ye, X., & Qi, L. (2011). *Nano Today, 6*, 608.
Yin, Y., Lu, Y., & Xia, Y. (2001). *Journal of the American Chemical Society, 123*, 771.
Yin, Y., & Xia, Y. (2001). *Advanced Materials, 13*, 267.
Zhang, H., Bu, X., Yip, S., Liang, X., & Ho, J. C. (2020). *Advanced Intelligent Systems, 2*, 1900085.
Zhang, J., Li, Y., Zhang, X., & Yang, B. (2010). *Advanced Materials, 22*, 4249.
Zhong, Y., Li, B., & Haynie, D. T. (2006). *Biotechnology Progress, 22*, 126.
Zou, J., & Kim, F. (2014). *Nature Communications, 5*, 5254.

CHAPTER 3

Biomimetic coatings for orthopedic implants

Muhammad Awais[1], Safee Ullah Chaudhary[2] and Muhammad Sohail Zafar[3,4,5]

[1]Department of Industrial Engineering, Faculty of Engineering, Taibah University, Madinah, Saudi Arabia
[2]Biomedical Informatics & Engineering Research Laboratory, Department of Life Sciences, Lahore University of Management Sciences, Lahore, Pakistan
[3]Department of Restorative Dentistry, College of Dentistry, Taibah University, Madinah, Saudi Arabia
[4]Center of Medical and Bio-allied Health Sciences Research, Ajman University, Ajman, United Arab Emirates
[5]Department of Dental Materials, Islamic International Dental College, Riphah International University, Islamabad, Pakistan

3.1 Introduction

Biomimetic coatings applied to metallic or nonmetallic surfaces refer to surface treatments or coatings that mimic the properties found in nature (Zafar, 2020). These coatings are designed to reproduce certain functionalities or characteristics found in natural materials or living organisms, such as self-cleaning (Yao, 2022), self-healing (Diesendruck et al., 2015), antifouling (Selim et al., 2020), antireflective (Jiao et al., 2023), and superhydrophobic (Liu, 2017) properties. By mimicking the nature, biomimetic coatings aim to augment the performance and functional durability of metallic or nonmetallic surfaces.

The development of biomimetic coatings involves understanding the unique features and structures found in nature, such as the self-cleaning ability of lotus leaves (Collins & Safiuddin, 2022) or the resistance of shark skin to biofouling (Pu et al., 2016). Researchers have attempted to replicate these features on substrate surfaces by using various methods, materials, and techniques.

Some commonly used biomimetic coating techniques include the following.

1. Self-assembly: In this approach, coatings are created by allowing molecules to self-assemble into organized structures. For example, nanostructures on a lotus leaf surface have been created by researchers to form a specific pattern by arranging molecules similar to that of a leaf (Collins & Safiuddin, 2022).

Smart Biomimetic Coatings
DOI: https://doi.org/10.1016/B978-0-443-21738-8.00003-5

2. Surface texturing: In surface texturing, specific patterns or structures are created on the surface of substrate materials to achieve the desired properties. For instance, replicating the rough texture found on shark skin can reduce biofouling and drag (Pu et al., 2016).
3. Functional material deposition: In this technique, functional materials are developed on surfaces with hydrophobic or superhydrophobic properties that prevent water, oil, or other liquids from sticking to the surface, or by preparing antireflective materials that reduce glare (Jiao et al., 2023; Liu, 2017).
4. Bioinspired coatings: Bioactive or bioinspired coatings have been developed that mimic the chemical composition or properties of natural materials, such as proteins or human blood plasma, to achieve specific functionalities (Adawy & Abdel-Fattah, 2013; Ananth et al., 2015; Arafat et al., 2011; Forsgren et al., 2007; Habibovic et al., 2002; Koju et al., 2017; Tas, 2000). For example, bioactive coatings mimic the natural mineralization process that occurs during bone tissue formation. These coatings typically involve the deposition of bone-like materials, such as calcium phosphate (CaP), onto the surface of a substrate to enhance its biocompatibility and promote interactions with biological tissues.

Bioactive coatings used for the development of biomedical implants are extremely important for quick healing in orthopedic and dental applications. Most implants have weak osteointegration and often cause interfacial displacement due to the development of a fibrous collagenous capsule around the implant, which eventually provokes toxic effects in the body due to the release of metal cations. Conversely, nonmetallic degradable implants are required to have a well-regulated degradation rate and sustained mechanical stability (Montazerian et al., 2022). Incidentally, bioactive coatings are extremely beneficial when applied to biomedical implants to improve direct bonding with the host bone (Gu, 2023). There are several coating techniques, including mechanical, physical, chemical, and biological techniques, to prepare implants for biomedical applications. These coating techniques are used to prepare metal oxide, bioactive glass, silicate-based, nitride, carbon-based, and CaP coatings for applications in the human body. Hydroxyapatite (HA) is the most common CaP phase used for such applications, and in this chapter, one of the wet deposition techniques (the so-called biomimetic) is discussed to prepare bioactive HA coatings. Nature-inspired coatings are extremely important for improving the functionality of orthopedic implants.

The application of biomimetic coatings onto implant surfaces using simulated body fluid (SBF) has gained popularity since 1998, following the breakthrough work of Kokubo (1998). In fact, he coined the term SBF'. Since then, many research groups have utilized this strategy, with some improvements in implant preparation. It is required that this artificially created medium should perform like body fluids with the limitation of lacking organic biomolecules such as amino acids and proteins. Thus the words biomimicry and SBF were similar. This approach has the key benefit of avoiding any harsh treatment of processing at a high temperature. In contrast, plasma spraying applies a high processing temperature, which may damage the implant substrates during the process of deposition. In addition, high-temperature processing cannot be used for coating heat-sensitive materials such as low-melting-point polymers, which are frequenting used for various biomedical applications, including orthopedics and bone tissue engineering scaffolds (Koju et al., 2017).

3.2 Reaction mechanism of biomimetic coatings

Fig. 3.1 shows the reaction mechanisms that occur during the biomimetic process (Zhou et al., 2013). The pretreatment of the substrate is an essential step in the biomimetic coating process. It is necessary to modify the surface of the polymer substrate to facilitate the nucleation and growth of the HA layer.

Various pretreatment methods can be employed including: (Fig. 3.2)

1. Surface activation: The surface is treated to enhance its reactivity, often by techniques such as plasma treatment, corona discharge, or chemical etching using acids or alkalis. These methods introduce functional groups or create microstructures on the surface, which promotes the adhesion and nucleation of CaP.
2. Surface roughening: Mechanical methods such as sandblasting, or abrasion can be used to roughen the surface. The increased surface roughness provides more sites for nucleation and improves the mechanical interlocking between the polymer and coating.
3. Surface functionalization: The substrate surface can be modified by introducing functional groups that facilitate interactions with calcium ions or provide binding sites for nucleation. This can be achieved through chemical or heat treatment.

In summary, It involves a brief surface treatment using either activation, roughening, or surface functionalization, followed by soaking in an

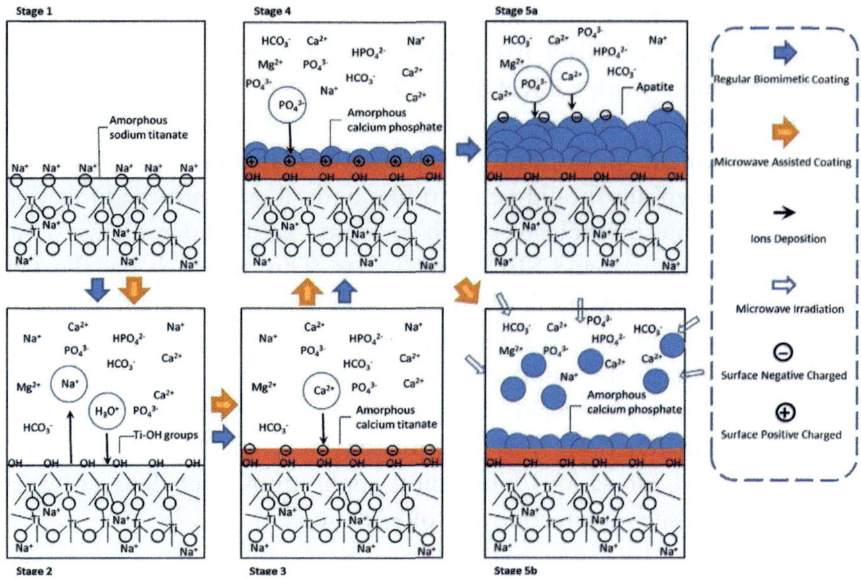

Figure 3.1 Comparison of conventional and microwave-assisted processes (Zhou et al., 2013). *From Zhou, H., Nabiyouni, M., & Bhaduri, S. B. (2013). Microwave assisted apatite coating deposition on Ti6Al4V implants.* Materials Science and Engineering C, *33(7), 4435–4443. https://doi.org/10.1016/j.msec.2013.06.043.*

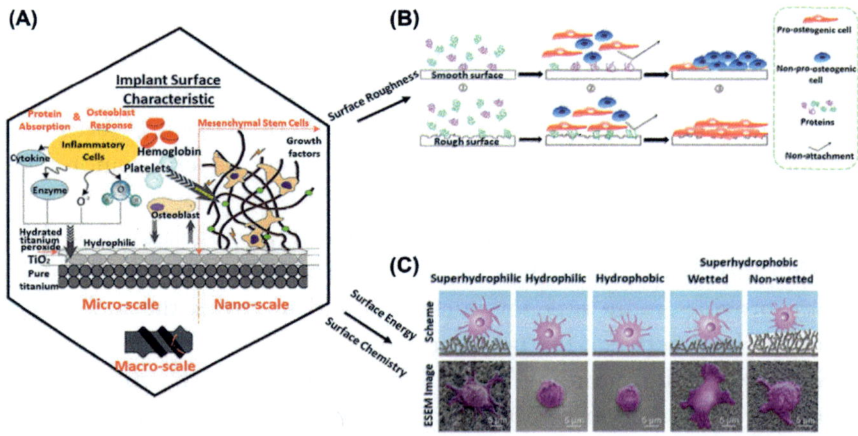

Figure 3.2 Protein adsorption on the substrate from (A) nano-to-macro level which is dependent on several factors. (B) Surface roughness. (C) Surface chemistry and surface energy (Liu et al., 2021). *Open source*

SBF under ambient conditions of temperature (37°C) and pH (7.4) using buffer solutions for approximately 3 weeks. During soaking, heterogeneous nucleation and growth of bone-like calcium-deficient carbonated hydroxyapatite (CDHA) forms on the surface of implant (Koju et al., 2017).

To demonstrate the procedure using a titanium-based metallic implant as an illustration, the process begins with an alkali pretreatment that results in the deposition of an amorphous sodium titanate layer on the implant's surface. This sodium titanate layer then interacts with SBF, leading to the formation of Ti–OH groups. These Ti–OH groups subsequently undergo a reaction with the calcium ions present in the SBF, giving rise to the development of an amorphous calcium titanate layer. This amorphous calcium titanate layer, in turn, undergoes a transformation into amorphous calcium phosphate (ACP), characterized by a calcium-to-phosphate (Ca/P) ratio of approximately 1.4. Finally, this ACP further evolves into a bone-like CDHA with a Ca/P ratio of approximately 1.65, closely resembling the composition of natural bone (Koju et al., 2017).

3.3 Compositions of simulated body fluid

Fig. 3.3 presents detailed information regarding the various compositions of SBFs (Koju et al., 2017). The inspiration for the development of SBFs can be traced back to two commonly used culture media including Hanks' balanced salt solution (HBSS) and Earle's balanced salt solution (Earle, 1943; Liu et al., 2021), which are derived from the physiological saline through Ringer (Hanks & Wallace, 1949). As discussed, the main objective behind formulating SBFs is to closely replicate the composition of human plasma, maintaining a physiological pH of 7.4; buffers are commonly used for this purpose. TRIS (tris-hydroxymethyl-aminomethane)–HCl (Ringer, 1882) and HEPES (2-(4-(2-hydroxyethyl)-1-piperazinyl) ethane sulfonic acid)–NaOH (Bigi et al., 2000; Takadama et al., 2001) are commonly used buffers.

However, both TRIS and HEPES buffers have limitations. TRIS buffer may form soluble complexes engaging various cations, such as Ca^{2+}, which restricts the availability of free Ca^{2+} ions for CaP coating (Koju et al., 2017). These limitations were not observed with HEPES buffer. In contrast, Dorozhkina and Dorozhkin (2002) reported that HEPES is less stable than TRIS and may lose certain amount of the initially dissolved carbonates, which is crucial for the composition of SBF and maintain an appropriate HCO_3^- concentration of 27 mM, resembling that of blood plasma. However, conventional SBF derives from

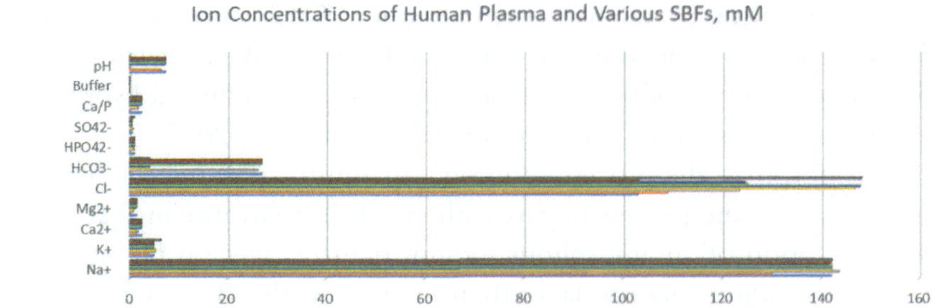

	Na+	K+	Ca2+	Mg2+	Cl-	HCO3-	HPO42-	SO42-	Ca/P	Buffer	pH
Muller-SBF	142	6.5	2.5	1.5	148	4.2	1	1	2.5	0	0
r-SBF	142	5	2.5	1.5	103	27	1	0.5	2.5	0	7.4
Bigi-SBF	141.5	5	2.5	1.5	124.5	27	1	0.5	2.5	0	7.4
Tas- SBF	142	5	2.5	1.5	125	27	1	0.5	2.5	0	7.4
c- SBF	142	5	2.5	1.5	147.8	4.2	1	0.5	2.5	0	7.4
HBSS	142.1	5.33	1.26	0.9	146.8	4.2	0.78	0.41	1.62	0	0
EBSS	143.5	5.37	1.8	0.8	123.5	26.2	1	0.8	1.8	0	0
Ringer	130	4	1.4	0	109	0	0	0	0	0	6.5
Blood Plasma	142	5	2.5	1.5	103	27	1	0.5	2.5	0	7.4

Figure 3.3 Ion concentrations of human plasma and various SBFs, mM (Koju et al., 2017). *SBF*, Stimulated body fluid. *From Koju, N., Sikder, P., Ren, Y., Zhou, H., & Bhaduri, S. B. (2017). Biomimetic coating technology for orthopedic implants.* Current Opinion in Chemical Engineering, 15, *49–55. https://doi.org/10.1016/j.coche.2016.11.005.*

HBSS and contains a lower concentration of HCO_3^- (~ 4.2 mM) (Kokubo, 1998). Tas reported an increase in the concentration of carbonate ion in a Tris–HCl-buffered SBF (~27 mM) (Tas, 2000), while Bigi et al. (2000) demonstrated similar findings in a HEPES–NaOH-buffered SBF.

3.4 Strategies used for accelerating coating kinetics

The slow kinetics is the main challenge faced by biomimetic coatings using SBFs. There are two strategies reported to address this issue by relaxing strict biomimetic conditions. The first strategy involves the use of higher-concentration SBFs. Typically, solutions with increased ionic concentrations of SBF are used. For example, Wang and Sun (2009) and Miyaji et al. (1999) prepared solutions twice as strong, whereas Habibovic et al. (2002) prepared five times concentrated solutions. These stronger SBF-like solutions were created without buffering agents and by removing certain ions such as K^+ and SO_2^{-4}. Tas and Bhaduri (2004) used 10× SBF-like solution (10 mM HPO_2^{-4} and 25 mM Ca^{2+}) and reported promising results for surface coating of Ti6A14V at room temperature in a short period of time. However, it is important to note that highly concentrated solutions, such as solutions with 5 or 10 times the strength of SBF, tend to precipitate with greater carbonate content or off-stoichiometric Ca/P molar ratios (Koju et al., 2017). The second strategy utilizes a microwave-assisted approach to accelerate formation kinetics (Tas & Bhaduri, 2004; Wang & Sun, 2009). For example, SBF is referred to a supersaturated biomimetic fluid, indicating that by altering the biomimetic conditions, the fluids get supersaturated with relevant ions however without exact replication plasma ions composition. A comparison between microwave-assisted and conventional is shown in Fig. 3.1 (Koju et al., 2017). The coating process involved multiple stages, including the formation of sodium titanate in stage-1, followed by the deposition of Ti—OH groups on the surface, which were responsible for the nucleation of CaP in the second stage. In stages 3 and 4, the coating grew from initial nuclei. In the following phase, a contrast becomes evident between the traditional approach and the microwave-assisted procedures. As illustrated in Fig. 3.1, the Ti6Al4V surface exhibited complete coverage with an interconnected network of Ca/P globules, forming a thicker apatite coating. In the microwave-assisted technique, two noteworthy phenomena emerge. Initially, the rate of coating deposition accelerates significantly, typically occurring within about 5 minutes, thanks to the elevated temperature of the aqueous solution. Second, a multitude of Ca/P nuclei forms across the entire Ti6Al4V surface instead of the typical formation of an apatite coating (Koju et al., 2017). Similarly, (Barrere et al., 2002). synthesized coatings within 24 hours using a microwave-assisted process, while Ghorbani et al. (2018) achieved the formation of biomimetic HA within 8 hours using the emission of microwave energy.

3.5 Biomimetic coatings on metallic implants

Metallic substrates, with their inherent properties, such as high fracture toughness, good ductility, favorable strength-to-weight ratio, and biocompatibility, are valuable for fabricating orthopedic and dental implants.

3.5.1 Nonbiodegradable metallic substrates

3.5.1.1 Titanium and related alloys

Ti alloys are widely used in implant applications in the human body. However, the bioactivity of these materials can be further improved in laboratory settings (in vitro) as well as within living organisms (in vivo) by applying coatings of bone-like apatite. To promote osseointegration, specific coating methods, such as plasma spray and sol—gel, are commonly employed on titanium substrates. However, these techniques have certain drawbacks, including nonuniform coating thickness, insufficient adherence to the substrate, and high processing temperatures. To address the challenges associated with titanium-based implants, biomimetic routes, either by the first or second strategy (some groups used both strategies), have been utilized by many research groups. For instance, Habibovic et al. (2002) used two-step biomimetic process to produce CaP coatings onto Ti6Al4V implant. First, a thin but uniform CaP layer was produced by immersion in 5 × SBF. Second, immersion in SBF with decreased crystal growth inhibitors (i.e., Mg^{2+} and HCO_3^-) improved the Ca/P precipitation. Song et al. (2004) used 1.5 × SBF, which resulted in less time for the formation and apatite induction, and film surface oxidation was obtained at a low voltage of 350 V. Tas and Bhaduri (2004) to achieve a 65 μm thick CaP layer with a 10 × SBF solution onto a Ti6Al4V implant. Linear and fast deposition kinetics were observed using this process. Kodama et al. (2009) also observed the fast deposition kinetics with 10 × SBF with the addition of TiO_2 nanotubes. Oliveira et al. (2003) utilized sodium silicate gel precursor before immersing the substrates in an SBF solution, resulting in apatite formation after just 6 hours. Liu and Ma used 1.5 × SBF solution to prepare CaP layer whereas Forsgren (Forsgren et al., 2007) used phosphate-buffered saline (PBS) instead of SBF to prepare similar HA layer; however, it took up to 7 days to get it. Zhou et al. (2013) suggested the benefits of microwave-assisted deposition in producing rapid CaP layer in SBF. Barrère et al. (Barrère, 1999; Barrere, 2002; Barrere, 2004; Oliveira et al., 2003; Yang, 2001) worked extensively to improve the formation of CaP coatings on Ti6Al4V surfaces by adding Ca^{2+}, Mg^{+}, Mg^{2+}, HCO_3^-, and HPO_4^- ions and under 5 × SBF. With only Ca^{2+} and HPO_4^- ions, epitaxial octacalcium phosphate (OCP) crystal growth was observed, whereas Ca-deficient SBF was formed instead of OCP, with Mg^{+} and B-carbonated apatite deposited using HCO_3^- ions. The formation of the CaP layer was achieved within 24 hours using 5 × SBF and microwave energy; thus, both strategies were utilized to improve the reaction kinetics.

3.5.1.2 Metallic biodegradable substrates

Magnesium and related alloys

Magnesium (Mg) and its alloys have emerged as feasible biomaterials for implants (Staiger et al., 2006; Barrere et al., 2004). Their combination of characteristics, including high strength-to-weight ratio, low Young's modulus, biodegradability, and biocompatibility, made them significant. However, rapid degradation limits their clinical applications. To overcome this issue, various types of surface coatings such as polymeric films and CaP have been developed to control the rate of magnesium alloy degradation. These coatings enable the alloys to maintain their mechanical integrity until the complete healing of the fractured bones. For example, Cui et al. (2008) were able to control the degradation rate and improve the bioactivity of a Mg-alloy (AZ31) using a biomimetic technique. By adjusting the immersion time, they were able to produce 10–20 μm thick CaP coatings. Similarly, Zhang et al. (2009) improved the corrosion rate of Mg substrates by creating apatite coatings via SBF immersion. Keim et al. (2011) prepared a biomimetic layer on a Mg substrate with CaP and carbon on it, using a cell culture medium, resulting in a remarkable reduction of Mg release and improved cell adhesion. Gray-Munro et al. (2009) used several surface modification layers onto Mg alloy to minimize the formation of toxic by-products. The corrosion rate of the surface-modified Mg alloy in descending order was as follows: Clean > acid etched > CaP coated > poly(lactic acid) coated > poly(DTH carbonate) coated. Li et al. (2004) found no mass loss, when 99.99% pure magnesium Mg substrates (alkali and heat treated) were immersed for 180 days in SBF with high and low concentration of Cl^- ions. They found no effect on marrow cell growth owing to apatite coating, which hindered the corrosion of Mg substrates. Witte et al. (2005) also found the same effect on Mg substrates when immersed in SBF, even when bone cell activation was performed at high Mg concentrations. No formation of bone was observed in the adjacent tissues; however, gas pockets were observed with no adverse effects on the bone tissue and implant surfaces.

Biomimetic coatings on polymer surfaces

The enhanced biocompatibility offered by the development of a CaP layer on the polymer substrates has become significant. Various techniques have been employed for coating, including biomimetic coating, laser deposition, spray coating, coupling, and low-temperature precipitation processes. Among these methods, biomimetic coating is the most frequently used approach. Similar to metallic substrates, polymers are also found in nonbiodegradable and biodegradable grades and are applied in the human body according to their applications and usage (Koju et al., 2017).

3.6 Nonbiodegradable polymer substrates

3.6.1 Polyetheretherketone and polyetherketoneketone

Polyetheretherketone (PEEK) (Khurshid, 2020) and polyetherketoneketone (PEKK) (Alqurashi et al., 2021) are nonbiodegradable polymers, which have been investigated for various biomedical applications. To enhance the bioactivity, Yu et al. (2005) obtained HA/PEEK composite coatings using biomimetic techniques and reported a direct relationship between HA volume fraction and crystal quantity. In addition, the crystal size was enlarged with prolonged immersion times. Chi et al. (2013) reported that biomimetic immersion led to crystalline and columnar (rutile or anatase phase) for R-TiO_2/PEEK substratess, with enhanced formation of HA and osteocompatibility. Zheng et al. (2014) used plasma polymerization of acrylic acid to attach carboxyl groups on the PEEK surface. Subsequently, these plasma-carboxylated PEEK specimens were immersed in SBF for 4 weeks to obtain surface deposition of bone-like apatite and retaining its bulk mechanical properties. Zhou et al. (2014) used rapid microwave-assisted biomimetic technique to produce bioactive apatite coating onto PEEK substrates. Kakinuma et al. (2015) produced HA film on the acid-treated PEEK by immersing using SBF, urea, and urease. HA-coated specimens were immersed in an inositol phosphate solution and silver nitrite solution, which provided both antibacterial activity and biocompatibility. Yuan et al. (2022) developed a porous PEKK scaffold using biomimetics with enhanced osteoinductivity.

3.6.2 Biodegradable polymer substrates

3.6.2.1 Poly(ε-caprolacetone)

Yang et al. (2001) were able to produce a uniform fiber coating of calcium-deficient apatite after 7 days SBF immersion onto poly(ε-caprolacetone) (PCL) substrates with higher scaffold surface density. Zhang et al. (2005) observed bone marrow stromal cell infiltration into electrospun PCL of up to 48 μm and PCL/gelatin scaffolds of up to 114 μm. Oyane et al. (2005) used two-dimensional (2D) and three-dimensional (3D) structures of PCL substrates and produced a thin layer of interconnected porous apatite with good adhesion and uniformity. Arafat et al. (2011) achieved enhanced bone marrow mesenchymal stromal cells using CHA/gelatin-coated scaffolds onto PCL substrates with good adhesion and higher compressive modulus. Araujo et al. (2008) noticed an increase in the crystallinity of CaP coatings onto PCL substrate with the increase in socking time in SBF solution. Huang et al. (2015) found an increased wound healing rate using PCL/cellulose acetate substrate modified using collagen and chitosan.

3.6.2.2 Poly(lactic acid)/poly(lactic-co-glycolide)

Kim et al. (Huang, 2015) studied in vivo transplantation of poly(lactic-*co*-glycolide) (PLGA)/HA composites and observed satisfactory osteoconductivity, wherein, fibrin gel, BMP-2 released up to 8 weeks. Yang et al. (2001) demonstrated very good adhesion and growth of human osteoprogenitors on 3D biodegradable PLGA scaffolds polymer films with excellent differentiation and cell proliferation. Shi et al. (2014) and Kim (2008) used micropatterning biomimetic technique on PLGA nanosheets and found protein and gene expression with direct cellular alignment.

3.6.2.3 Opportunities and challenges

Additive manufacturing (AM) techniques such as 3D printing have improved manufacturing owing to less waste, customization, difficulty in producing complex geometries, greater design freedom, and a rapid production rate (Shi, 2014). Furthermore, the investigation of various manufacturing properties through AM has led to the study of bioinspired structures, encompassing the imitation of plants, animals, and insects (Fig. 3.4) (Bourell, 2017).

There is a huge opportunity to utilize biomimetic 3D printing materials with improved physical and mechanical properties (Chaturvedi et al., 2022; Yan, 2021). 3D printed bioinspired coating can be further investigated in two separate categories: (1) single-material bioinspired reinforced structures that are manufactured by 3D printing using a single material, such as polymers, metals, and graphene. In addition, honeycomb structures can be produced by an AM technique called fused deposition modeling, which is a process accomplished by directly extruding the

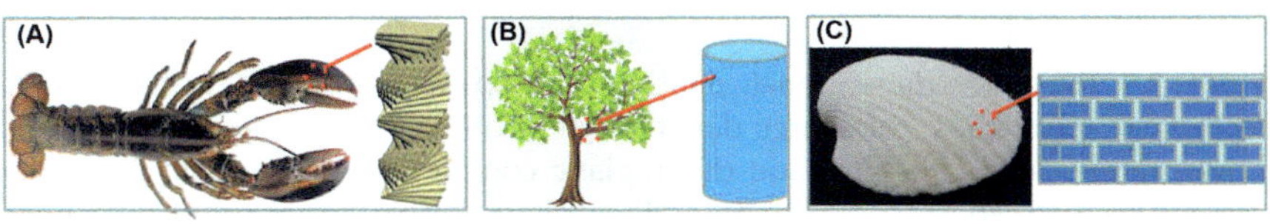

Figure 3.4 Schematic diagram shows the biomimetic structures: (A) Bouligand structure from lobster claw; (B) aligned fiber in balsa wood; (C) brick-and-mortar structure in natural nacre (Bourell, 2017). *From Bourell, D. et al. (2017). Materials for additive manufacturing.* CIRP Annals, *66(2), 659–68, open source.*

materials with a heated printing nozzle (Fig. 3.5) (Bourell, 2017). (2) Multimaterials: numerous 3D-printed constructions such as those stimulated by the Bouligand structure, balsa wood structure, and other structures capable of shape-changing (Zhu, 2021).

For example, the Bouligand structure in a lobster claw improves the toughness and impact resistance of the material by increasing the difficulty of crack propagation (Bourell, 2017). Similarly, the aligned fiber in a balsa wood structure strengthens the structure, which further enhances the wind resistance capability of the produced materials. The brick-and-mortar structure in natural nacre leads to increased impact resistance owing to crack deflection and energy dissipation. For instance, (Compton and Lewis, 2014) prepared a biomimetic structure of balsa wood produced by 3D direct ink writing, which oriented milled carbon fibers in epoxy resin along the print direction (Zimmermann, 2013). Nature provides excellent models that can be further adjusted to develop products that best suit real-life applications. Coincidentally, rapid advancements in

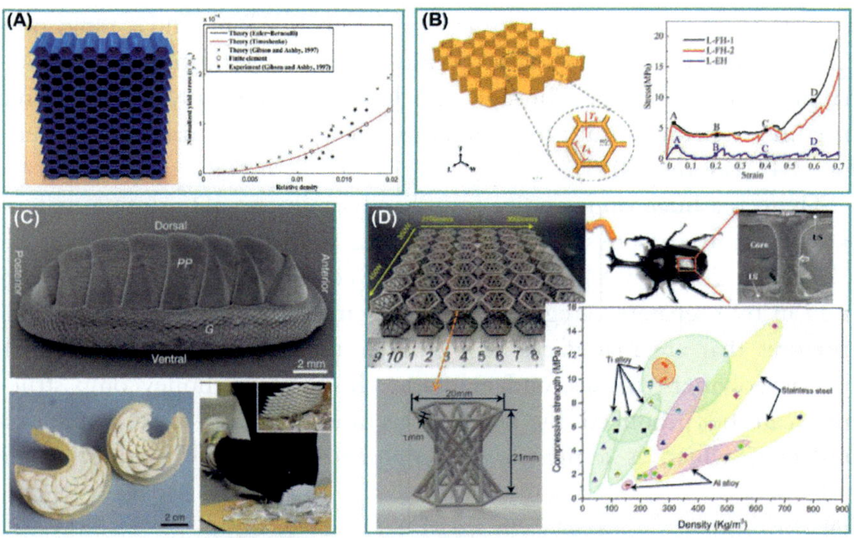

Figure 3.5 The three-dimensional printing bioinspired reinforced structures: (A) Mechanical properties of three-dimensional printed thick honeycombs; (B) honeycomb-inspired structures and the in-plane compressive stress-strain curves for different layer thicknesses; (C) chiton scale-inspired flexible armor using rigid polymers; (D) the adult Allomyrina dichotoma beetle-inspired structure with the metal lattice structure fabricated by selective laser melting (Bourell, 2017). *From Bourell, D. et al. (2017). Materials for additive manufacturing.* CIRP Annals, 66*(2), 659–68, open source.*

current manufacturing techniques are driving progress in bioinspired 3D printing technology (Bourell, 2017). To achieve this objective, we still need further push towards next-generation nature-inspired structures utilizing innovative materials and 3D printing techniques that are environmentally sustainable, cost-effective, powered by renewables, and asserting improvement in structural design. Understanding the mechanisms of natural structures more can serve as inspiration for shaping 3D printing processes crucial to forthcoming engineering applications.

3.7 Conclusion

In this chapter, we have discussed various biomimetic approaches for applying CDHA coatings to metallic or nonmetallic orthopedic implants. Such biomimetic coatings demonstrate properties similar to that of natural bone tissues and promote osseointegration. Additional biomimetic approaches such as surface pretreatment of metallic implants (such as acid etching, or heat treatment) prior to soaking in SBF can potentially reduce implant rejection and improve the overall outcomes of biomimetic coated implants. In contrast, other techniques such as plasma spraying involve harsh conditions of high temperature, which may damage the underlying substrate and compromise the clinical performance of implants.

References

Adawy, A., & Abdel-Fattah, W. I. (2013). An efficient biomimetic coating methodology for a prosthetic alloy. *Materials Science and Engineering C*, *33*(3), 1813–1818. Available from https://doi.org/10.1016/j.msec.2012.12.056.

Alqurashi, H., Khurshid, Z., Syed, A. U. Y., Habib, S. R., Rokaya, D., & Zafar, M. S. (2021). Polyetherketoneketone (PEKK): An emerging biomaterial for oral implants and dental prostheses. *Journal of Advanced Research*, *28*, 87–95.

Ananth, K. P., Jose, S. P., Nathanael, A. J., Oh, T. H., Mangalaraj, D., & Ballamurugan, A. M. (2015). Biomimetic ion substituted hydroxyapatite coating on surgical grade 316L SS for implant applications. *Advanced Materials Letters*, *6*(11), 984–989. Available from https://doi.org/10.5185/amlett.2015.5913.

Arafat, M. T., Lam, C. X., Ekaputra, A. K., Wong, S. Y., Li, X., & Gibson, I. (2011). Biomimetic composite coating on rapid prototyped scaffolds for bone tissue engineering. *Acta Biomaterialia*, 7(2), 809–820.

Araujo, J., Martins, A., Leonor, I., Pinho, E. D., Reis, R., & Neves, N. (2008). Surface controlled biomimetic coating of polycaprolactone nanofiber meshes to be used as bone extracellular matrix analogues. *Journal of Biomaterials Science. Polymer Edition*, *19* (10), 1261–1278.

Barrere, F., Snel, M. M. E., Van Blitterswijk, C. A., De Groot, K., & Layrolle, P. (2004). Nano-scale study of the nucleation and growth of calcium phosphate coating on titanium implants. *Biomaterials, 25*(14), 2901–2910. Available from https://doi.org/10.1016/j.biomaterials.2003.09.063.

Barrere, F. V., Van Blitterswijk, C., De Groot, K., & Layrolle, P. (2002). Nucleation of biomimetic Ca–P coatings on Ti6Al4V from a SBF × 5 solution: Influence of magnesium. *Biomaterials, 23*(10), 2211–2220.

Barrère, F., Layrolle, P., Van Blitterswijk, C. A., & De Groot, K. (1999). Biomimetic calcium phosphate coatings on Ti6Al4V: A crystal growth study of octacalcium phosphate and inhibition by Mg^{2+} and HCO_3. *Bone, 25*(2 Suppl. 1), 107S–111S. Available from https://doi.org/10.1016/s8756-3282(99)00145-3.

Bigi, A., Boanini, E., Panzavolta, S., & Roveri, N. (2000). Biomimetic growth of hydroxyapatite on gelatin films doped with sodium polyacrylate. *Biomacromolecules, 1*(4), 752–756.

Bourell, D., Kruth, J., Leu, M., Levy, G., Rosen, D., Beese, A., & Clare, A. (2017). Materials for additive manufacturing. *CIRP Annals, 66*(2), 659–681. Available from https://doi.org/10.1016/j.cirp.2017.05.009.

Chaturvedi, I., Jandyal, A., Wazir, I., Raina, A., & Ul Haq, M. I. (2022). Biomimetics and 3D printing – Opportunities for design applications. *Sensors International, 3*, 100191. Available from https://doi.org/10.1016/j.sintl.2022.100191.

Chi, M.-H., Tsou, H.-K., Chung, C.-J., & He, J.-L. (2013). Biomimetic hydroxyapatite grown on biomedical polymer coated with titanium dioxide interlayer to assist osteocompatible performance. *Thin Solid Films, 549*, 98–102.

Collins, C. M., & Safiuddin, M. (2022). Lotus-leaf-inspired biomimetic coatings: Different types, key properties, and applications in infrastructures. *Infrastructures*, 7(4), 46.

Cui, F., Yang, J., Jiao, Y., Yin, Q., Zhang, Y., and., & Lee, I.-S. (2008). Calcium phosphate coating on magnesium alloy for modification of degradation behavior. *Frontiers of Materials Science China, 2*, 143–148.

Diesendruck, C. E., Sottos, N. R., Moore, J. S., & White, S. R. (2015). Biomimetic self-healing. *Angewandte Chemie International Edition, 54*(36), 10428–10447.

Dorozhkina, E. I., & Dorozhkin, S. V. (2002). Surface mineralisation of hydroxyapatite in modified simulated body fluid (mSBF) with higher amounts of hydrogencarbonate ions. *Colloids and Surfaces A: Physicochemical and Engineering Aspects, 210*(1), 41–48.

Earle, W. R. (1943). Production of malignancy in vitro. I. Method of cleaning glassware. *Journal of the National Cancer Institute, 4*(2), 131–133.

Forsgren, J., Svahn, F., Jarmar, T., & Engqvist, H. (2007). Formation and adhesion of biomimetic hydroxyapatite deposited on titanium substrates. *Acta Biomaterialia, 3*(6), 980–984.

Ghorbani, F., Zamanian, A., Behnamghader, A., & Joupari, M. D. (2018). Microwave-induced rapid formation of biomimetic hydroxyapatite coating on gelatin-siloxane hybrid microspheres in 10X-SBF solution. *e-Polymers, 18*(3), 247–255.

Gray-Munro, J. E., Seguin, C., & Strong, M. (2009). Influence of surface modification on the in vitro corrosion rate of magnesium alloy AZ31. *Journal of Biomedical Materials Research Part A, 91*(1), 221–230.

Gu, Y., Liu, Y., Jacobs, R., Wei, L., Sun, Y., Tian, L. Liu, Y., & Politis, C. (2023). BMP-2 incorporated into a biomimetic coating on 3D-printed titanium scaffold promotes mandibular bicortical bone formation in a beagle dog model. *Materials & Design, 228*, 111849. Available from https://doi.org/10.1016/j.matdes.2023.111849.

Habibovic, P., Barrère, F., Van Blitterswijk, C. A., De Groot, K., & Layrolle, P. (2002). Biomimetic hydroxyapatite coating on metal implants. *Journal of the American Ceramic Society, 85*(3), 517–522. Available from https://doi.org/10.1111/j.1151-2916.2002.tb00126.x.

Hanks, J. H., & Wallace, R. E. (1949). Relation of oxygen and temperature in the preservation of tissues by refrigeration. *Proceedings of the Society for Experimental Biology and*

Medicine, *71*(2), 196–200. Available from https://doi.org/10.3181/00379727-71-17131.

Huang, R., et al. (2015). Biomimetic LBL structured nanofibrous matrices assembled by chitosan/collagen for promoting wound healing. *Biomaterials*, *53*, 58–75.

Jiao, Z., Wang, Z., Wang, Z., & Han, Z. (2023). Multifunctional biomimetic composite coating with antireflection, self-cleaning and mechanical stability. *Nanomaterials*, *13* (12), 1855.

Kakinuma, H., Ishii, K., Ishihama, H., Honda, M., Toyama, Y., Matsumoto, M., & Aizawa, M. (2015). Antibacterial polyetheretherketone implants immobilized with silver ions based on chelate-bonding ability of inositol phosphate: Processing, material characterization, cytotoxicity, and antibacterial properties. *Journal of Biomedical Materials Research Part A*, *103*(1), 57–64.

Keim, S., Brunner, J. G., Fabry, B., & Virtanen, S. (2011). Control of magnesium corrosion and biocompatibility with biomimetic coatings. *Journal of Biomedical Materials Research Part B, Applied Biomaterials*, *96*(1), 84–90.

Khurshid, Z., Saudah, H., Samet, T., Syed, R. H., Rizwan, U., Farshid S., & Muhammad, S. Z. (2020). *Titanium, zirconia, and polyetheretherketone (PEEK) as a dental implant material*. In *S.N. Khan, Z. Farshid SefatKhurshid, S. Hafeji, S. Tekin, S.R. Habib, R. Ullah, F. Sefat, & M.S. Zafar (Eds.), Dental implants* (pp. 5–35). Woodhead Publishing.

Kim, S. S. (2008). Orthotopic bone formation by implantation of apatite-coated poly (lactide-co-glycolide)/hydroxyapatite composite particulates and bone morphogenetic protein-2. *Journal of Biomedical Materials Research Part A*, *87*, 245–253.

Kodama, A., Bauer, S., Komatsu, A., Asoh, H., Ono, S., and., & Schmuki, P. (2009). Bioactivation of titanium surfaces using coatings of TiO_2 nanotubes rapidly pre-loaded with synthetic hydroxyapatite. *Acta Biomaterialia*, *5*(6), 2322–2330.

Koju, N., Sikder, P., Ren, Y., Zhou, H., & Bhaduri, S. B. (2017). Biomimetic coating technology for orthopedic implants. *Current Opinion in Chemical Engineering*, *15*, 49–55. Available from https://doi.org/10.1016/j.coche.2016.11.005.

Kokubo, T. (1998). Apatite formation on surfaces of ceramics, metals and polymers in body environment. *Acta Materialia*, *46*(7), 2519–2527.

Li, L., Gao, J., and., & Wang, Y. (2004). Evaluation of cyto-toxicity and corrosion behavior of alkali-heat-treated magnesium in simulated body fluid. *Surface and Coatings Technology*, *185*(1), 92–98.

Liu, J., Mohd Rafiq, N. B., Wong, L. M., and., & Wang, S. (2021). Surface treatment and bioinspired coating for 3D-printed implants. *Frontiers in Chemistry*, *9*. Available from https://doi.org/10.3389/fchem.2021.768007, https://www.frontiersin.org/articles/.

Liu, Y., et al. (2017). One-step fabrication of biomimetic superhydrophobic surface by electrodeposition on magnesium alloy and its corrosion inhibition. *Journal of Colloid and Interface Science*, *491*, 313–320. Available from https://doi.org/10.1016/j.jcis.2016.12.022.

Miyaji, F., Kim, H.-M., Handa, S., Kokubo, T., and., & Nakamura, T. (1999). Bonelike apatite coating on organic polymers: Novel nucleation process using sodium silicate solution. *Biomaterials*, *20*(10), 913–919.

Montazerian, M., Hosseinzadeh, F., Migneco, C., Fook, M. V. L., & Baino, F. (2022). Bioceramic coatings on metallic implants: An overview. *Ceramics International*, *48*(7), 8987–9005. Available from https://doi.org/10.1016/j.ceramint.2022.02.055.

Oliveira, A., Malafaya, P., & Reis, R. L. (2003). Sodium silicate gel as a precursor for the in vitro nucleation and growth of a bone-like apatite coating in compact and porous polymeric structures. *Biomaterials*, *24*(15), 2575–2584.

Oyane, A., Onuma, K., Ito, A., Kim, H., Kokubo, T., and., & Nakamura, T. (2003). Formation and growth of clusters in conventional and new kinds of simulated body fluids. *Journal of Biomedical Materials Research Part A*, *64*(2), 339–348.

Oyane, A., Uchida, M., Yokoyama, Y., Choong, C., Triffitt, J., & Ito, A. (2005). Simple surface modification of poly(ε-caprolactone) to induce its apatite-forming ability. *Journal of Biomedical Materials Research Part A*, *75*(1), 138–145. Available from https://doi.org/10.1002/jbm.a.30397.

Pu, X., Li, G., & Huang, H. (2016). Preparation, anti-biofouling and drag-reduction properties of a biomimetic shark skin surface. *Biology Open*, *5*(4), 389–396.

Ringer, S. (1882). Concerning the influence exerted by each of the constituents of the blood on the contraction of the ventricle. *The Journal of Physiology*, *3*(5–6), 380.

Selim, M. S., El-Safty, S. A., Shenashen, M. A., Higazy, S. A., & Elmarakbi, A. (2020). Progress in biomimetic leverages for marine antifouling using nanocomposite coatings. *Journal of Materials Chemistry B*, *8*(17), 3701–3732.

Shi, X., Fujie, T., Saito, A., Takeoka, S., Hou, Y., Shu, Y., Mingwei, C., Hongkai, W., & Ali, K. (2014). Periosteum-mimetic structures made from freestanding microgrooved nanosheets. *Advanced Materials*, *26*(20), 3290–3296.

Song, W.-H., Jun, Y.-K., Han, Y., & Hong, S.-H. (2004). Biomimetic apatite coatings on micro-arc oxidized titania. *Biomaterials*, *25*(17), 3341–3349.

Staiger, M. P., Pietak, A. M., Huadmai, J., & Dias, G. (2006). Magnesium and its alloys as orthopedic biomaterials: A review. *Biomaterials*, *27*(9), 1728–1734.

Takadama, H., Kim, H., Kokubo, T., & Nakamura, T. (2001). TEM-EDX study of mechanism of bonelike apatite formation on bioactive titanium metal in simulated body fluid. *Journal of Biomedical Materials Research*, *57*(3), 441–448.

Tas, A. C. (2000). Synthesis of biomimetic Ca-hydroxyapatite powders at 37°C in synthetic body fluids. *Biomaterials*, *21*(14), 1429–1438.

Tas, A. C., & Bhaduri, S. B. (2004). "Rapid coating of Ti6Al4V at room temperature with a calcium phosphate solution similar to 10× simulated body fluid. *Journal of Materials Research*, *19*(9), 2742–2749.

Wang, M., & Sun, T. (2009). Electrochemical deposition of apatite/collagen composite coating on NiTi shape memory alloy and coating properties. *MRS Online Proceedings Library (OPL)*, *1239*, 1239–VV02-07. Available from https://doi.org/10.1557/PROC-1239-VV02-07.

Witte, F., Kaese, V., Haferkamp, H., Switzer, E., Meyer-Lindenberg, A., Wirth, C. J., & Windhagen, H. (2005). In vivo corrosion of four magnesium alloys and the associated bone response. *Biomaterials*, *26*(17), 3557–3563.

Yan, X., Brandon, B., Hengxi, C., Siqi, X., Shuang, L., Brian, T., Laiming, J., & Yang, Y. (2021). Recent advancements in biomimetic 3D printing materials with enhanced mechanical properties. *Frontiers in Materials*, *8*. Available from https://doi.org/10.3389/fmats.2021.518886.

Yang, X., Roach, H. I., Clarke, N. M. P., Howdle, S. M., Quirk, R., Shakesheff, K. M., & Oreffo, R. O. C. (2001). Human osteoprogenitor growth and differentiation on synthetic biodegradable structures after surface modification. *Bone*, *29*(6), 523–531.

Yao, Y., Dang, X., Qiao, X., Li, R., Chen, J., Huang, Z., & Gong, Y. K. (2022). Crosslinked biomimetic coating modified stainless-steel-mesh enables completely self-cleaning separation of crude oil/water mixtures. *Water Research*, *224*, 119052.

Yu, S., Hariram, K. P., Kumar, R., Cheang, P., & Aik, K. K. (2005). In vitro apatite formation and its growth kinetics on hydroxyapatite/polyetheretherketone biocomposites. *Biomaterials*, *26*(15), 2343–2352.

Yuan, B., Zhang, Y., Zhao, R., Lin, H. Yang, X., Zhu, X. Zhang, K., Mikos, A. G., & Zhang, X. (2022). A unique biomimetic modification endows polyetherketoneketone scaffold with osteoinductivity by activating cAMP/PKA signaling pathway. *Science Advances*, *8*(40), eabq7116.

Zafar, M. S., Amin, F., Fareed, M. A., Ghabbani, H., Riaz, S., Khurshid, Z., & Kumar, N. (2020). Biomimetic aspects of restorative dentistry biomaterials. *Biomimetics*, *5*(3), 34.

Zhang, Y., Venugopal, J., Huang, Z.-M., Lim, C., & Ramakrishna, S. (2005). Characterization of the surface biocompatibility of the electrospun PCL-collagen nanofibers using fibroblasts. *Biomacromolecules*, *6*(5), 2583–2589.

Zhang, Y., Zhang, G., & Wei, M. (2009). Controlling the biodegradation rate of magnesium using biomimetic apatite coating. *Journal of Biomedical Materials Research Part B Applied Biomaterials*, *89*(2), 408–414.

Zheng, Y., Xiong, C., & Zhang, L. (2014). Formation of bone-like apatite on plasma-carboxylated poly (etheretherketone) surface. *Materials Letters*, *126*, 147–150.

Zhou, H., Goel, V. K., & Bhaduri, S. B. (2014). A fast route to modify biopolymer surface: A study on polyetheretherketone (PEEK). *Materials Letters*, *125*, 96–98.

Zhou, H., Nabiyouni, M., & Bhaduri, S. B. (2013). Microwave assisted apatite coating deposition on Ti6Al4V implants. *Materials Science and Engineering C*, *33*(7), 4435–4443.

Zhu, Y., Dylan, J., Weitong, S., Yiyu, C., Jiahui, R., Hanyu, Z., Siqi, X., & Xiangjia, L. (2021). 3D printing biomimetic materials and structures for biomedical applications. *Bio-Design and Manufacturing*, *4*(2), 405–428. Available from https://doi.org/10.1007/s42242-020-00117-0.

Zimmermann, E. A., Gludovatz, B. Schaible, E., Dave, N. K. N., Yang, W., Meyers, M. A., & Ritchie, R. O. (2013). Mechanical adaptability of the Bouligand-type structure in natural dermal armour. *Nature Communications*, *4*(1), 2634.

CHAPTER 4

Biomimetic coatings for the dental implants

Naresh Kumar[1], Faiza Amin[1], Nazrah Maher[1], Muhammad Amber Fareed[2,3] and Muhammad Sohail Zafar[3,4,5]

[1]Department of Science of Dental Materials, Dow University of Health Sciences, Karachi, Pakistan
[2]Clinical Sciences Department, College of Dentistry, Ajman University, Ajman, United Arab Emirates
[3]Center of Medical and Bio-allied Health Sciences Research, Ajman University, Ajman, United Arab Emirates
[4]Department of Restorative Dentistry, College of Dentistry, Taibah University, Madinah, Saudi Arabia
[5]Department of Dental Materials, Islamic International Dental College, Riphah International University, Islamabad, Pakistan

4.1 Introduction

Biomimetic surface modifications refer to developing and applying materials and techniques that mimic the properties and structures found in nature (Kumar et al., 2022). Scientists and engineers can create synthetic materials with enhanced properties and improved performance by studying and emulating the designs and functions of biological surfaces. In recent years, extensive research has been conducted on the bioactive and biomimetic coating design of dental implant surfaces (Cruz et al., 2022; Dua et al., 2023; Mathur et al., 2022) enhancing the bioactive properties of dental implants (Cruz et al., 2022). In this chapter, several biomimetic approaches and manufacturing processes that have been historically and potentially employed to improve the characteristics of dental implant coatings are discussed.

There are various ways in which biomimetic surface modifications can be achieved as shown in Table 4.1.

The functionalization of biomimetic implant coatings containing organic or bioactive molecules promotes the adhesion of various bone-forming cells (Zafar et al., 2020). Titanium and its alloys are the most used implant materials and represent gold standards for dental implant fabrication because of their exceptional combination of high corrosion resistivity, favorable mechanical properties, and biocompatibility (Gil et al., 2021; Li et al., 2021; Sánchez-Bodón et al., 2022). Although titanium dental implants have been reported to have the highest success rate, some

Smart Biomimetic Coatings
DOI: https://doi.org/10.1016/B978-0-443-21738-8.00004-7

Table 4.1 Strategies for biomimetic surface modifications.

No.	Surface modification techniques	Description	Mechanism	References
1.	Surface texturing	To replicate the micro- and nanoscale structures found on the surfaces of dental implant materials	By mimicking these structures, superhydrophobic coatings have been developed	Cruz et al. (2022), Accioni et al. (2022), Knaus et al. (2020)
2.	Bioinspired coatings	To develop implant coatings that mimic the properties of natural materials	By recreating these structures, adhesive coatings have developed that can be used for various applications	Dua et al. (2023), Accioni et al. (2022), Knaus et al. (2020)
3.	Surface functionalization	Involves modifying the surface chemistry of materials to replicate the properties of natural surfaces.	This effect has been replicated by creating textured surfaces and modifying surface chemistry	Mathur et al. (2022), Knaus et al. (2020), Knaus et al. (2020)
4.	Bioactive surfaces	Biomimetic surface modifications involved incorporating biological molecules onto surfaces to enhance the bonding between the implant and surrounding tissue	Mimic the structure of bone to improve dental implant integration by encouraging cell growth	Mathur et al. (2022), Accioni et al. (2022), Knaus et al. (2020)
5	Protein-based coatings	Utilize natural proteins, such as collagen or fibronectin, to mimic the Extracellular Matrix (ECM) found in tissues to enhance cell attachment and promote tissue integration.	Provide a reservoir for growth factors and bioactive molecules, further enhancing the regenerative potential of the implant.	Cruz et al. (2022), Accioni et al. (2022), Knaus et al. (2020)
6.	Biomimetic antibacterial coatings	Inspired by natural antimicrobial properties, which are designed to inhibit bacterial growth, and prevent infections.	Based on antimicrobial peptides, silver nanoparticles, or other materials antimicrobial activity.	Cruz et al. (2022), Accioni et al. (2022), Knaus et al. (2020)

complications due to titanium hypersensitivity and immune reactions still occur, in addition to osseointegration problems in patients with bone-related diseases (Gil et al., 2021). Moreover, biomimetic coatings improve the corrosion resistance, biocompatibility, and bioactivity of dental implants using a variety of collagen, bioglass, titanium dioxide, and inorganic coatings (dicalcium phosphate, tricalcium phosphate, hydroxyapatite (HA), and nano-HA) to promote and accelerate bone formation around dental implants (Li et al., 2021; Najeeb et al., 2017; Zafar et al., 2019). By combining scientific understanding with advanced materials and techniques, biomimetic implant coatings aim to provide patients with restorations that closely resemble their natural teeth, both in appearance and function. Therefore there is a need for continuous improvement of dental implant surfaces to achieve this essential goal, particularly implant coating material characteristics, such as biomimetic coating design, to ensure the long-term success of osseointegration of dental implants.

4.2 Biomimetic approaches in clinical dentistry and dental implants

Biomimetics is a multidisciplinary field that combines biology, materials science, and engineering principles to develop innovative dental treatments and materials to focus on the tooth structure to achieve a more harmonious integration and enhance functionality (Graeff et al., 2021). Biomimetic approaches in clinical dentistry involve the application of principles and techniques that mimic the natural structures, functions, and properties of teeth and oral tissues (Paryani et al., 2023; Zafar et al., 2010). The goal is to achieve dental restorations that closely resemble natural teeth in terms of esthetics, strength, and durability. Biomimetics in dentistry represents a paradigm shift in restorative dentistry, focusing on preserving tooth structure, achieving long-lasting results, and mimicking the natural properties of teeth (Paryani et al., 2023; Shinya, 2023).

4.3 Biomimetic coatings for dental implants

Biomimetic coatings are specialized materials or surface modifications that are designed to mimic and replicate the properties and functions of natural biological systems. The purpose of biomimetic coatings is to enhance the performance, integration, and longevity of various biomedical implants, including dental implants (Choi et al., 2013). These coatings aim to promote biological responses, such as cell adhesion, tissue growth, and integration, by emulating the characteristics found in natural tissues and organs (Dua et al., 2023; Stewart et al., 2019). However, biomechanical properties, surface properties, and biocompatibility play a crucial role in the effectiveness of biomimetic coatings in enhancing osseointegration of dental implants. The surface properties, including surface roughness, topography, chemistry, and wettability of biomimetic coatings, determine their interaction with the surrounding biological environment (Zhang et al., 2020). By introducing nano-surface structures, these coatings can mimic the natural roughness of bone, facilitating cell attachment and growth (Sachin et al., 2022). Biomimetic surface coatings promote desirable cell adhesion, proliferation, and differentiation to help create an environment that facilitates the integration of implants with the surrounding biological tissues, whereas the biocompatibility of biomimetic coatings enables them to coexist harmoniously (Gadallah et al., 2022) with the host tissues, promoting tissue healing, regeneration, and integration that closely resemble the composition and surface characteristics of natural bone tissue. Thus enhanced biocompatibility of the biomimetic implant surface reduces the risk of adverse reactions and promotes favorable cellular responses for the attachment and proliferation of bone cells, leading to better integration with the implant (Mathew et al., 2020).

In the context of dental implants, biomimetic coatings play a crucial role in improving the success rate and long-term stability of the implants by enhancing the osseointegration, implant stability, and reduced chances of complications. Thus osseointegration is critical in dental implants' long-term success and stability. Biomimetic coatings can significantly enhance osseointegration by mimicking the properties and structure of natural tissues. Moreover, some biomimetic coatings have inherent bioactive properties, releasing ions or growth factors (GFs) that are beneficial for bone regeneration and integration (Liu et al., 2021; Zafar et al., 2020). For example, coatings containing HA or bioactive glasses (BAGs) can release calcium and phosphate ions, promoting the formation of a bone-like apatite layer on the implant surface (Sousa et al., 2017). This layer acts as a bridge between the implant and the surrounding alveolar bone, enhancing osseointegration. Biomimetic coatings can optimize the stress distribution between the implant and the surrounding bone. By mimicking the natural structures and properties of bone, these coatings can improve load transfer and distribution, reducing stress concentration and potential implant failure. This aspect is crucial for long-term implant stability and success. Thus biomimetic coatings play a vital role in enhancing osseointegration by improving biocompatibility, modifying surface properties, and creating an environment that promotes cellular responses and tissue integration. By mimicking the natural characteristics of bone, these coatings can optimize the implant's interaction with the host tissue, leading to improved stability, functionality, and longevity of dental implants (Kravania et al., 2022; Liu et al., 2021).

4.4 Biomimetic approaches in dental implants

Dental patients often lose dentition because of disease, trauma, and developmental anomalies. Traditionally, fixed prostheses or removable dentures are used to restore functions and esthetics; however, these treatment options have certain limitations, including compromised durability of the prosthesis, fracture of teeth, questionable biocompatibility of the restorative materials, restricted occlusal forces, gradual loss of residual alveolar bone, and secondary caries (Davarpanah et al., 2000). Alternatively, numerous types of dental implants have been introduced to replace lost dentition, which include endosteal implants, subperiosteal, and transosteal for the rehabilitation of fully or partially edentulous patients: implant treatment has become a foremost treatment option (Assaf et al., 2023; Elani et al., 2018; Papaspyridakos et al., 2012). In clinical practice, endosteal implants have been regarded as the most reliable implant system because of their adequate occlusal force distribution, excellent esthetics, clinical outcomes, and minimum surgical morbidity (Elani et al., 2018; Gallardo et al., 2019).

At the moment, dental implants are dependable options for long-term use as abutments in a broad spectrum of scenarios (Gulati et al., 2014). In optimal conditions, high survival and success rates are reported. However, patients with compromised health conditions like diabetes, poor bone quality, and osteoporotic disabilities are undergoing frequent clinical failures. However, in these cases, implant stability can be maintained by enhanced bone formation, and as a result, good mechanical implant-bone fixation can be achieved. Nevertheless, this success can only be possible with the selection of an appropriate dental implant by professional assessment of available bone quality and dimensions of the residual edentulous ridge (Iacono, 2000). During selecting the implant system and patient, it should be kept in mind that the implant surface microtopography can affect the migration and orientation of osteoblasts, which may result in compromised osseointegration of dental implants (Schneider et al., 2004). Fig. 4.1 summarizes the different biomimetic approaches to dental implants.

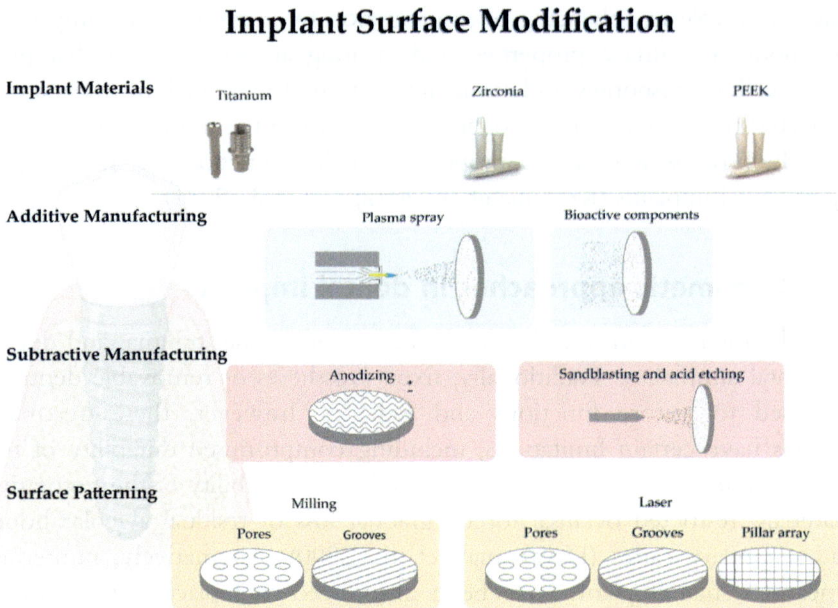

Figure 4.1 Approaches in biomimetic dental implants coatings. *Reproduced from Cruz, M. B., Silva, N., Marques, J. F., Mata, A., Silva, F. S., & Caramês, J. (2022). Biomimetic implant surfaces and their role in biological integration—A concise review.* Biomimetics, *7, 74.*

4.4.1 Additive manufacturing

Additive manufacturing (AM) is a fabrication method that involves accumulation of materials and establishes a 3D form. Customized design solutions, rapid prototyping in combination with computer-aided design (CAD), made this technique the most popularized among the other manufacturing methods. AM allows the evaluation of the materials that may be too intricate for the conventional fabrication technique. However, with the growing popularity of this technique, the accessibility of the treatment can be enhanced (Kim et al., 2023).

4.4.2 Plasma spraying

Sir Crooke identified plasma in 1879 (Crookes, 1883) and the name was given by Langmuir in 1929. In the late 1850s, Simens used the first plasma discharge to create the ozone layer. In recent times, the study of plasma has advanced rapidly and expanded its scope to encompass various domains such as agriculture, aerospace technology, biomedicine, environmental science, and defense (Heinlin et al., 2011). For the fabrication and disinfection process of dental instruments, Eva Stoffels used plasma in dentistry (Sladek et al., 2004). In the plasma spraying technique, during the coating process of dental implants, the feedstock requires to be melted at high temperature. This process needs argon or argon/hydrogen mixture as a carrier molecule. The implant surface should be prepared onto which the molten and semimolten particles are propelled (Fauchais & Montavon, 2007). The plasma stream that is produced during the process can reach temperatures of 8000 K or higher and this level of heat is adequate for melting refractory materials as well as metallic and nonmetallic that has a high melting point (Erne & Kolar, 2012). For coating on implant substrate, plasma spraying can be broadly divided into thermal and no thermal as well as radio frequency discharges and direct current arcs-generated plasmas. Thermal plasmas are natural phenomena that are used for coating flames, detonation guns high-velocity oxy-fuel flames, high-velocity air-fuel flames (HVAF), and wire arcs, whereas nonthermal plasmas, also known as nonthermal atmospheric pressure plasma (NTAPP), cold atmospheric plasma, or low-temperature atmospheric pressure plasma, constructed from artificial sources and due to which, the temperature and composition can be changed (Fauchais & Montavon, 2007). NTAPP is also used as a surface treatment in the form of chairside applications (Laroussi & Lu, 2005).

Plasma spray process through HA deposition increases the surface roughness of the implant substrate (Becker et al., 2016; Huang et al., 2017). At high temperatures, plasma torch is bombarded with the particles of plasma and then particles are condensed merged and projected onto the implant surface. Before the projection of particles, sand blasting is carried out on the surface to ensure excellent durability. The thickness of the surface obtained through this process can range from a few micrometers to millimeters (Laroussi & Lu, 2005). Nevertheless, delamination and marginal bone resorption are the common complications reported with plasma spraying process (Åstrand et al., 2000; Becker et al., 2016).

4.4.3 Subtractive manufacturing

Manufacturers usually use subtractive techniques particularly for the metals that involve the elimination of the materials from initially crude shaped parts like bar, slab, forgoing, and casting. The basic objective is to achieve the desired shape and dimensions of the final product. The chief examples of this technique are acid etching, anodizing, blasting, laser, milling, patterning, and sand blasting (Cao et al., 2010). The recent innovation in the contemporary subtractive technique is the introduction of digital control that involves integration of several processes into a single machine. The advantage of this technique is that it skips the loading and unloading of the workpiece between the different steps of the process (Hutchings & Shipway, 2017).

4.4.4 Anodizing, blasting, and acid etching

Previously, at the time of introduction of implants by Branemark, implant surfaces were produced by milling, turning, or polishing techniques, and they were designated as machined implants (Brånemark et al., 1983). Depending on the quality of the bone and anatomical location, these machined implants require a long healing time period on an average from 3 to 6 months. The literature has reported that after osseointegration, long-term survival rates of these machined implant surfaces (Albrektsson et al., 1981; Jemt et al., 2015; Wennerberg et al., 2018) were higher than nonmachined implant surfaces. However, the failure of these implants might be because of insufficient surface roughness, which results in limited attachment of osteogenic cells, inadequate bone deposition, and insufficient bone—implant interface. Therefore, to promote osseointegration, surface roughness in the range of 1—2 μm is required (Albrektsson & Wennerberg, 2004). In recent clinical studies, it was found by the researchers that machined implants demonstrated poor prognosis in terms of osseointegration, when compared with rough surface implants (Chrcanovic et al., 2016; Karl & Albrektsson, 2017; Lang & Jepsen, 2009; Lennerås et al., 2015; Omar et al., 2011; Research, 2015; Wennerberg et al., 2018) (Fig. 4.2). It was revealed that Implant stability was enhanced, enabling the use of immediate and early loading protocols when there is an increase in the surface roughness of implants as they increase contact osteogenesis, and bone ingrowth (Wennerberg & Albrektsson, 2009).

These subtractive procedures were introduced in dentistry in the early 1900s and can be used either individually or simultaneously in combination with each other (Bowers et al., 1992). Anodization is an electrochemical modality in which implant surface undergoes electrolytic process. This electrolytic process involves treating the implant surface with strong acids such as hydrofluoric acid (HF), nitric acid (HNO_3), sulfuric acid (H_2SO_4), and phosphoric acid (H_3PO_4). The outcome of this technique is to increase the

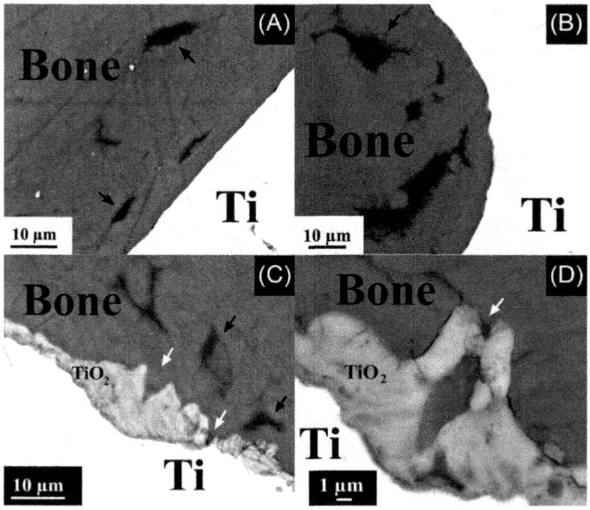

Figure 4.2 Backscattered SEM illustrations of (A and B) machined implant and (C and D) oxidized implant. The black and white arrows highlight some osteocyte lacunae and bone ingrowth, respectively. *Reproduced from Omar, O. M., Lennerås, M. E., Suska, F., Emanuelsson, L., Hall, J. M., Palmquist, A., & Thomsen, P. (2011). The correlation between gene expression of proinflammatory markers and bone formation during osseointegration with titanium implants.* Biomaterials, 1*(32), 374-386.*

thickness of the titanium oxide layer on implant surface (Hall, 2000). Anodization technique modifies the implant surface and increases the oxide layer formation and surface roughness using strong acids such as HF, nitric acid (HNO_3), sulfuric acid (H_2SO_4), and phosphoric acid (H3PO4). Higher bone-to-implant contact (BIC) was reported in anodization-treated implant surface in comparison with the machined implant surfaces in animal and human studies (Rocci et al., 2013; Traini et al., 2018). When sand blasting and acid etching process were combined Sub-acute Bacterial Endocarditis (SABE), an excellent adhesion for proteins and mechanical fixation was obtained as this combination of treatment produced excellent surface roughness (Al-Nawas et al., 2008). In this combination method, the rough surface was created on machined implant by projecting high-velocity particles through a nozzle. These particles were in range of 10 to several 100 μm. This process was followed by bombardment with Al_2O_3 and TiO_2 or calcium phosphates particles (Le Guéhennec et al., 2007). To remove the remnants and contaminants, these implant surfaces were immersed in strong acids at elevated temperature. This process removed blasted particles from the surface and also improved the topography and chemistry of the surface. The roughness of machined implant surface was increased from an average (Sa) of $\leq 0.5\ \mu m$ to Sa of $1-2\ \mu m$ following anodization and Sandblasted Acid Etched (SA) process. It was demonstrated that the long-term survival rate of implant surface was increased by 98.5% and 96.7% after anodization and SA processes, respectively, compared to 96.4% previously (Wennerberg et al., 2018), It was found that sand blasting and acid etching implants demonstrated a greater resistance against reverse torque as well as the highest osteoblastic differentiation in vivo when compared to implant surfaces processed with different surface treatments (Cho & Park, 2003; Hirano et al., 2015; Kim et al., 2015) (Fig. 4.3). However, the limitation of this process is that even after acid etching, the remnants or contaminants of the particles were not able to clean properly and act as a major contamination which adversely affects the properties. Moreover, it was noteworthy that the reported literature is mostly based on the coating applied on titanium implants and there is a dearth of literature on zirconia-based coatings (Ehrenfest MDC & Kang, 2014; Senna et al., 2015).

4.4.5 Biomimetic surface patterning

Surface patterning was initially used on titanium surfaces as surface coating by utilizing biologically inspired topographies to control the epithelial cell

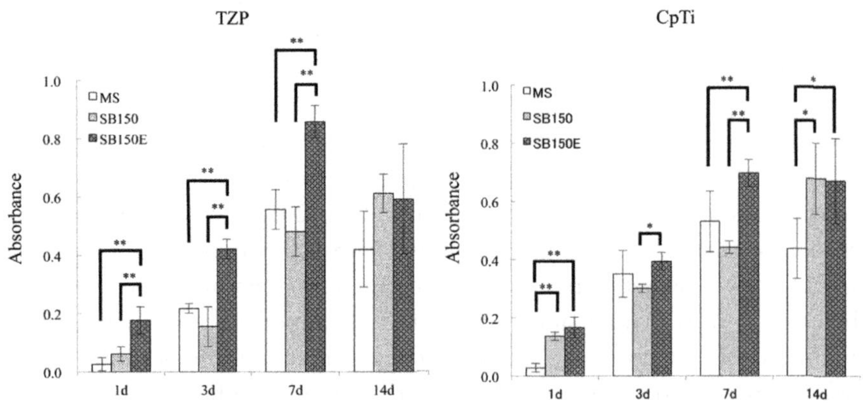

Figure 4.3 Highlights the cell proliferation ability on different surfaces of zirconia (TZP) and titanium (CpTi). In both TZP and CpTi, a relatively greater cell proliferation was observed on the blasted and etched surface (SB150E) as compared to the mirror-polished (MS) and blasted only (SB150) surfaces. *Reproduced from Hirano, T., Sasaki, H., Honma, S., Furuya, Y., Miura, T., Yajima, & Y, et al. (2015). Proliferation and osteogenic differentiation of human mesenchymal stem cells on zirconia and titanium with different surface topography.* Dental Materials Journal, 34, *872-880.*

migratory behavior (Senna et al., 2015). This technique is considered a promising approach in the literature, demonstrating a clear relationship between patterning surface topography and cell adhesion and behavior (Ketabi & Deporter, 2013; Mendoza-Arnau et al., 2016; Taniguchi et al., 2016; Wang et al., 2003). Chehroudi and co-workers concluded in their in vitro and in vivo studies that greater epithelial cell adhesion was found at the depth of 10μm grooves when patterning surface was compared with the smooth titanium surfaces (Chehroudi et al., 1988). The existing research in this field has primarily focused on the titanium surfaces and a limited amount of work has been done and published on the implant surfaces based on zirconia. Moreover, there is a lack of unanimity among the studies about optimal shape and dimensions of these macro patterns (Delgado-Ruíz et al., 2016; Nadeem et al., 2013; Stangl et al., 2001).

4.4.6 Milling

On the industrial scale, milling is an effective, adaptable, and precision cutting technology used to alter the shape of the material by removing the substrate material. Presently, with the advancement in the technique, pores or holes can also be processed. There are several types of milling cutting tools like drills and milling cutters. However, it is noteworthy that the effectiveness and efficiency of the milling process can be compromised, if the machinability technique is not properly utilized. There are many factors that should be considered before the milling process like the tools used for cutting, surface finish, the type of chips formed, machining power, and the volume of chips removed per time interval (Ghalandari et al., 2021). It was demonstrated that a good bone-to-implant interface will be created through these imperfections and milled surfaces as these surfaces allowed osteogenic cells to attach and deposit bone, though these treatments showed inconsistent results on cell behavior. Milling technique has an impact on osteoblast cellular differentiation; however, it does not promise cell proliferation (Brunette, 1986)

4.4.7 Laser

Laser technology is used to promote surface characteristics at macro, micro, and nanolevels. The material is heated, melted, and sublimated at high temperature and density (De Tullio et al., 2020; Lee & Bance, 2019). Among all the surface treatments of implants, this is the only method that operates without risk of contamination and allows the speedy

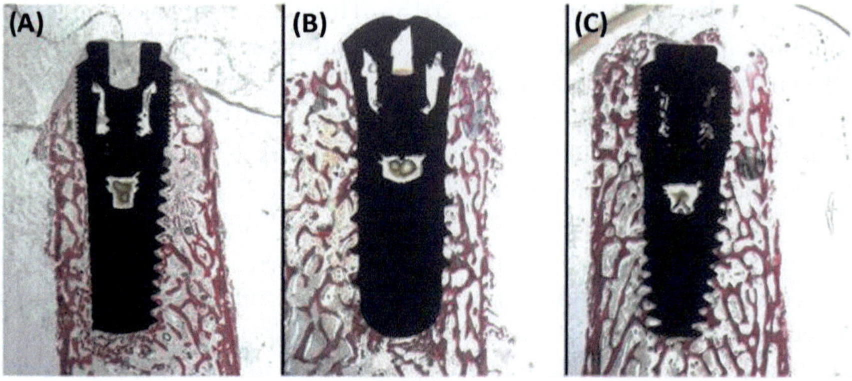

Figure 4.4 The optic microscopic illustrations of (A) machined implant, (B) sandblasted and acid-etched implant and (C) laser-treated implant after 30 days of their placement. Both (B) and (C) implants exhibit more osteogenesis areas and mineralization nuclie compared to (A) implant. *Reproduced from De Tullio, I., Berardini, M., Di Iorio, D., Perfetti, F., Perfetti, G. (2020). Comparative evaluation among laser-treated, machined, and sandblasted/acid-etched implant surfaces: An in vivo histologic analysis on sheep.* International Journal of Implant Dentistry, *6, 1-8.*

and precise formation of grooves (De Tullio et al., 2020; Pellegrini et al., 2018) (Fig. 4.4). To create surface roughness on zirconia implant surfaces, Nd: YAG and CO_2 lasers are more frequently used. However, many different types of lasers have been introduced, including free-electron lasers, gas lasers (CO_2 and excimer), semiconductor lasers (quantum cascade laser and diode laser) solid-state lasers (Nd:YAG, Ti: sapphire and fiber laser), liquid lasers (organic dye liquid). Lasers can operate in both continued and paused mode (De Tullio et al., 2020; SAMANT, 1976). It is noteworthy that the laser treatment did not affect the crystalline structure of the zirconia but significantly increased the surface roughness. At the same time, laser technology keeps the surface clean and homogenous (Delgado-Ruiz et al., 2014; Rompen et al., 2006). According to literature, osseointegration was potentially increased after the laser treatment. When titanium implants were placed in human, studies demonstrated that apical migration of epithelium was inhibited along with a reduction in crestal bone (Wang et al., 2003). Moreover, cell colonization after the placement of zirconia implants, the surfaces of which have been treated by different techniques and patterns, is not evident scientifically. Besides, superior cell behavior was observed in Nd:YAG laser-patterned zirconia surfaces when compared with nontextured surfaces (Stangl et al., 2001).

4.5 Biomimetic coatigs for dental implants

Surface modification of the dental implant has also been done by coating its surface with biological bioactive molecules that imitate the living tissue or structure and enhance the bonding between implant and surrounding tissue by promoting cell growth (Javed et al., 2020; Saleem et al., 2020).

4.5.1 Biological coating

Osseointegration of endosseous implant can be improved by coating the surface with biomolecules that can present adhesive factors to cells, and one approach is to use bioactive cell adhesion peptides present in the components of the ECM like fibronectin (FN), collagen, peptides, and laminin, etc.

4.5.2 Collagen

Collagen, a primary protein in the bone ECM, consists of 3 α-chains, tightly wrapped into a triple helix of polypeptides, and forms the striated fibril by the self-aggregation process. Type 1 collagen constitutes 90% of the total bone collagen, providing a backbone for bone formation. Collagen contains an Arginine-Glycine-Aspartate, RGD amino acid sequence (arginine—glycine—aspartate) that adheres with the specific surface integrin receptors on the osteoblast. This interaction supports the attachment, differentiation, and proliferation of osteoblastic cells (Itoh et al., 2002; Moursi et al.,1997; Puleo & Bizios, 1991). Thus collagen is the crucial ECM protein for implant research and studies.

Successful osseointegration and stability of implants depend on the early osteoblast attachment and its dissemination on the implant surface. The implants coated with collagen compared to uncoated ones have revealed higher osteoblastic adhesion and proliferation (Geißler et al., 2000). Micro-CT and histological evaluation in an in vivo study demonstrated the presence of mature bone in proximity with the coated surface at 15, 30, and 60 days with no signs of inflammation, bone resorption, and destruction (Fig. 4.5). It also found significant differences in the bone area inner thread, BIC, and bone area outer thread between coated and uncoated surfaces, indicating its ability to promote early osteogenesis (Scarano et al., 2019). Collagen-coated nano-topographical implants can stimulate the process of in vitro osteogenesis by significantly enhancing the osteoblastic proliferation, Alkaline Phosphatase (ALP) activity, ECM mineralization, the release of bone sialoprotein (BSP), and the gene

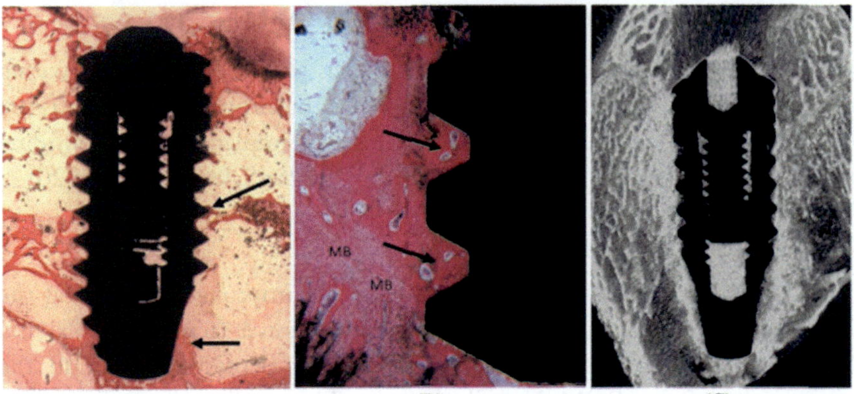

(A) (B) (C)

Figure 4.5 (A and B) Histological evaluation and (C) micro-CT evaluation showing mature trabecular bone in close proximity with the collagen-coated implant. *Reproduced from Scarano, A., Lorusso, F., Orsini, T., Morra, M., Iviglia, G., & Valbonetti, L. (2019). Biomimetic surfaces coated with covalently immobilized collagen type I: An X-ray photoelectron spectroscopy, atomic force microscopy, micro-CT and histomorphometrical study in rabbits.* International Journal of Molecular Sciences, 20, *724*

expression of osteoblastic cell survival markers (Coll1a, OSX, OC, and BAX genes) (Costa et al., 2017). Collagen fibril coating, because of its high surface/volume ratio, adheres better to the implant surface and increases the gene expression involved in osteoblastic differentiation (Bougas et al., 2012; Wolf-Brandstetter, 2004). An experimental study revealed that the phenolic-enriched collagen fibril coating promoted osteogenic differentiation by enhancing the COL1A1 and BGLAP genes and reducing the expression of proinflammatory cytokines (Mieszkowska et al., 2020). The combination of collagen and HA coating showed higher BIC and bone development in the peri-implant area, contrary to only collagen-coated (Lee et al., 2014)

Implant failure can also occur due to soft tissue defects around the implant, and collagen, being the main constituent of the gingival fibroblast ECM, can solve these problems by improving cell—implant interaction. An experimental study revealed that the fibroblast cells better adhered and proliferated on the collagen1-coated implant (Ti/Col-1) with optimized ECD (electrochemical disposition) conditions (Fig. 4.6) (Truc et al., 2018). Three-dimensional mesh-like collagen nanofiber-coated dental implant was used in a preclinical pilot study, and the results showed that the nanofiber yielded improved gingival tissue adhesion to titanium as gingival collagen fiber penetrated the mesh structure resulting in tight

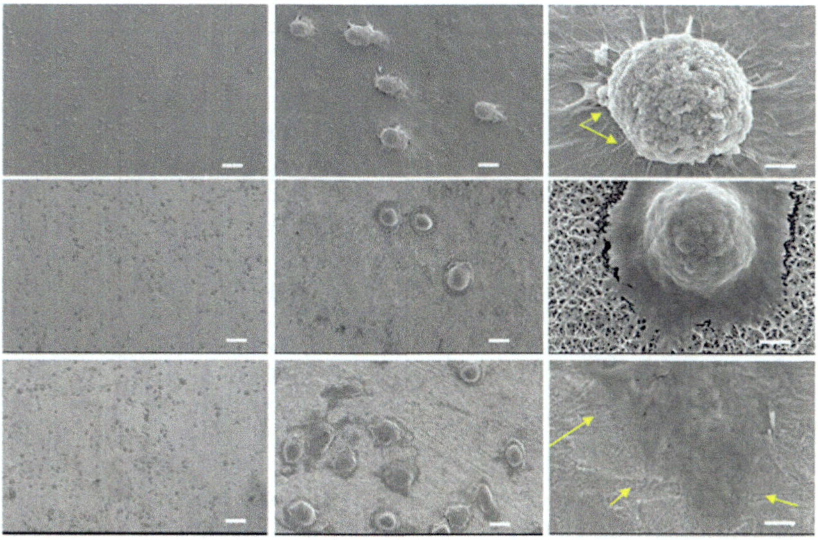

Figure 4.6 Scanning electron microscopy images showing fibroblast cell attachment on (A) untreated Ti, (B) porous TiO_2, (C) collagen-coated Ti at various magnifications. *Reproduced from Truc, N. T., Minh, H. H., Khanh, L. L., Thuy, V. M, Van Toi, V., Van Man, T, Nam, H. C., Quyen, T. N., Hiep, N. T. (2018). Modification of type I collagen on TiO_2 surface using electrochemical deposition.* Surface and Coatings Technology, 25*(344), 664-672.*

contact. (Raita et al., 2015). The articles that covered collagen coatings on dental implant surfaces are summarized in Table 4.2.

4.5.3 Fibronectin

FN is the most abundant noncollagenous ECM protein that also regulates various interactions between extracellular and intracellular environments via the RGD sequence that binds to integrin receptors. (Pearson et al., 1988) It is a multifunctional, dimeric, high molecular weight(400 kDa) extracellular glycoprotein composed of two homologous polypeptides held by di-sulfide covalent bond at their carboxyl termini (Pankov & Yamada, 2002). It is released in the initial phases of osteogenesis and plays a key part in osteoblast cell attachment, growth, and proliferation. (García et al., 1998)

It has been immobilized onto the implant surface by various methods and has demonstrated early osteoblast adhesion (Hayakawa et al., 2005). When the FN was immobilized on the implant fixture using the Tresyl chloride activation technique in the rabbit tibiae, the histological and

Table 4.2 Surface modifications of dental implant with collagen proteins.

No.	Surface Modification	Results	References
1	Collagen type I-coated implant surfaces	Collagen-coated implants showed improved BIC, BAIT, BOAT, and osseointegration at 15, 30, and 60 days compared to controls.	Scarano et al. (2019)
2	Collagen coating on titanium implants with nano-topography	Enhanced cell proliferation, ALP activity, ECM mineralization, the release of BSP, and expression of Coll1a, OSX, OC, and BAX genes	Costa et al. (2017)
3	Implants coated with HA (hydroxyapatite), CH (collagen plus HA), and CHB (bone morphogenetic protein2 with collagen and HA)	The CH group showed notably higher bone development and BIC than HA and CHB groups.	Lee et al. (2014)
4	Titanium coated with phenolic-enriched collagen fibrillar	Promoted osteogenic differentiation by increasing the COL1A1, and BGLAP relative expressions. Also, reduced the inflammatory response by decreasing the inflammatory cytokines and MMP2 gene expressions.	Mieszkowska et al. (2020)
5	Modification of collagen Type 1 on Ti surface by utilizing ECD (electrochemical deposition) method	Col-1 coated Ti demonstrated the quick and highest amount of fibroblast adhesion, the capacity of spreading, viability, and proliferation compared with the uncoated Ti.	Truc et al. (2018)
6	Collagen nanofiber-coated dental implants using electrospray deposition technique (ESD) technique	Gingival connective tissue attachment (percentage) for Coll- nanofiber: 45.7%—Coll: 25.3%—Ti: 20.7%	Raita et al. (2015)

histomorphometric observations revealed a marked improvement in bone mass, bone adaptation, and BIC after 12 weeks, then uncoated control (Hirota et al., 2015). Implants grafted with FN by glow discharge plasma not only increased the implant surface topography, hydrophilicity, and osteogenic differentiation. (Chang et al., 2016) but also increased the implant stability, bone mass, and BIC due to early osteoblast cells attachment on the implant surface (Fig. 4.7) (Chang et al., 2016). According to biomolecular and histological analysis, the ability of FN and rhBMP-7 to early control the expression of TGF- superfamily cytokines (BMP-4, BMP-7, and TGF-2) led to stronger neo-osteogenesis and antiinflammatory properties than collagen 1-coated (Schierano et al., 2021). A preclinical experimental study showed that the peptides derived from FN also enhanced osteogenic induction by upregulating Runx2, BSP, and OC gene expressions (Pramono et al., 2016).

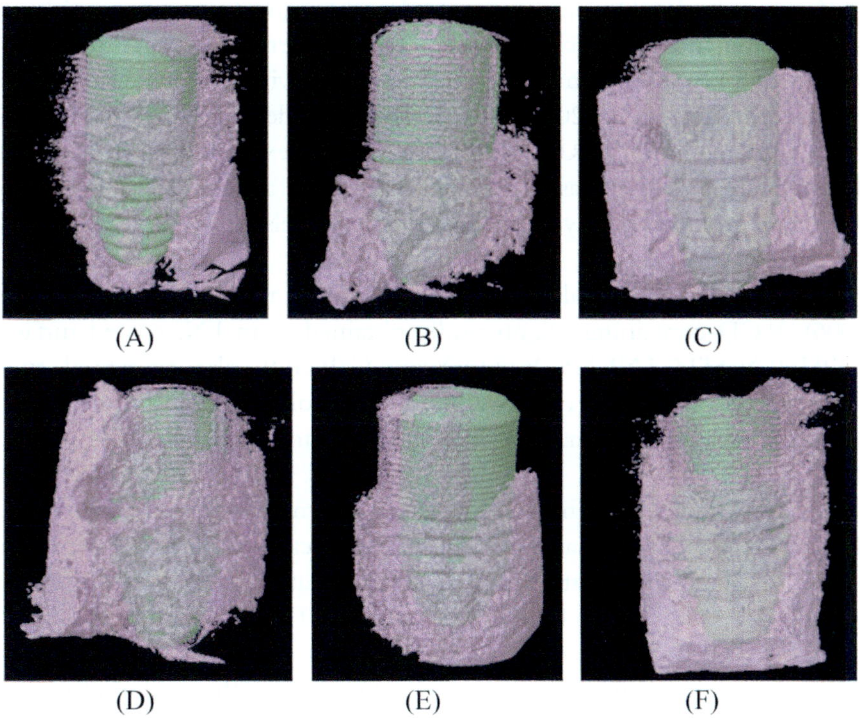

Figure 4.7 Early osteoblastic adhesion and differentiation around fibronectin-coated implants (D, E, F) compared to uncoated (A, B, C). *Reproduced from Chang, Y. C., Lee, W. F., Feng, S. W., Huang, H. M., Lin, C. T., Teng, N. C., Chang, W.J. (2016). In vitro analysis of fibronectin-modified titanium surfaces.* PLoS One, *11,* e0146219.

FN can also promote soft connective tissue attachment to the implant fixture, as in an experimental study, it exhibited more human gingival fibroblast adhesion, spread, and proliferation, particularly on the micro-grooved implant surface compared to smooth (Jian et al., 2017). Table 4.3 describes the papers that discussed FN coatings on dental implant surfaces.

4.5.4 RGD peptides

Research has recently been focused on developing and incorporating RGD-containing peptides to support early osteoblast cell adhesion because the majority of ECM components in bones, such as FN, collagen, and osteopontin, possess RGD amino acid sequences that are significant mediators of cell adhesion stages (Itoh et al., 2002). These peptides are preferred over whole ECM molecules due to their availability in vast quantities, easy maneuvering, decreased antigenicity, and stability.

Among the RGD-sequenced peptides, those produced from FN have received the most research attention. FN fragment has successfully imitated native FN in human osteoblast-like cell activities and its related gene expressions (Kim et al., 2007). FN-derived peptides GRGDSP, PHSRN, and a combination of GRGDSP/PHSRN, in an experimental study, have shown increased osteoblast-like cell MC3T3-E1 attachment, differentiation, and proliferation by expressing higher levels of Runx2, BSP, and OC, ALP activity, and matrix mineralization. However, GRGDSP/PHSRN-coated Ti revealed the most promising results (Pramono et al., 2006). RGD-containing oligopeptide, obtained from FN, coated surface (DPHSRN-SITGTNLTPGYTITVYAVTG-RGD), also presented two times greater osteoblastic cell attachment and proliferation in vitro and significantly greater bone mass in vivo than the uncoated ones (Kim et al., 2007).

RGD peptides exist in two different conformations, linear and cyclic; the two forms have variations in their biological behavior. (Al-Noaman et al., 2012) Preclinical studies have shown that compared to the linear peptide (l-RGD), cyclic RGD peptide (c-RGD) significantly and positively influenced the osteoblast, endothelial cells, and platelets behavior by inhibiting the aggregation of platelets, promoting the endothelial and osteoblast cells adhesion and differentiation (Kämmerer et al., 2011; Kim et al., 2005; Verrier et al., 2002). Histological examination in an in vitro study also demonstrated increased BIC and vertical bone apposition in the c-RGD-coated surface (Heller et al., 2018).

Table 4.3 Surface modification of dental implant with fibronectin proteins.

No.	Surface modification	Results	References
1	Dental implants coated with collagen type 1, fibronectin, rhBMP-7	Fibronectin and rhBMP-7 demonstrated osteogenic and antiinflammatory effects by early regulating the expression of cytokines (BMP-4, BMP-7, TGF-β2) from the TGF-β superfamily.	Schierano et al. (2021)
2	Fibronectin-coated titanium disk using tresyl chloride activation technique	New bone formation, BIC, and bone mass (BM) were significantly higher for Fn/Ti	Hirota et al. (2015)
3	Fibronectin-grafted titanium dental implants using GDP	GDP-fib displayed significantly greater implant stability quotient and bone volume/total volume ratio compared to Ar-GDP at 2 and 4 weeks.	Chang et al. (2016)
4	Fibronectin-modified titanium surfaces	GDP-fib promoted osteoblast-like cell (MG-63 cell) attachment, spreading, and differentiation on the surface of titanium	Chang et al. (2016)
5	FN (fibronectin) and FN-derived peptides coated Ti	FN and FN-derived peptides enhanced the osteogenic differentiation of MC3T3-E1 cells, mineralization of ECM, ALP activity, and Runx2, BSP, and OS gene expression.	Pramono et al. (2016)
6	Fibronectin-coated micro-grooved titanium plate	Ti with micro-grooved structure (35 m in width, 15 m in bridge, and 10 m in depth) coated with FN caused human gingival fibroblasts (HGFs) to arrange alongside the grooves and promoted cell dissemination, adhesion, and differentiation compared to a smooth surface.	Jian et al. (2017)

4.5.5 Non-RGD peptides

Osteoblast adhesion occurs through two distinct mechanisms: the first involves the RGD sequence interaction with the integrin receptor, and the second, less well-understood, process is the interaction of osteoblastic cell—membrane heparan sulfate with heparin-binding domain of ECM proteins. (Dalton et al., 1995; Xiao & Truskey, 1996). Non-RGD peptides are osteoblast-specific and promote adhesion, differentiation, and proliferation through the second mechanism. The following heparin-binding domains have recently been identified in ECM proteins: REDRV sequences in FN, IKVAV sequences in laminin, and DGEA sequences in Type 1 collagen (Rezania & Healy, 1999).

The experimental study evaluated the bioactivity level for RGD (GRGDSP) and non-RGD peptides (HVP) through osteoblastic cell adhesion and detachment assay, and the results revealed that although the RGD-sequenced was the most active in improving cell adhesion strength, the HVP showed a similar adhesion capacity due to its osteoblast-specific nature (Bagno et al., 2007). Multidomain peptide (LA2) containing IKVAV amino acid sequences and heparin-binding domain induced the osteo-differentiation by supporting the adhesion of MC3T3-E1 (osteoblast cell line) and production of ALP in in vitro testing and, when grafted subcutaneously in mice, the improved tissue integration was observed, without inflammation and unwanted side effects (Lin et al., 2006). Hence, these non-RGD sequenced peptides can be promising bioactive molecules for biomimetic titanium surface modification, which requires considerable research in the future. The publications that reported RGD and non-RGD coatings on dental implant surfaces are described in Table 4.4.

4.5.6 Growth factors

GFs constitute a diverse range of proteins that play a crucial role in numerous biological processes, encompassing cell differentiation, chemotactic, and cell proliferation (Delgado-Ruiz et al., 2014). In today's era, the combination of dental implant surfaces and GF proteins has become increasingly significant. In promoting bone formation, the osteogenic potential of these GFs has been utilized by many researchers (Table 4.5). Nevertheless, the activity of these biologically active proteins and locally delivered at the site of application is yet to be identified (Thomson & Lotze, 2003). Bone formation will be enhanced when GFs are deposited

Table 4.4 Surface modification of dental implant with RGD and non-RGD peptides.

NO.	Surface Modification	Results	References
RGD PEPTIDES			
1	Fibronectin and fibronectin fragment including Arg-Gly-Asp sequence (RGD) and Pro–His–Ser–Arg–Asn sequence (PHSRN)-coated implants	Fibronectin fragment, at a suitable concentration of $\geq 1\ \mu M$, successfully replicated natural FN in human osteoblast-like cell activities and its associated genes regulation.	Kim et al. (2003)
2	RGD-containing oligopeptide-coated surface (DPHSRNSITGTNLTPGYTITVYAVTG-RGD)	Increased osteoblastic cell attachment and proliferation in vitro and statistically significantly higher bone mass in vivo.	Kim et al. (2007)
3	Pretreated Ti surface modified with Linear and cyclic RGD peptides (l-RGD and c-RGD)	c-RGD peptides coated surface showed the highest endothelial cell coverage and proliferation.	Kämmerer et al. (2011)
4	linear and cyclic RGD peptides (c and l-RGD) immobilized on titanium surfaces	c and l-RGD promoted osteogenic differentiation in vitro. In vivo, improved VBA and BIC were observed for c-RGD.	Heller et al. (2018)
NON-RGD PEPTIDES			
1	Multidomain peptide (LA2) containing cell and heparin binding domains	LA2 on porous titanium implants showed improved adaptation of bone cells onto the implant surface	Lin et al. (2006)
2	(GRGDSP)4 K (RGD Peptide)and (351–359)HVP (non-RGD peptide) coated implants	HVP peptide showed an adhesion capacity that is comparable to the RGD-grafted one	Bagno et al. (2007)

Table 4.5 Surface modifications of dental implants with growth factors.

Author	Surface modification	Findings
Anitua (2006)	Titanium implant surface coated with plasma-rich growth factor	Higher percentage of BIC in 99.6% coated implants
Lan et al. (2006)	rhBMP-2 coated with (rhbFGF) or (rhIGF-1)	Enhance new bone formation To improve osseointegration operate synergistically with rhbFGF and rhIGF-1
Park et al. (2006)	Ti implants coated with FGF-FN.	Improved osseointegration.
Nikolidakis et al. (2009)	TGF-β1 coated around the implant.	During the early post-implantation healing phase detrimental effect on the placement of oral implants in trabecular bone.
Schouten et al. (2009)	TGF-β1 on implant surface	Insignificant results
Lee et al. (2010)	Ti surface coated with the combination of PLGA and bFGF	Improved peri-implant bone formation
Ramazanoglu et al. (2011)	Recombinant human vascular endothelial growth factor I65 (rhVEGFI65) and rhBMP-2 coated implants	Increases Bone Density but no effect on BIC
Schliephake et al. (2015)	sandblasted acid-etch implants; coated with DNA oligonucleotide hybridized with rhVEGF-	Enhanced BIC

BIC, Bone implant contact; BD, bone density; TGF-β1, transforming growth factor; bFGF, basic fibroblast growth factor; rhBMP-2, recombinant human bone morphogenetic protein-2; rhbFGF, human basic fibroblast growth factor; rhIGF-1, recombinant human insulin-like growth factor 1; FGFFN, fibroblast growth factor-fibronectin; TGF-β1, transforming growth factor; PLGA, poly (lactide-co-glycolide); BFGF, basic fibroblast growth factor; rhVEGFI65, recombinant human vascular endothelial growth factor I65; VEGF, vascular endothelial growth factor.

on the implant surfaces through immobilization techniques. This bone formation induced differentiation of large number of osteogenic cells without a widespread systemic release and become attached to the surface. (Kim et al., 2008).

To induce cell differentiation, cell migration, and cell proliferation, the attachment of osteoblast cells to the ECM is the key requirement for the GFs (Mazor et al., 2004). Due to the high content of GFs in plasma-rich proteins, it is used in many treatment modalities in oral and maxillofacial surgery (Mazor et al., 2004). Coating the implant with plasma-rich protein can be very effective as these proteins boost the regeneration process that is facilitated by the releasing of GFs. These GFs are present inside the granules of platelets, which include transforming GFs (TGF), platelet-derived GFs, and insulin-like GF-1 (IGF-1).

Although there are a lot of uncertainties about the coating of implants with platelet-rich proteins (PRP) treatment. The foremost challenge is to evenly distribute GFs to the implant surface. Moreover, the basic requirement of biomimetic coating agents is that they should have a long half-life so that they properly release their effect. Therefore one of the major limitations of the PRP impregnated on implant surface is that GFs have very short half-life (Freymiller & Aghaloo, 2004). Further studies are required to develop effective methods of incorporating GFs and control their actions, in the target area further studies are required.

4.5.7 Bone morphogenetic proteins

Bone morphogenetic proteins (BMPs) belong to the proteins family discovered in the 1960s. The significant role of BMPs is in the formation and induction of bone and cartilage on areas where it normally would not form. Naturally, in minute amounts (1 g/kg dry weight of bone) are found in bone material. They are synthesized by many tissues, including bone, cartilage, and central nervous system. In the development and maintenance of skeletal, these BMPs play a major and critical role (Christiansen et al., 2000). Twenty types and subtypes of BMPs have been described to date. All BMPs belong to the TGF superfamily except for BMP-1 that comes under metalloproteinase class (Urist et al., 1983). An identical sequence of 114 amino acids is found in humans, mice, and rats of BMP-2 proteins. BMP-7 comprising 139 amino acids also known as osteogenic protein-1 or Vg-1 is identical mouse and human proteins. Over the last decade, recombinant human BMPs (rhBMP-2) have been identified to be used as coadjuvant therapy in dentistry and other biomedical fields. rhBMP-2 acts as a bone-modulating agent (Boyne, 2001). After the placement of the implants coated with rh-BMP-2, researchers found the long-term stability due to the ample amount of bone formation around the intraosseous implants (Wikesjö et al., 2001). When placed in supraalveolar areas, it should be noteworthy that a BMP carrier must not only be capable of resisting compression forces but also simultaneously it should be dimensionally stable. It was also demonstrated that during clinical, any addition process that required should not change the properties of these molecules. When rh-BMP-2-coated implant is used clinically as biomimetic agent, it was observed by the researchers that the features and properties of an implant influenced the release and action of this protein. In a study, Puleo et al. (2002) demonstrated that on the surface of implant, a contemporary material that is allylamine is used instead of silane method to immobilize BMPs. The combination of the implants with BMPs can be successfully used to repair mandibular segmental defects and alveolar bone defects (Fiorellini et al., 2001; Marukawa et al., 2002). There are many benefits of using these proteins such as very well adhering to physiologic pH and temperature condition; therefore they remain unaltered and retain their properties until their therapeutic use. They can be used as a biomimetic coating agent on all types of implant materials, including polymers and metals. Moreover, small doses of these proteins are sufficient to produce periimplant osteogenesis as these BMPs have high osteogenic potential (Tatakis et al., 2002). However, the major disadvantages of BMPs include uncontrolled bone formation at ectopic sites and their high cost. For biomimetic applications, BMPs have the highest bioactive capacity and are the most favorable group with the highest beneficial prospective (Table 4.6). Nevertheless, for the commercial availability of BMP-enriched implants, further experimental research is needed.

4.5.8 Fibroblast growth factors

Fibroblast growth factors (FGFs) are the protein GFs that are derived from mesoderm and neuroderm and play a significant role in cell-simulating properties (Rodan et al., 1989). FGFs increase the growth of the cells that are capable of synthesizing bone collagen which in turn results in enhance bone formation (Aspenberg & Lohmander, 1989). In the course of implant treatment, bone healing is a prime procedure. These FGFs have angiogenic properties that speed up the bone healing process. Increase bone formation was found, when FGFs was incorporated with the demineralized bone, and then implanted the bone and FGFs combination in rats (Park et al., 2006). Miniosmotic pump along with grafting with FGFs also enhances the bone growth incorporation (Wang & Aspenberg, 1994).

Table 4.6 Surface modification of dental implants with bone morphogenetic proteins.

Author	Surface modification	Findings
Becker et al. (2006)	Sand-blasted and acid-etched	Both BIC and bone density were improved.
Lan et al. (2007)	rhBMP-2	Implant-bone osseointegration was improved by rhBMP-2
Wikesjo et al. (2008)	rhBMP-2 on titanium implants	Successful bone formation and osseointegration at 8 weeks due to induction of dose dependent peri-implant bone remodeling
Huh et al. (2012)	Anodized implants coated with rhBMP-2	Improved bone formation and implant stability
Hunziker et al. (2012)	The capacity of BMP-2 to induce peri-implant bone formation can be influenced by its mode of delivery	the osteoinductive efficacy increased
Kim et al. (2015)	rhBMP-2 on osseointegration in dogs (0.1, 0.5, and 1 mg/mL) were applied to sandblasted and acid etched (SLA) implants	Enhancing osseointegration in SLA implants coatings

These FGFs also aid the in vitro osteoblasts proliferation and in vivo bone repair. (Kawaguchi et al., 2001). In MG63 human osteoblastic cells, FGF enhances FN-mediated adhesion by the activation of extracellular regulated kinase (ERK). This activation occurs by the interaction of recombinant human FN peptide (hFNIII9−10) with integrin, resulted in cascade of signaling pathways (Jang et al., 2002).

4.5.9 Natural silk

Natural silks are protein-based polymers that are whirled into fibers under ambient conditions by silkworms and spiders, although silkworm produces most of the natural silk (Hoffman et al., 2012; Zarkoob et al., 2004). Silk fiber consists of an inner protein component called fibroin and an external protective layer called Sericin, which protects the fiber from microbial and environmental degradation. Since sericin can cause hypersensitive and autoimmune reactions, it is extracted from the fiber before any biological application, and only the fibroin portion of the silk is utilized (Hakimi et al., 2007).

Natural silk has been used for many years in medical sciences for various applications due to its excellent biocompatibility, nontoxic nature, and superior mechanical properties (Zuo et al., 2006; Gosline et al., 1999). It degrades slowly in the biological environment (Hakimi et al., 2007). It has a long history in the medical field as surgical suture material and, recently, it is utilized in other biomedical applications such as drug delivery, tissue engineering, and scaffolds. Furthermore, depending upon the application, it can be manipulated to form films, fibers, hydrogels, foams, and coatings on other materials (Hardy et al., 2008).

The coating of silk fibroin has also been employed for dental implants owing to its favorable biocompatibility and physicomechanical characteristics. Elia, Michelson, Perera, Brunner, et al. (2015) developed silk electrogels coatings for Ti implants, and the purpose was to produce a biocompatible and biodegradable coating that can withstand the mechanical forces during implant insertion. Two innovative coating methods were created to coat the implant surface uniformly with silk fibroin. One technique included electrodepositing silk directly onto the titanium surface, while the other involved melting electrogels and using the molten gels to coat the titanium substrate. Coating reproducibility and adhesive strength were evaluated, and the results showed that both the coating procedures produced uniform, controlled coatings with adequate adhesion and mechanical strength to withstand implantation force (Elia, Michelson, Perera, Harsono, et al., 2015). The study also assessed these coatings potential for drug release, mechanical strength, and reproducibility, and the results showed that these approaches produced coatings with adequate adhesive strength and reproducibility and also allowed for the inclusion of medicines and their controlled release (Elia, Michelson, Perera, Harsono, et al., 2015).

In a preclinical study, multifunctional coating (a combination of vancomycin, silk fibroin, and tricalcium phosphate) was developed to coat the implant surface by electrophoretic deposition. The antibacterial assay, cell viability of the MC3T3-E1 cells, and the osteogenic differentiation of multifunctional coating were thoroughly evaluated, and the results revealed that the silk fibroin enabled a controlled release of bioactive substances [vancomycin and Tri-calcium Phosphate (TCP)] on-site and the liberation of vancomycin from the coating resulted in a notable decrease bacterial adhesion at various time intervals. The release of TCP increased the MC3T3-E1 cell line survival, spreading, and proliferation for up to 28 days. (Karaji et al., 2020). Thus natural silk can be a promising bioactive agent for implant coating which requires more extensive research.

4.6 Bioceramic coatings

Different bioceramic materials, such as calcium phosphate, HA, and calcium silicate, can be used as implant coatings while keeping the biomimetic approach in mind and taking into account the properties of bone ECMs (Mohammadi & Sepantafar, 2016).

4.6.1 Hydroxyapatite

Calcium apatite, also known as HA Ca5 (PO4)3(OH), is a mineral that occurs naturally. $Ca_{10}(PO4)_6(OH)_2$ is a crystal unit cell consisting of two different entities that are frequently used in HA formula.

As time has passed, the titanium (Ti) implants have been coated with HA crystals with promising and encouraging results (Joos et al., 2011). The extensively recorded osteoconductive activity of HA promotes bone repair and results in positive bone-implant interactions (Xie et al., 2016). There is evidence of accelerated bone repair surrounding HA-coated implants from several experimental in vivo trials. In terms of HA's direct interaction with bone, the biointegration of HA-coated implants is also obvious. To determine the exact mechanism of HA adhesion with bone, Jemat et al. (2015) and Novaes et al. (2010) recommended further biological and clinical research.

The absence of detectable implant mobility in bone is a positive clinical indicator of osseointegration and is wanted for the duration of the patient's life (Möller et al., 2012). The specific processes underlying the complementary osseointegration and biointegration of HA-covered implants are still unknown. Based on findings in published studies, osseointegration and biointegration between an implant and bone are comparable to the ankylosis of alveolar bone with natural teeth. The biointegrated interface in ceramic-coated metallic implants was noticed by Albrektsson et al. (1981); however, due to degradation over time, the strength of this contact was questioned. In comparison to titanium implants that are not coated, research found that HA coating can speed up implant healing (Porter et al., 2004). Consequently, HA coating has been used frequently because titanium implants have increased bioactivity. In clinical trials, cellular differentiation and proliferation have shown that the HA coating on the titanium implant surface is biocompatible (Bodhak et al., 2009). According to Kuroda et al. (2006) and Choi et al. (2013), HA implant coatings have superior osteoconductivity and osteoinductivity. The early period required for cell differentiation and proliferation can be influenced by HA surface through signal transduction pathways. An osteoinductive milieu is produced when mesenchymal stem cells differentiate into osteoblasts in the presence of cell GFs (Goto et al., 2004). It is now possible to create HA at the nanoscale owing to the development of nanotechnology. For the manufacture of these HA coatings, the "bottom-up" method is most frequently used. It is thought that the surface area and reactivity of these nanostructured HA are higher. Exceptional characteristics were found when nano-HA was used to coat implants in a variety of biological applications, including dentistry. Through chemical interaction and bonding with bone, these nanostructured HAs promote osseointegration and biological fixation (Heiland & Ebker, 2016; Jafari et al., 2016). A perfect environment for the deposition of new bone is also created by these materials (Parnia et al., 2017). Additionally, according to a study, nanoparticles increase the density of osteoblast cells on the implant, which contributes to the stability of the implant (Van Rijt & Habibovic, 2017).

The HA coatings have been found to have many benefits in research investigations (Amini et al., 2012; Joos et al., 2011; Xie et al., 2016); however, Johnson (1992) also noted that they are more susceptible to bacterial colonization than real teeth or titanium implants. Since HA coatings' propensity for increased plaque deposition has been connected to their roughened surfaces, the possibility of periimplantitis cannot be discounted (Rams et al., 1991). Additionally, the mobility of dental implants and subsequent loss has been linked to HA layer degradation (Cranin et al., 1994). According to many scientists (Nancollas & Tucker, 1994; Takeshita et al., 1996), the disintegration or fracture of the HA coating at the coating–titanium interface is another cause of coating failure. After 16 weeks of implantation, a study team observed 65% resorption of the 50-m-thick HA covering and subsequent movement in implants (van Blitterswijk et al., 1985). Due to weak fatigue and shear strength characteristics of the HA layer, it may sustain damage and resorption (Lemons, 1988).

4.6.2 Calcium silicate

As a biocompatible material that has the ability to stimulate osteoblast proliferation and differentiation due to its bioactivity, calcium silicate

(Ca-Si) can be used as a covering for titanium implants (Mohammadi & Sepantafar, 2016).

Since these coatings have similar coefficient of thermal expansion to Ti-6Al-4V, it has a better interfacial bonding than HA does. However, these benefits come at the expense of Ca-Si's poorer strength, faster rate of deterioration, and chemical instability. Implant surface interaction with proteins has been facilitated by the silica layer created by the Ca-Si coating (Mohammadi & Sepantafar, 2016). Several changes have been performed to enhance the properties of Ca-Si. For instance, the integration of trace elements and the addition of PVA-gel improved both the mechanical and biological properties of Ti6Al4V implants and improved the adhesion of coating to them (Azam et al., 2016). CaO-SiO_2 coatings are modified using zirconium, titanium, and magnesium zinc. The roughness of CaO-ZrO_2-SiO_2 CZS makes it similar to HA and promotes the growth of marrow stem cells. In comparison to CaO-ZrO_2-SiO_2, baghdadite, also known as $Ca_3ZrSi_2O_9$, is a modified calcium silicate that exhibits more roughness and weaker bonding. Other calcium silicate minerals also have comparable qualities, such as $Ca_2MgSi_2O_7$ (akermanite) and $CaMgSi_2O_6$ (diopside); however, akermanite shows a faster rate of degradation (Najafinezhad et al., 2017). In a study, when Ti-6Al-4V implants were coated with bioactive $Sr_2ZnSi_2O_7$ (strontium, zinc, and silicon), evaluators found inhibition of fibrosis, inflammatory cytokines, osteoclastic, and osteoclastogenesis events. In contrast to HA coating, $Sr_2ZnSi_2O_7$ bonding strength was found to be greater (Chen et al., 2014).

4.6.3 Bioactive glass

BAG is a class of material that has numerous uses outside orthopedics and dentistry, including controlled drug administration, tissue engineering, regeneration, and the treatment of cancer (Skallevold et al., 2019).

In the late 1960s, the first BAG material was introduced by Prof. Larry Hench and is known as 45S5 Bioglass. Since its widespread application began in 1985, orthopedics and dentistry have benefited greatly from its use (Baino et al., 2016a). Because Bioglass 45S5 could not be removed from bone without causing damage, this was deemed evidence of an extremely strong link between the two materials. This bonding is because of hydroxycarbonate apatite layer that formed on the glass' surface during its early disintegration (Jones, 2013).

BAG has been widely used as a coating for dental implants (Alkhayyat & Hill, 2014). Both the implant material and BAG are thought to be capable of forming a strong chemical interaction with bone quickly (Mistry et al., 2016). Researchers compared implants with HA coating to implants with BAG coating, finding that HA has significantly less bioactivity than BAG (Mesquita-Guimarães et al., 2018). A coating of BAG is highly corrosion resistant in addition to being bioactive, which limits the release of metallic ions and creates a suitable environment for the osseointegration of implants.

Additionally, BAG permits matrix deposition and has the ability to promote cell adhesion and proliferation. Although the strength of BAG-coated implants is thought to be satisfactory, it is insufficient to withstand the stresses in a load-bearing area. Not only is the adhesion of BAG-coated implant to the surrounding tissue important, but it also needs to tolerate stresses. To get the best adherence, a 100–200 nm layer of BAG-coating must be applied to implants (Lopez-Esteban et al., 2003). When an in vitro research was conducted by Schrooten and Helsen (2000), researchers found that 75.5 and 43.6 MPa, respectively, were observed when the plasma-sprayed BAG coating on metallic implants was done. This implies that the coating can increase the load-bearing capacity of implants. According to Al-Noaman et al. (2012), BAG may become the preferred coating for dental implants due to its many advantageous qualities.

4.7 Conclusions

It appears that the interest of researchers is inclined towards the utilization of biomimetic concepts in the dental implants so as to improve their clinical performance and enhance their durability. By thoroughly looking into the relevant research work, the following meaningful conclusions can be drawn:

1. All strategies, namely, surface texturing, functionalization, bioactivity, and provision of bioinspired, biological, and antibacterial coatings on the surface of dental implants are responsible for various useful features.
2. The coatings of natural proteins, such as collagen or FN, have potential to mimic the ECM found in tissues which ultimately enhances cell attachment and promotes tissue integration.
3. The biological coatings also provide a reservoir for GFs and bioactive molecules which enhance the regenerative potential of the dental implant.

4. The HA coating is commonly employed on the surface of the dental implant and it mimics the structure of bone and improves dental implant integration by encouraging cell growth.
5. Overall, relevant in vitro studies have frequently been conducted, and the results are highly promising. However, long clinical trials should be conducted on the dental implants coated with biological factors so as to know about their survival rate.

References

Accioni, Francesca, Vázquez, Juan, Merinero, Manuel, Begines, Belén, & Alcudia, Ana (2022). Latest trends in surface modification for dental implantology: Innovative developments and analytical applications. *Pharmaceutics*, *14*(2). Available from https://doi.org/10.3390/pharmaceutics14020455.

Albrektsson, T., & Wennerberg, A. (2004). Oral implant surfaces: Part 1-review focusing on topographic and chemical properties of different surfaces and in vivo responses to them. *International Journal of Prosthodontics*, *17*(5), 536–543.

Albrektsson, T., Brånemark, P.I., Hansson, H.A., Lindström, J. (1981). Osseointegrated titanium implants: Requirements for ensuring a long-lasting, direct bone-to-implant anchorage in man. *Acta Orthopaedica Scandinavica*, 52(2), 155-170.

Al-Nawas, B., Groetz, K. A., Goetz, H., Duschner, H., & Wagner, W. (2008). Comparative histomorphometry and resonance frequency analysis of implants with moderately rough surfaces in a loaded animal model. *Clinical Oral Implants Research*, *19* (1), 1–8. Available from https://doi.org/10.1111/j.1600-0501.2007.01396.x.

Al-Noaman, A., Rawlinson, S. C. F., & Hill, R. G. (2012). The role of MgO on thermal properties, structure and bioactivity of bioactive glass coating for dental implants. *Journal of Non-Crystalline Solids*, *358*(22), 3019–3027. Available from https://doi.org/10.1016/j.jnoncrysol.2012.07.039.

Amini, A. R., Laurencin, C. T., & Nukavarapu, S. P. (2012). Bone tissue engineering: Recent advances and challenges. *Critical Reviews in Biomedical Engineering*, *40*(5), 363–408.

Anitua, E. A. (2006). Enhancement of osseointegration by generating a dynamic implant surface. *The Journal of Oral Implantology*, *32*(2), 72–76. Available from https://doi.org/10.1563/736.1.

Aspenberg, P., & Lohmander, L. S. (1989). Fibroblast growth factor stimulates bone formation bone induction studied in rats. *Acta Orthopaedica*, *60*(4), 473–476. Available from https://doi.org/10.3109/17453678909149323.

Assaf, A., & Saad, M. (2023). Use of narrow-diameter implants in the posterior segments of the jaws: A retrospective observational study of 2 to 11 years. *The Journal of Prosthetic Dentistry*, *130*(6), 840–848.

Åstrand, Per, Anzén, Bengt, Karlsson, Ulf, Sahlholm, Sten, Svärdström, Pia, & Hellem, S. ölve (2000). Nonsubmerged implants in the treatment of the edentulous upper jaw: A prospective clinical and radiographic study of ITI Implants—Results after 1 year. *Clinical Implant Dentistry and Related Research*, *2*(3), 166–174. Available from https://doi.org/10.1111/j.1708-8208.2000.tb00008.x.

Azam, F. A. A., Ismail, H., Shamsudin, R., Zainuddin, Z., & Hamid, M. A. A. (2016). Characterizations on morphology and adhesion of calcium silicate coating on Ti6Al4V substrate. *Key Engineering Materials*, *694*, 83–87.

Bagno, A., Piovan, A., Dettin, M., Chiarion, A., Brun, P., Gambaretto, R., Fontana, G., Di Bello, C., Palù, G., & Castagliuolo, I. (2007). Human osteoblast-like cell adhesion on titanium substrates covalently functionalized with synthetic peptides. *Bone, 40*, 693–699, Albrektsson & Wennerberg, 2004.

Baino, F., Novajra, G., Miguez-Pacheco, V., Boccaccini, A. R., & Vitale-Brovarone, C. (2016a). Bioactive glasses: special applications outside the skeletal system. *Journal of Non-Crystalline Solids, 432*, 15–30.

Becker, J., Kirsch, A., Schwarz, F., et al. (2006). Bone apposition to titanium implants bio-coated with recombinant human bone morphogenetic protein-2 (rhBMP-2). A pilot study in dogs. *Clinical Oral Investigations, 10*, 217–224.

Becker, S. T., Beck-Broichsitter, B. E., Rossmann, C. M., Behrens, E., Jochens, A., & Wiltfang, J. (2016). Long-term survival of straumann dental implants with TPS surfaces: A retrospective study with a follow-up of 12 to 23 years. *Clinical Implant Dentistry and Related Research, 18*, 480–488. (Albrektsson & Wennerberg, 2004).

Bodhak, S., Bose, S., & Bandyopadhyay, A. (2009). Role of surface charge and wettability on early stage mineralization and bone cell–materials interactions of polarized hydroxyapatite. *Acta Biomaterialia, 5*, 2178–2188, Anitua, 2006.

Bougas, K., Jimbo, R., Xue, Y., Mustafa, K., & Wennerberg, A. (2012). Novel implant coating agent promotes gene expression of osteogenic markers in rats during early osseointegration. *International Journal of Biomaterials.*

Bowers, K. T., Keller, J. C., Randolph, B. A., Wick, D. G., & Michaels, C. M. (1992). Optimization of surface micromorphology for enhanced osteoblast responses in vitro. *The International Journal of Oral & Maxillofacial Implants*, 7. (Albrektsson & Wennerberg, 2004).

Boyne, P. J. (2001). Application of bone morphogenetic proteins in the treatment of clinical oral and maxillofacial osseous defects. *JBJS, 83*, S146–S150. (Accioni et al., 2022).

Brånemark, P. I., Adell, R., Albrektsson, T., Lekholm, U., Lundkvist, S., & Rockler, B. (1983). Osseointegrated titanium fixtures in the treatment of edentulousness. *Biomaterials, 4*, 25–28. (Accioni et al., 2022).

Brunette, D. (1986). Spreading and orientation of epithelial cells on grooved substrata. *Exp. Cell Res., 167*, 203–217. (Accioni et al., 2022).

Cao, Y., Zeng, X., Cai, Z., & Duan, J. (2010). *Laser micro/nano-fabrication techniques and their applications in electronics. Adv. Laser Mater. Processing* (pp. 629–670). Woodhead Publishing, Jan 1.

Chang, Y. C., Lee, W. F., Feng, S. W., Huang, H. M., Lin, C. T., Teng, N. C., & Chang, W. J. (2016). In vitro analysis of fibronectin-modified titanium surfaces. *PLoS One, 11*, e0146219. (Accioni et al., 2022).

Chehroudi, B., Gould, T., & Brunette, D. (1988). Effects of a grooved epoxy substratum on epithelial cell behavior in vitro and in vivo. *J. Biomed. Materials Res., 22*, 459–473. (Anitua, 2006).

Chen, Z., Yi, D., Zheng, X., Chang, J., Wu, C., & Xiao, Y. (2014). Nutrient element-based bioceramic coatings on titanium alloy stimulating osteogenesis by inducing beneficial osteoimmmunomodulation. *Journal of Materials Chemistry B, 2*(36), 6030–6043.

Cho, S.-A., & Park, K.-T. (2003). The removal torque of titanium screw inserted in rabbit tibia treated by dual acid etching. *Biomaterials, 24*(20), 3611–3617.

Choi, A. H., Ben-Nissan, B., Matinlinna, J. P., & Conway, R. C. (2013). Current perspectives: Calcium phosphates nanocoatings and nanocomposite coatings in dentistry. *Journal of Dental Research, 92*, 853–859.

Chrcanovic, B., Albrektsson, T., & Wennerberg, A. (2016). Turned versus anodised dental implants: A meta-analysis. *Journal of Oral Rehabilitation, 43*(9), 716–728.

Christiansen, J. H., Coles, E. G., & Wilkinson, D. G. (2000). Molecular control of neural crest formation, migration and differentiation. *Current Opinion in Cell Biology, 12*, 719–724. (Anitua, 2006).

Costa, D. G., Ferraz, E. P., Abuna, R. P., de Oliveira, P. T., Morra, M., Beloti, M. M., & Rosa, A. L. (2017). The effect of collagen coating on titanium with nanotopography on in vitro osteogenesis. *Journal of Biomedical Materials Research: Part A, 105*(10), 2783–2788.

Cranin, A. N., Mehrali, M., & Baraoidan, M. (1994). Hydroxyapatite-coated endosteal implants from the clinicians' perspective. *The Journal of Oral Implantology, 20*, 235–239.

Crookes, W. (1883). On radiant matter spectroscopy: A new method of spectrum analysis. *Journal of the Franklin Institute, 116*, 118–128. (Albrektsson et al., 2009).

Cruz, M. B., Silva, N., Marques, J. F., Mata, A., Silva, F. S., & Caramês, J. (2022). Biomimetic implant surfaces and their role in biological integration—A concise review. *Biomimetics*, 7, 74. (Albrektsson et al., 2009).

Dalton, B. A., McFarland, C. D., Underwood, P. A., & Steele, J. G. (1995). Role of the heparin binding domain of fibronectin in attachment and spreading of human bone-derived cells. *Journal of Cell Science, 108*, 2083–2092.

Davarpanah, M., Martinez, H., Tecucianu, J. F., Fromentin, O., & Celletti, R. (2000). To conserve or implant: which choice of therapy? *International Journal of Periodontics & Restorative Dentistry., 20*. (Al-Nawas et al., 2008).

Delgado-Ruiz, R. A., Calvo-Guirado, J. L., Abboud, M., Ramirez-Fernandez, M. P., Mate-Sanchez, J. E., Negri, B., et al. (2014). Histologic and histomorphometric behavior of microgrooved zirconia dental implants with immediate loading. *Clinical Implant Dentistry and Related Research., 16*, 856–872. (Anitua, 2006).

Delgado-Ruíz, R. A., Gomez Moreno, G., Aguilar-Salvatierra, A., Markovic, A., Mate-Sánchez, J. E., & Calvo-Guirado, J. L. (2016). Human fetal osteoblast behavior on zirconia dental implants and zirconia disks with microstructured surfaces. An experimental in vitro study. *Clinical Oral Implants Research, 27*(11), e144–e153.

De Tullio, I., Berardini, M., Di Iorio, D., Perfetti, F., & Perfetti, G. (2020). Comparative evaluation among laser-treated, machined, and sandblasted/acid-etched implant surfaces: An in vivo histologic analysis on sheep. *International Journal of Implant Dentistry., 6*, 1–8. (Accioni et al., 2022).

Dua, R., Vadivel, J., Khurana, I., Karim, E.T., Mutreja, I., Kumar, D., Shankar, M.R. (2023). Development of smart metallic orthopedic and dental implants based on biomimetic design.

Ehrenfest MDC, D. M. D., & Kang, B.-S. (2014). Identifcation card and codifcation of the chemical and morphological characteristics of 62 dental implant surfaces. Part 3: sandblasted/acid-etched (SLA type) and related surface (Group 2A, main subtractive process). *POSEIDO, 2*. (Accioni et al., 2022):37-5.

Elani, H. W., Starr, J. R., Da Silva, J. D., & Gallucci, G. O. (2018). Trends in dental implant use in the US, 1999–2016, and projections to 2026. *Journal of Dental Research, 97*(13), 1424–1430.

Elia, R., Michelson, C. D., Perera, A. L., Brunner, T. F., Harsono, M., Leisk, G. G., Kugel, G., & Kaplan, D. L. (2015). Electrodeposited silk coatings for bone implants. *Journal of Biomedical Materials Research Part B: Applied Biomaterials, 103*(8), 1602–1609.

Elia, R., Michelson, C. D., Perera, A. L., Harsono, M., Leisk, G. G., Kugel, G., & Kaplan, D. L. (2015). Silk electrogel coatings for titanium dental implants. *Journal of Biomaterials Applications, 29*(9), 1247–1255.

Erne, M., & Kolar, D. (2012). *Thermal spraying of oxide ceramic and ceramic metallic coatings*. Rijeka, Croatia: InTech.

Fauchais, P., & Montavon, G. (2007). Plasma spraying: from plasma generation to coating structure. *Advances in Heat Transfer, 40*, 205–344.

Fiorellini, J. P., Buser, D., Riley, E., & Howell, T. H. (2001). Effect on bone healing of bone morphogenetic protein placed in combination with endosseous implants: a pilot study in beagle dogs. *International Journal of Periodontics & Restorative Dentistry, 21*, 41–48. (Accioni et al., 2022).

Freymiller, E. G., & Aghaloo, T. L. (2004). Platelet-rich plasma: ready or not? *Journal of Oral and Maxillofacial Surgery, 62*, 484–488. (Al-Nawas et al., 2008).

Gadallah, M. A., Darwish, R. M, Alshimy, A. M., Gepreel, M. A, & Marei, M. K. (2022). Biomimetic coating of titanium surface using bioactive glass nanoparticles. *International Journal of Oral & Maxillofacial Implants, 37*(1), 86–97.

Gallardo, Y. N., da Silva-Olivio, I. R., Gonzaga, L., Sesma, N., & Martin, W. (2019). A systematic review of clinical outcomes on patients rehabilitated with complete-arch fixed implant-supported prostheses according to the time of loading. *Journal of Prosthodontics, 28*(9), 958–968.

García, A. J., Ducheyne, P., & Boettiger, D. (1998). Effect of surface reaction stage on fibronectin-mediated adhesion of osteoblast-like cells to bioactive glass. *Journal of Biomedical Materials Research, 40*, 48–56.

Geißler, U., Hempel, U., Wolf, C., Scharnweber, D., Worch, H., & Wenzel, K. W. (2000). Collagen type I-coating of Ti6A14V promotes adhesion of osteoblasts. *Journal of Biomedical Materials Research, 51*, 752–760.

Ghalandari, V., Esmaeilpour, M., Payvar, N., & Reza, M. T. (2021). A case study on energy and exergy analyses for an industrial-scale vertical roller mill assisted grinding in cement plant. *Advanced Powder Technology., 32*, 480–491, Feb 1.

Gil, Javier, et al. (2021). Mineralization of titanium surfaces: Biomimetic implants. *Materials, 14*(11), 2879.

Gosline, J. M., Guerette, P. A., Ortlepp, C. S., & Savage, K. N. (1999). The mechanical design of spider silks: from fibroin sequence to mechanical function. *Journal of Experimental Biology, 202*(23), 3295–3303.

Goto, T., Yoshinari, M., Kobayashi, S., & Tanaka, T. (2004). The initial attachment and subsequent behavior of osteoblastic cells and oral epithelial cells on titanium. *Biomedical Materials and Engineering, 14*, 537–544. (Al-Nawas et al., 2008).

Graeff, Eliot, et al. (2021). Biomimetics from practical feedback to an interdisciplinary process. *Research in Engineering Design, 32*, 349–375.

Gulati, M., Govila, V., Anand, V., & Anand, B. (2014). Implant maintenance: a clinical update. *International Scholarly Research Notices*, 2014.

Hakimi, O., Knight, D. P., Vollrath, F., & Vadgama, P. (2007). Spider and mulberry silkworm silks as compatible Biomater. *Composites Part B: Engineering, 38*, 324–337.

Hall, J. (2000). Properties of a new porous oxide surfase on titanium implants. *Applied Osseointegration Research, 1*, 5–8.

Hardy, J. G., Römer, L. M., & Scheibel, T. R. (2008). Polymeric materials based on silk proteins. *Polymer, 49*, 4309–4327.

Hayakawa, T., Nagai, M., Yoshinari, M., Makimura, M., & Nemoto, K. (2005). Cell-adhesive protein immobilization using tresyl chloride-activation technique for the enhancement of initial cell attachment. *Journal of Oral Tissue Engineering, 2*, 14–24.

Heiland, M., & Ebker, T. (2016). Impact of dental implant surface modifications on osseointegration. *BioMed Research International*. Available from https://doi.org/10.1155/2016/6285620, 6285620.

Heinlin, J., Isbary, G., Stolz, W., Morfill, G., Landthaler, M., Shimizu, T., et al. (2011). Plasma applications in medicine with a special focus on dermatology. *Journal of the European Academy of Dermatology and Venereology, 25*, 1–11. (Accioni et al., 2022).

Heller, M., Kumar, V. V., Pabst, A., Brieger, J., Al-Nawas, B., & Kämmerer, P. W. (2018). Osseous response on linear and cyclic RGD-peptides immobilized on titanium surfaces in vitro and in vivo. *Journal of Biomedical Materials Research: Part A., 106*, 419–427. (Albrektsson et al., 2009).

Hirano, T., Sasaki, H., Honma, S., Furuya, Y., Miura, T., Yajima, Y., et al. (2015). Proliferation and osteogenic differentiation of human mesenchymal stem cells on zirconia and titanium with different surface topography. *Dental Materials Journal, 34*, 872–880. (Anitua, 2006).

Hirota, M., Shimpo, H., Ohkubo, C., Umegaki, T., Toyama, T., & Hayakawa, T. (2015). Bone adaptation of fibronectin-immobilized titanium implants using a tresyl chloride-activated method. *Journal of Hard Tissue Biology, 24*, 341–346. (Al-Nawas et al., 2008).

Hoffman, A. S., Schoen, F. J., Lemons, J. E., & Ratner, B. D. (Eds.), (2012). *Biomaterials science: An introduction to materials in medicine*. Academic Press, Dec 31.

Huang, Y., McGowan, T., Lee, R., & Ivanovski, S. (2017). 7.23 dental implants: Biomaterial properties influencing osseointegration. *Comprehensive Biomaterials II, 7*, 444–466.

Huh, J. B., Kim, S. E., Kim, H. E., et al. (2012). Effects of anodized implants coated with *Escherichia coli*-derived rhBMP-2 in beagle dogs. *International Journal of Oral and Maxillofacial Surgery, 41*, 1577–1584.

Hunziker, E. B., Enggist, L., Küffer, A., Buser, D., & Liu, Y. (2012). Osseointegration: The slow delivery of BMP-2 enhances osteoinductivity. *Bone, 51*, 98–106.

Hutchings, I., & Shipway, P. (2017). *Tribology: friction and wear of engineering materials*. Butterworth-heinemann, Apr 13.

Iacono, V. (2000). Dental implants in periodontal therapy. *Journal of Periodontology, 71*(12), 1934–1942.

Itoh, D., Yoneda, S., Kuroda, S., Kondo, H., Umezawa, A., Ohya, K., et al. (2002). Enhancement of osteogenesis on hydroxyapatite surface coated with synthetic peptide (EEEEEEEPRGDT) in vitro. *Journal of Biomedical Materials Research, 62*, 292–298.

Jafari, S., Maleki-Dizaji, N., Barar, J., Barzegar-Jalali, M., Rameshrad, M., & Adibkia, K. (2016). Methylprednisolone acetate-loaded hydroxyapatite nanoparticles as a potential drug delivery system for treatment of rheumatoid arthritis: In vitro and in vivo evaluations. *European Journal of Pharmaceutical Sciences: Official Journal of the European Federation for Pharmaceutical Sciences, 91*, 225–235.

Jang, J.-H., Ku, Y., Chung, C.-P., & Heo, S.-J. (2002). Enhanced fibronectin-mediated cell adhesion of human osteoblast by fibroblast growth factor, FGF-2. *Biotechnology Letters, 24*, 1659–1663.

Javed, F., Akram, Z., Khan, J., & Zafar, M. S. (2020). *Growth factors and guided bone regeneration. Dental implants* (pp. 133–143). Woodhead Publishing, Jan 1.

Jemat, A., Ghazali, M. J., Razali, M., & Otsuka, Y. (2015). Surface modifications and their effects on titanium dental implants. *BioMed Research International*. Available from https://doi.org/10.1155/2015/791725.

Jemt, T., Olsson, M., & Franke Stenport, V. (2015). Incidence of first implant failure: A retroprospective study of 27 years of implant operations at one specialist clinic. *Clinical Implant Dentistry and Related Research, 17*, e501–e510.

Jian, X., Huang, W., Wu, D., You, D., Lin, Z., & Chen, J. (2017). Effect of fibronectin-coated micro-grooved titanium surface on alignment, adhesion, and proliferation of human gingival fibroblasts. *Medical Science Monitor: International Medical Journal of Experimental and Clinical Research, 23*, 4749.

Johnson, B. W. (1992). HA-coated dental implants: Long-term consequences. *Journal of the California Dental Association, 20*, 33–41.

Jones, J. R. (2013). Review of bioactive glass: from Hench to hybrids. *Acta Biomaterialia, 9*, 4457–4486.

Joos, U., Wiesmann, H. P., Neunzehn, J., & Meyer, U. (2011). Applications of biomaterials in alveolar and maxillofacial bone reconstruction. *Preprosthetic and Maxillofacial Surgery*, 175–184.

Kämmerer, P. W., Heller, M., Brieger, J., Klein, M. O., Al-Nawas, B., & Gabriel, M. (2011). Immobilisation of linear and cyclic RGD-peptides on titanium surfaces and their impact on endothelial cell adhesion and proliferation. *European Cells & Materials, 21*, 364–372, Apr 11.

Karaji, Z. G., Jahanmard, F., Mirzaei, A. H., Van der Wal, B., & Yavari, S. A. (2020). A multifunctional silk coating on additively manufactured porous titanium to prevent implant-associated infection and stimulate bone regeneration. *Biomedic. Mater., 15*, 065016, Sep 24.

Karl, M., & Albrektsson, T. (2017). Clinical performance of dental implants with a moderately rough (TiUnite) surface: A meta-analysis of prospective clinical studies. *The International Journal of Oral & Maxillofacial Implants, 32*.

Kawaguchi, H., Nakamura, K., Tabata, Y., Ikada, Y., Aoyama, I., Anzai, J., et al. (2001). Acceleration of fracture healing in nonhuman primates by fibroblast growth factor-2. *Journal of Clinical Endocrinology, 86*, 875–880.

Ketabi, M., & Deporter, D. (2013). The effects of laser microgrooves on hard and soft tissue attachment to implant collar surfaces: A literature review and interpretation. *International Journal of Periodontics & Restorative Dentistry, 33*.

Kim, T. I., Lee, G., Jang, J. H., Chung, C. P., & Ku, Y. (2007). Influence of RGD-containing oligopeptide-coated surface on bone formation in vitro and in vivo. *Biotechnology Letters, 29*, 359–363.

Kim, H.-K., Woo, K. M., Shon, W.-J., Ahn, J.-S., Cha, S., & Park, Y.-S. (2015). Comparison of peri-implant bone formation around injection-molded and machined surface zirconia implants in rabbit tibiae. *Dental Materials Journal, 34*, 508–515. (Al-Nawas et al., 2008).

Kim, J., Hong, S. Y., Park, H. S., Kim, D. S., & Lee, W. (2005). Structure and function of RGD peptides derived from disintegrin proteins. *Moland Cells, 19*, 205–211.

Kim, J., Yang, Z., Ko, H., Cho, H., & Lu, Y. (2023). Deep learning-based data registration of melt-pool-monitoring images for laser powder bed fusion additive manufacturing. *Journal of Manufacturing Processes, 68*, 117–129, Jun 1.

Kim, T. I., Jang, J. H., Chung, C. P., & Ku, Y. (2003). Fibronectin fragment promotes osteoblast-associated gene expression and biological activity of human osteoblast-like cell. *Biotechnology Letters, 25*, 2007–2011.

Kim, T. I., Jang, J. H., Kim, H. W., Knowles, J. C., & Ku, Y. (2008). Biomimetic approach to dental implants. *Current Pharmaceutical Design, 14*(22), 2201–2211.

Knaus, Jennifer, Schaffarczyk, Dietmar, & Cölfen, Helmut (2020). On the future design of bio-inspired polyetheretherketone dental implants. *Macromolecular Bioscience, 20*(1), 1900239.

Kumar, N., Maher, N., Amin, F., Ghabbani, H., Zafar, M. S., Rodríguez-Lozano, F. J., & Oñate-Sánchez, R. E. (2022). Biomimetic approaches in clinical endodontics. *Biomimetics*, 7, 229, Dec 6.

Kuroda, K., Nakamoto, S., Miyashita, Y., Ichino, R., & Okido, M. (2006). Osteoinductivity of HAp films with different surface morphologies coated by the thermal substrate method in aqueous solutions. *Materials Transactions, 47*, 1391–1394.

Lan, J., Wang, Z., Wang, Y., Wang, J., & Cheng, X. (2006). The effect of combinant human bone morphogenetic protein-2 and basic fibroblast growth factor or insulin-like growth factor-I on dental implant osseointegration by confocal laser scanning microscopy. *The Journal of Periodontology*, 77, 357–363.

Lan, J., Wang, Z. F., Shi, B., Xia, H. B., & Cheng, X. R. (2007). The influence of recombinant human BMP-2 on bone-implant osseointegration: biomechanical testing and histomorphometric analysis. *International Journal of Oral and Maxillofacial Surgery, 36*, 345–349.

Lang, N. P., & Jepsen, S. (2009). Implant surfaces and design (Working Group 4). *Clinical Oral Implants Research*, *20*, 228–231.

Laroussi, M., & Lu, X. (2005). Room-temperature atmospheric pressure plasma plume for biomedical applications. *Applied Physics Letters*, *87*(11), 113902.

Le Guéhennec, L., Soueidan, A., Layrolle, P., & Amouriq, Y. (2007). Surface treatments of titanium dental implants for rapid osseointegration. *Dental Materials*, *23*(7), 44–54.

Lee, J. W. Y., & Bance, M. L. (2019). Physiology of osseointegration. *Otolaryngologic Clinics of North America*, *52*, 231–242. (Albrektsson et al., 2009).

Lee, S. W., Hahn, B. D., Kang, T. Y., Lee, M. J., Choi, J. Y., Kim, M. K., & Kim, S. G. (2014). Hydroxyapatite and collagen combination-coated dental implants display better bone formation in the peri-implant area than the same combination plus bone morphogenetic protein-2–coated implants, hydroxyapatite only coated implants, and uncoated implants. *Journal of Oral and Maxillofacial Surgery*, *72*, 53–60, Jan 1.

Lee, S. Y., Koak, J. Y., Heo, S. J., Kim, S. K., Lee, S. J., & Nam, S. Y. (2010). Osseointegration of anodized titanium implants coated with poly(lactide-co-glycolide)/basic fibrobalst growth factor by electrospray. *The International Journal of Oral & Maxillofacial Implants*, *25*, 315–320.

Lemons, J. E. (1988). Hydroxyapatite coatings. *Clinical Orthopaedics and Related Research*, *235*, 220–223.

Lennerås, M., Palmquist, A., Norlindh, B., Emanuelsson, L., Thomsen, P., & Omar, O. (2015). Oxidized titanium implants enhance osseointegration via mechanisms involving RANK/RANKL/OPG regulation. *Clinical Implant Dentistry & Related Research*, *17*, e486–e500, Oct.

Li, J., et al. (2021). Innovative surface modification procedures to achieve micro/nano-graded ti-based biomedical alloys and implants. *Coatings*, *11*(6), 647.

Lin, X., Takahashi, K., Liu, Y., & Zamora, P. O. (2006). Enhancement of cell attachment and tissue integration by a IKVAV containing multi-domain peptide. *Biochimica et Biophysica Acta (BBA)-General Subjects*, *1760*(9), 1403–1410, Sep 1.

Liu, Ziqian, Liu, Xiaoling, & Ramakrishna, Seeram (2021). Surface engineering of biomaterials in orthopedic and dental implants: Strategies to improve osteointegration, bacteriostatic and bactericidal activities. *Biotechnology Journal*, *16*(7)2000116.

Lopez-Esteban, S., Saiz, E., Fujino, S., Oku, T., Suganuma, K., & Tomsia, A. P. (2003). Bioactive glass coatings for orthopedic metallic implants. *Journal of the European Ceramic Society*, *23*(15), 2921–2930.

Marukawa, E., Asahina, I., Oda, M., Seto, I., Alam, M., & Enomoto, S. (2002). Functional reconstruction of the non-human primate mandible using recombinant human bone morphogenetic protein-2. *International Journal of Oral and Maxillofacial Surgery*, *31*, 287–295. (Albrektsson & Wennerberg, 2004).

Mathew, Anil, Babu, Anna Serene, & Keepanasseril, Arun (2020). Biomimetic properties of engineered periodontal ligament/cementum in dental implants. *Contemporary Clinical Dentistry*, *11*(4), 301.

Mathur, A., Kharbanda, O. P., Koul, V., Dinda, A. K., Anwar, M. F., & Singh, S. (2022). Fabrication and evaluation of antimicrobial biomimetic nanofiber coating for improved dental implant bioseal: An in vitro study. *The Journal of Periodontology*, *93* (10), 1578–1588.

Mazor, Z., Peleg, M., Garg, A. K., & Luboshitz, J. (2004). Platelet-rich plasma for bone graft enhancement in sinus floor augmentation with simultaneous implant placement: patient series study. *Implant Dentistry*, *13*, 65–72. (Accioni et al., 2022).

Mendoza-Arnau, A., Vallecillo-Capilla, M.-F., Cabrerizo-Vílchez, M.-Á., & Rosales-Leal, J.-I. (2016). Topographic characterisation of dental implants for commercial use. *Medicina Oral, Patologia Oral y Cirugia Bucal*, *21*, e631.

Mesquita-Guimarães, J., Henriques, B., & Silva, F. (2018). Bioactive glass coatings. *Bioactive Glasses, 2,* 103–118, Elsevier.

Mieszkowska, A., Beaumont, H., Martocq, L., Koptyug, A., Surmeneva, M. A., Surmenev, R. A., Naderi, J., Douglas, T. E., & Gurzawska-Comis, K. A. (2020). Phenolic-enriched collagen fibrillar coatings on titanium alloy to promote osteogenic differentiation and reduce inflammation. *International Journal of Molecular Sciences, 21* (17), 6406, Sep 3.

Mistry, S., Roy, R., Kundu, B., Datta, S., Kumar, M., Chanda, A., & kundu, D. (2016). Clinical outcome of hydroxyapatite coated, bioactive glass coated, and machined Ti6Al4V threaded dental implant in human jaws: a short-term comparative study. *Implant Dentistry, 25,* 252–260.

Mohammadi, H., & Sepantafar, M. (2016). Ion-doped silicate bioceramic coating of Ti-based implant. *Iranian Biomedical Journal, 20,* 189.

Möller, B., Terheyden, H., Açil, Y., Purcz, N. M., Hertrampf, K., Tabakov, A., et al. (2012). A comparison of biocompatibility and osseointegration of ceramic and titanium implants: an in vivo and in vitro study. *International Journal of Oral and Maxillofacial Surgery, 41,* 638–645. (Al-Noaman et al., 2012).

Moursi, A. M., Globus, R. K., & Damsky, C. H. (1997). Interactions between integrin receptors and fibronectin are required for calvarial osteoblast differentiation in vitro. *Journal of Cell Science, 110,* 2187–2196.

Nadeem, D., Sjostrom, T., Wilkinson, A., Smith, C. A., Oreffo, R. O., Dalby, M. J., et al. (2013). Embossing of micropatterned ceramics and their cellular response. *Journal of Biomedical Materials Research: Part A., 101*(11), 3247–3255.

Najafinezhad, A., Abdellahi, M., Ghayour, H., Soheily, A., Chami, A., & Khandan, A. (2017). A comparative study on the synthesis mechanism, bioactivity and mechanical properties of three silicate bioceramics. *Materials Science and Engineering: C, 72,* 259–267.

Najeeb, S., Zafar, M. S., Khurshid, Z., Zohaib, S., Hasan, S. M., & Khan, R. S. (2017). Bisphosphonate releasing dental implant surface coatings and osseointegration: A systematic review. *Journal of Taibah University Medical Sciences., 12,* 369–375. (Al-Noaman et al., 2012).

Nancollas, G. H., & Tucker, B. E. (1994). Dissolution kinetics characterization of hydroxyapatite coatings on dental implants. *The Journal of Oral Implantology, 20,* 221–226.

Nikolidakis, D., Meijer, G. J., Oortgiesen, D. A., Walboomers, X. F., & Jansen, J. A. (2009). The effect of a low dose of transforming growth factor β1 (TFG-β1) on the early bone-healing around oral implants inserted in trabecular bone. *Biomaterials, 30,* 94–99.

Novaes, A. B., Jr., Souza, S. L. S. D., Barros, R. R. M. D., Pereira, K. K. Y., Iezzi, G., & Piattelli, A. (2010). Influence of implant surfaces on osseointegration. *Brazilian Dental Journal, 21,* 471–481. (Anitua, 2006).

Omar, O. M., Lennerås, M. E., Suska, F., Emanuelsson, L., Hall, J. M., Palmquist, A., & Thomsen, P. (2011). The correlation between gene expression of proinflammatory markers and bone formation during osseointegration with titanium implants. *Biomaterials, 32,* 374–386, Jan 1.

Pankov, R., & Yamada, K. M. (2002). Fibronectin at a glance. *Journal of Cell Science, 115,* 3861–3863.

Papaspyridakos, P., Chen, C. J., Singh, M., Weber, H. P., & Gallucci, G. O. (2012). Success criteria in implant dentistry: A systematic review. *Journal of Dental Research, 91* (3), 242–248.

Park, J. M., Koak, J. Y., Jang, J. H., Han, C. H., Kim, S. K., & Heo, S. J. (2006). Osseointegration of anodized titanium implants coated with fibrobalst growth factor-fibronectin (FGF-FN) fusion protein. *The International Journal of Oral & Maxillofacial Implants, 21*, 859–866.

Parnia, F., Yazdani, J., Javaherzadeh, V., & Dizaj, S. M. (2017). Overview of nanoparticle coating of dental implants for enhanced osseointegration and antimicrobial purposes. *Journal of Pharmaceutical Sciences, 20*, 148–160.

Paryani, Meghna, et al. (2023). Evolution of biomimetic approaches for regenerative and restorative dentistry. *Cureus, 15*(1).

Pearson, B. S., Klebe, R. J., Boyan, B. D., & Moskowicz, D. (1988). Comments on the clinical application of fibronectin in dentistry. *Journal of Dental Research, 67*, 515–517.

Pellegrini, G., Francetti, L., Barbaro, B., & Del Fabbro, M. (2018). Novel surfaces and osseointegration in implant dentistry. *Journal of Investigative and Clinical Dentistry, 9*, e12349. (Al-Nawas et al., 2008).

Porter, A. E., Taak, P., Hobbs, L. W., Coathup, M. J., Blunn, G. W., & Spector, M. (2004). Bone bonding to hydroxyapatite and titanium surfaces on femoral stems retrieved from human subjects at autopsy. *Biomaterials, 25*(21), 5199–5208.

Pramono, S., Pugdee, K., Suwanprateep, J., & Koontongkaew, S. (2016). Sandblasting and fibronectin-derived peptide immobilization on titanium surface increase adhesion and differentiation of osteoblast-like cells (MC3T3-E1). *Journal of Dental Sciences, 11* (4), 427–436.

Puleo, D., Kissling, R., & Sheu, M.-S. (2002). A technique to immobilize bioactive proteins, including bone morphogenetic protein-4 (BMP-4), on titanium alloy. *Biomaterials, 23*(9), 2079–2087.

Puleo, D. A., & Bizios, R. (1991). RGDS tetrapeptide binds to osteoblasts and inhibits fibronectin-mediated adhesion. *Bone, 12*, 271–276.

Raita, Y., Komatsu, K., & Hayakawa, T. (2015). Pilot study of gingival connective tissue responses to 3-dimensional collagen nanofiber-coated dental implants. *Dental Materials Journal, 34*, 847–854, Nov 27.

Ramazanoglu, M., Lutz, R., Ergun, C., von Wilmowsky, C., Nkenke, E., & Schlegel, K. A. (2011). The effect of combined delivery of recombinant human bone morphogenetic protein-2 and recombinant human vascular endothelial growth factor 165 from biomimetic calcium-phosphate-coated implants on osseointegration. *Clinical Oral Implants Research, 22*, 1433–1439.

Rams, T. E., Roberts, T. W., Feik, D., Molzan, A. K., & Slots, J. (1991). Clinical and microbiological findings on newly inserted hydroxyapatite-coated and pure titanium human dental implants. *Clinical Oral Implants Research, 2*, 121–127.

Research (2015). 17, supplement 2:e486–e500.

Rezania, A., & Healy, K. E. (1999). Biomimetic peptide surfaces that regulate adhesion, spreading, cytoskeletal organization, and mineralization of the matrix deposited by osteoblast-like cells. *Biotechnology Progress, 15*, 19–32.

Rocci, A., Rocci, M., Rocci, C., Scoccia, A., Gargari, M., Martignoni, M., et al. (2013). Immediate loading of Brånemark system TiUnite and machined-surface implants in the posterior mandible, part II: a randomized open-ended 9-year follow-up clinical trial. *The International Journal of Oral & Maxillofacial Implants, 28*. (Albrektsson & Wennerberg, 2004).

Rodan, S. B., Wesolowski, G., Thomas, K. A., Yoon, K., & Rodan, G. A. (1989). Effects of acidic and basic fibroblast growth factors on osteoblastic cells. *Connective Tissue Research, 20*, 283–288. (Accioni et al., 2022; Albrektsson et al., 2009; Albrektsson & Wennerberg, 2004; Al-Nawas et al., 2008).

Rompen, E., Domken, O., Degidi, M., Farias Pontes, A. E., & Piattelli, A. (2006). The effect of material characteristics, of surface topography and of implant components and connections on soft tissue integration: A literature review. *Clinical Oral Implants Research, 17*, 55.

Sachin, Palekar Gouri, Uppoor, Ashita S., & Nayak, Sangeeta U. (2022). Nano-scale surface modification of dental implants—An emerging boon for osseointegration and biofilm control. *Acta Marisiensis – Seria Medica*, *68*(4), 154–158.

Saleem, M., Khurshid, Z., & Zafar, M. S. (2020). *Proteins and peptides coatings on the dental implant surface. Dental implants* (pp. 117–132). Woodhead Publishing, Jan 1.

Samant, S. (1976). *An improved method of calculating the tip vortex geometry for hovering rotors* (Ph.D. thesis).

Sánchez-Bodón, Julia, et al. (2022). Bioactive coatings on titanium: A review on hydroxylation, self-assembled monolayers (SAMs) and surface modification strategies. *Polymers*, *14*(1), 165.

Scarano, A., Lorusso, F., Orsini, T., Morra, M., Iviglia, G., & Valbonetti, L. (2019). Biomimetic surfaces coated with covalently immobilized collagen type I: An xX-ray photoelectron spectroscopy, atomic force microscopy, micro-CT and histomorphometrical study in rabbits. *International Journal of Molecular Sciences*, *20*, 724, Feb 8.

Schierano, G., Canuto, R. A., Mauthe von Degerfeld, M., Navone, R., Peirone, B., Preti, G., & Muzio, G. (2021). Role of rhBMP-7, fibronectin, and type I collagen in dental implant osseointegration process: An initial pilot study on minipig animals. *Materials.*, *14*(9), 2185.

Schliephake, H., Rublack, J., Förster, A., Schwenzer, B., Reichert, J., & Scharnweber, D. (2015). Functionalization of titanium implants using a modular system for binding and release of VEGF enhances bone-implant contact in a rodent model. *Journal of Clinical Periodontology*, *42*, 302–310.

Schneider, G. B., Zaharias, R., Seabold, D., Keller, J., & Stanford, C. (2004). Differentiation of preosteoblasts is affected by implant surface microtopographies. *Journal of Biomedical Materials Research. Part A: An Official J. of The Societ. Biomater., The Japanese Society for Biomater., and The Australian Society for Biomater. and the Korean Society for Biomater.*, *69*, 462–468.

Schouten, C., Meijer, G. J., van den Beucken, J. J., Spauwen, P. H., & Jansen, J. A. (2009). Effects of implant geometry, surface properties, and TFG-β1 on peri-implant bone response: an experimental study in goats. *Clinical Oral Implants Research*, *20*, 421–429.

Schrooten, J., & Helsen, J. (2000). Adhesion of bioactive glass coating to Ti6Al4V oral implant. *Biomaterials*, *21*, 1461–1469.

Senna, P., Antoninha Del Bel Cury, A., Kates, S., & Meirelles, L. (2015). Surface damage on dental implants with release of loose particles after insertion into bone. *Clinical Implant Dentistry & Related Research*, *17*, 681–692. (Al-Nawas et al., 2008).

Shinya, Akikazu (2023). Dental material research in prosthodontics—Towards developing better and efficient biomimetic materials. *Journal of Prosthodontic Research*, *67*(2), vi–vii.

Skallevold, H. E., Rokaya, D., Khurshid, Z., & Zafar, M. S. (2019). Bioactive glass applications in dentistry. *International Journal of Molecular Sciences*, *20*(23), 5960, Nov 27.

Sladek, R. E., Stoffels, E., Walraven, R., Tielbeek, P. J., & Koolhoven, R. A. (2004). Plasma treatment of dental cavities: a feasibility study. *IEEE Transactions on Plasma Science*, *32*, 1540–1543. (Al-Nawas et al., 2008).

Sousa, L. L., Ricci, V. P., Prado, D. G., Apolinario, R. C., Vercik, L. C., Rigo, E. C., Fernandes, M. C., & Mariano, N. A. (2017). Titanium coating with hydroxyapatite and chitosan doped with silver nitrate. *Materials Research*, *20*, 863–868.

Stangl, R., Rinne, B., Kastl, S., & Hendrich, C. (2001). The influence of pore geometry in cp Ti-implants—A cell culture investigation. *European Cells & Materials*, *2*, 1–9. (Albrektsson et al., 2009).

Stewart, Callum, et al. (2019). A review of biomimetic surface functionalization for bone-integrating orthopedic implants: Mechanisms, current approaches, and future directions. *Progress in Materials Science*, *106*100588.

Takeshita, F., Ayukawa, Y., Iyama, S., Suetsugu, T., & Kido, M. A. (1996). A histological evaluation of retrieved hydroxyapatite-coated blade-form implants using scanning electron, light, and confocal laser scanning microscopies. *Journal of Periodontology*, *67*, 1034–1040.

Taniguchi, Y., Kakura, K., Yamamoto, K., Kido, H., & Yamazaki, J. (2016). Accelerated osteogenic differentiation and bone formation on zirconia with surface grooves created with fiber laser irradiation. *Clinical Implant Dentistry & Related Research*, *18*, 883–894. (Al-Noaman et al., 2012).

Tatakis, D. N., Koh, A., Jin, L., Wozney, J. M., Rohrer, M. D., & Wikesjö, U. M. (2002). Peri-implant bone regeneration using recombinant human bone morphogenetic protein-2 in a canine model: A dose-response study. *Journal of Periodontal Research*, *37*, 93–100. (Albrektsson et al., 2009).

Thomson, A. W., & Lotze, M. T. (2003). *The Cytokine Handbook, Two-Volume Set*. Elsevier.

Traini, T., Murmura, G., Sinjari, B., Perfetti, G., Scarano, A., D'Arcangelo, C., et al. (2018). The surface anodization of titanium dental implants improves blood clot formation followed by osseointegration. *Coatings*, *8*, 252. (Aspenberg & Lohmander, 1989).

Truc, N. T., Minh, H. H., Khanh, L. L., Thuy, V. M., Van Toi, V., Van Man, T., Nam, H. C., Quyen, T. N., & Hiep, N. T. (2018). Modification of type I collagen on TiO2 surface using electrochemical deposition. *Surface and Coatings Technology.*, *344*, 664–672, Jun 25.

Urist, M. R., DeLange, R. J., & Finerman, G. (1983). Bone cell differentiation and growth factors. *Science (New York, N.Y.)*, *220*(4598), 680–686.

van Blitterswijk, C. A., Grote, J. J., Kuypers, W., Blok-vanHoek, C. J., & Daems, W. T. (1985). Bioreactions at the tissue/hydroxylapatite interface. *Biomaterials*, *6*, 243–251.

Van Rijt, S., & Habibovic, P. (2017). Enhancing regenerative approaches with nanoparticles. *Journal of the Royal Society Interface*, *14*(129).

Verrier, S., Pallu, S., Bareille, R., Jonczyk, A., Meyer, J., Dard, M., & Amedee, J. (2002). Function of linear and cyclic RGD-containing peptides in osteoprogenitor cells adhesion process. *Biomaterials*, *23*, 585–596.

Wang, J. H., Jia, F., Gilbert, T. W., & Woo, S. L. (2003). Cell orientation determines the alignment of cell-produced collagenous matrix. *Journal of Biomechanics*, *36*, 97–102. (Accioni et al., 2022).

Wang, J. S., & Aspenberg, P. (1994). Basic fibroblast growth factor increases allograf incorporation: Bone chamber study in rats. *Acta Orthopaedica Scandinavica*, *65*, 27–31, Jan 1.

Wennerberg, A., & Albrektsson, T. (2009). Effects of titanium surface topography on bone integration: a systematic review. *Clinical Oral Implants Research*, *20*, 172–184.

Wennerberg, A., Albrektsson, T., & Chrcanovic, B. (2018). Long-term clinical outcome of implants with different surface modifications. *European Journal of Oral Implantology*, *11*(suppl 1), S123–S136.

Wikesjo, U., Huang, Y., Xiropaidis, A., et al. (2008). Bone formation at recombinant human bone morphogenetic protein-2-coated tetanium implants in the posterior maxilla (Type IV bone) in non-human promates. *Journal of Clinical Periodontology*, *35*, 992–1000.

Wikesjö, U. M., Sorensen, R. G., & Wozney, J. M. (2001). Augmentation of alveolar bone and dental implant osseointegration: clinical implications of studies with rhBMP-2: A comprehensive review. *JBJS*, *83*, S136–S145.

Wolf-Brandstetter, C. (2004). Adsorptive Immobilisierung von Kollagen Typ I an Titanoxidoberflächen, Technische (Ph.D. thesis). Universität Dresden, Dresden, Germany.

Xiao, Y., & Truskey, G. A. (1996). Effect of receptor–ligand affinity on the strength of endothelial cell adhesion. *Biophysical Journal*, *71*, 2869–2884.

Xie, Y., Kocaefe, D., Chen, C., & Kocaefe, Y. (2016). Review of research on template methods in preparation of nanomaterials. *Journal of Nanomaterials*. Available from https://doi.org/10.1155/2016/2302595, 2302595.

Zafar, M. S., Farooq, I., Awais, M., Najeeb, S., Khurshid, Z., & Zohaib, S. (2019). *Bioactive surface coatings for enhancing osseointegration of dental implants. Biomedical, therapeutic and clinical applications of bioactive glasses* (pp. 313–329). Woodhead Publishing.

Zafar, Muhammad Sohail, et al. (2020). Biomimetic aspects of restorative dentistry biomaterials. *Biomimetics*, *5*(3), 34.

Zarkoob, S., Eby, R. K., Reneker, D. H., Hudson, S. D., Ertley, D., & Adams, W. W. (2004). Structure and morphology of electrospun silk nanofibers. *Polymer*, *45*(11), 3973–3977.

Zhang, Bingjun, et al. (2020). Bio-surface coated titanium scaffolds with cancellous bone-like biomimetic structure for enhanced bone tissue regeneration. *Acta Biomaterialia*, *114*, 431–448.

Zuo, B., Dai, L., & Wu, Z. (2006). Analysis of structure and properties of biodegradable regenerated silk fibroin fibers. *Journal of materials science*, *41*, 3357–3361.

CHAPTER 5

Biomimetic surface coatings for marine antifouling applications

Jeenat Aslam[1], Hilal Ahmad Parray[2] and Afroz Aslam[3]
[1]Department of Chemistry, College of Science, Taibah University, Yanbu, Al-Madina, Saudi Arabia
[2]Department of Pathology, University of Texas, Dallas, TX, United States
[3]Department of Chemistry, Constituent Government College, M.J.P. Rohilkhand University, Bareilly, Uttar Pradesh, India

5.1 Introduction

Living organisms growing on surfaces immersed in seawater are referred to as marine biofouling (Bloecher & Floerl, 2020; Fu et al., 2018). A major problem has been identified with the presence of macrofoulants (hydroids, barnacles, tubeworms, and macroalgae) and microfoulants (viruses, bacteria, fungus, diatoms, and algae) on marine structures like ships and buoys (Flemming et al., 2009). One significant effect of biofouling is that ships use more fuel, which raises carbon dioxide emissions (Hakim et al., 2019). To combat marine biofouling, antifouling (AF) paints have been developed. By releasing harmful substances into the nearby saltwater, these paints stop fouling organisms from adhering (Almeida et al., 2007a). The acrylic backbone polymers and ester connection to the tributyltin (TBT) side groups in tributyltin self-polishing copolymer (TBT-SPC) paint formulation have proven to be particularly effective among other formulations (Omae, 2003). At first, TBT-SPC paints offered long-lasting efficacy (>5 years) at a fair cost of manufacturing. This led to an estimated $60 billion in fuel savings annually and a decrease of 384 million tons of carbon dioxide emissions in the shipping sector (Demirel et al., 2018). But government regulations were tightened due to worries about TBT-SPC paints' toxicity and endurance, particularly with relation to mollusks. TBT-SPC paints were banned globally by the International Maritime Organization in October 2001 (Yebra et al., 2004). AF paints have shifted to contain biocides based on copper and zinc as a result of this ban. To increase efficacy against algae, biocides such as Irgarol 1051, zinc pyrithione, and Sea-Nine 211 were introduced (Flemming et al., 2009; Yebra et al., 2004). Regretfully, because of its extended half-life, current research

Smart Biomimetic Coatings
DOI: https://doi.org/10.1016/B978-0-443-21738-8.00005-9

has highlighted questions regarding Irgarol 1051 effects on marine plants (Okamura et al., 2000; Owen et al., 2002). Studying new ecologically friendly ways to solve biofouling problems has been prompted by the negative consequences of conventional AF coatings.

Microorganisms adhering to surfaces in a marine environment can improve cell survival (Flemming et al., 2009). Sedentary behavior is common in several marine phyla, and they all require surfaces to adhere to. These surfaces depict resources where individuals belonging to the same or distinct species are always in competition with one another (Bitton, 2002; Wahl, 1989). Diverse techniques for surface domination have evolved as a result of the competitive exclusion principle, which states that less suitable organisms must adapt or face extinction. Interestingly, the term "surface" refers to the outermost layer of any living organism that is essential to its survival, not just inorganic substrates (Amador & Hu, 2015). Different AF strategies are revealed by observing nature. To stop macroorganisms from colonizing them, microorganisms create chemical signals and biocides (Hellio et al., 2009; Lami, 2019). The superhydrophobic surface of lotus leaves reduces stickiness by utilizing micro and nanoarchitecture to repel water droplets (Feng & Jiang, 2006). On their wings, insects such as dragonflies and cicadas develop nanoprotrusions that rupture and destroy germs without sacrificing transparency (Ivanova et al., 2013; Kelleher et al., 2016). Setae are used by geckos to stick to surfaces, and persistent climbing aids in the removal of fouling macroparticles (Clemente et al., 2010; Hansen & Autumn, 2005). Mucus is secreted by fish, which coats their scales in a slimy coating to keep pollutants out (Liu et al., 2009; Xue et al., 2011; Zhang et al., 2017). As a result, nature has developed a variety of self-cleaning techniques and AF surfaces to maintain cleanliness throughout life. According to research on these natural situations, biomimetic techniques may provide useful information to develop nontoxic AF paints (Bixler & Bhushan, 2012; Ralston & Swain, 2011; Salta et al., 2010). To predict that choosing and combining efficient AF mechanisms from nature will soon lead to a new era of nontoxic AF paints, this study explores the current advancements in biomimetic AF surfaces.

5.2 Mechanism of attachment and fouling in marine organisms

The complex attachment process of marine fouling organisms involves the production of marine biofouling (Silverman & Roberto, 2007). Any object submerged in saltwater will accumulate organic materials on its surface, such as proteins, glycoproteins, and polysaccharides, due to electrostatic interactions, hydrogen bonds, and van der Waals forces. This will result in the formation of a reversible conditioned film, which can act as a food source for microorganisms that attach themselves (Jain & Bhosle, 2009). Microorganisms such as bacteria and diatoms cling to the conditioned coating within a single day of its forming. To aid in their adhesion to the material surface, these associated microbes produce viscous extracellular polymeric substances made of proteins, glycoproteins, and polysaccharides. The formation of a biofilm arises from the amalgamation of water, organic debris, bacteria, and extracellular metabolites (Lee et al., 2010). Biofilm offers plenty of food and nutrients for some protozoa and algal spores to cling to, which causes the surface to get covered in a mucus coating in a matter of days. A wide variety of macrofouling organisms, including macroalgae, mussels, and barnacles, attach and proliferate over the course of the next weeks to create intricate biotopes. This process leads to extensive fouling within a few months, illustrating a significant biofouling issue, as depicted in Fig. 5.1 (Abarzua & Jakubowski, 1995).

5.3 Biofouling in the maritime environment and its detrimental effects

A cutting-edge, dynamic, and complex challenge facing the shipping industry is biofouling. In the marine environment, it refers to the undesirable build-up of biotic and abiotic substances as well as micro and/or macroorganisms, plants, and animals (Carteaua et al., 2014; Schultz et al., 2010; Selim et al., 2017b). The three types of biofouling organisms are (1) biofilm, or conditioned film; (2) microfouling; and (3) macrofouling, as shown in Fig. 5.2A (Silverman & Roberto, 2007). There are three main

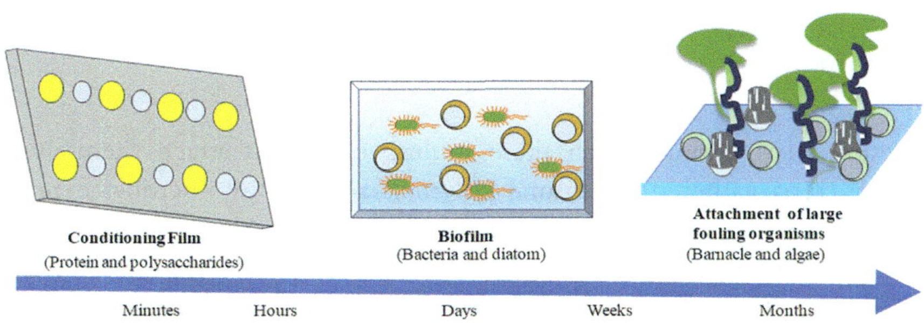

Figure 5.1 Illustration depicting the process of marine biofouling.

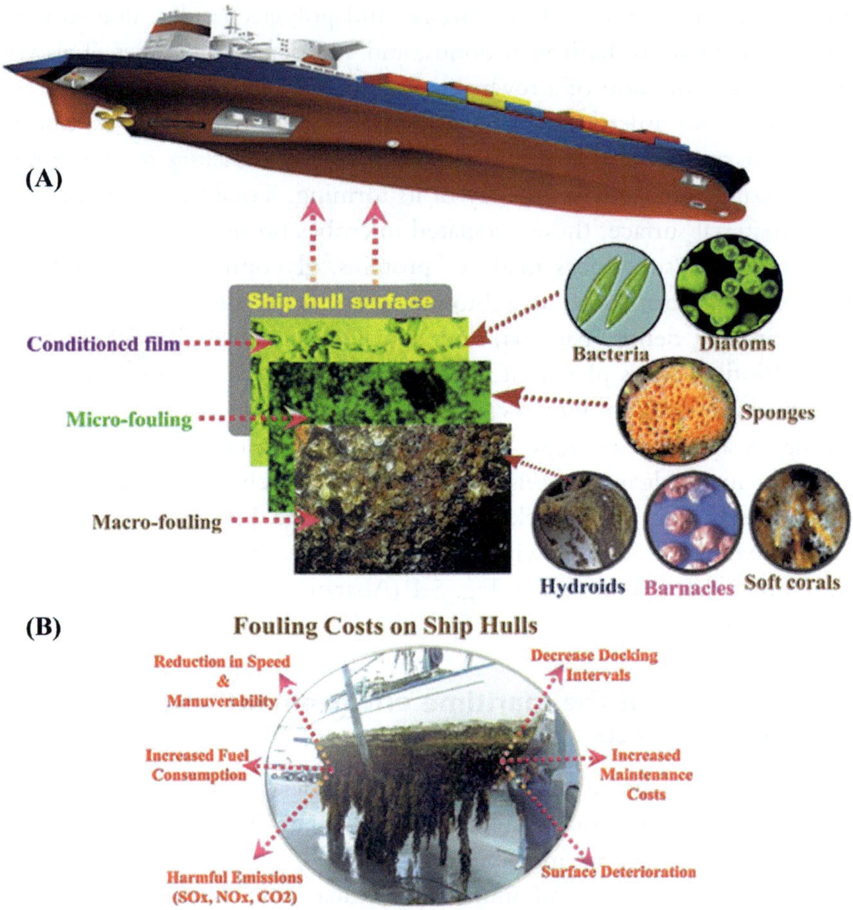

Figure 5.2 (A) An illustrated diagram showcasing the three typical fouling stages, encompassing molecular fouling (conditioned film), microfouling, and macrofouling. (B) The consequential fouling expenses resulting from the adherence to ship hulls, presenting significant challenges for the shipping industry. *Reproduced with permission Selim, M. S., Shenashen, M. A., El-Safty, S. A., Sakai, M., Higazy, S. A., Selim, M. M., Isago, H., & Elmarakbi, A. (2017b).* Progress in Materials Science, 87, *1–32, Copyright 2017, Elsevier.*

adhesion steps during which these fouling organisms attach themselves. First, bacteria gathered on natural polymers released by microbes expressing extracellular polymeric substances form the biofilm, also known as the conditioned film (Aslam et al., 2018; Maréchal & Hellio, 2009; Van Hullebusch et al., 2003). Two stages make up the second fouling organism, known as microfouling: (1) primary colonization, in which bacteria and diatoms physically adsorb onto the conditioned film and are easily detached (Detty et al., 2014); and (2) secondary colonization, in which macroalgal spores and protozoa form a microfilm with a mass that increases nonlinearly. Given its substantial influence on the hydrodynamic weight of the ship, macrofouling the third fouling organism is especially concerning (Compere et al., 2001).

Marine biofouling is a serious problem that costs the shipping industry billions of dollars in damages every year. Since shipping is essential to about 90% of world trade (Selim et al., 2017b), fouling adhesion is a factor in both environmental and economic problems, as Fig. 5.2B illustrates. The following happen when hull surfaces get fouled: (1) more drag resistance; (2) a decrease in ship velocity that makes maneuverability difficult; (3) more fuel consumption; and (4) more emission rates and amounts of polluting gases (like NO_x, CO_2, and SO_x) into the atmosphere. As a result, there is a reduction in drydocking intervals and an increase in overall voyage costs (Hoa & El-Safty, 2011; Soroldoni et al., 2018). Each year, the negative consequences of harmful emissions result in the loss of 60,000 lives and an estimated €200 billion in waste (Xue et al., 2014). As a result of these negative effects, cutting-edge technology is concentrating more and more on creating AF nanocomposite coatings. Previous methods used biocidal coatings to prevent fouling organisms, but these coatings were poisonous to creatures other than the intended target, such as fish and dolphins (Schultz, 2007). These coatings also encountered difficulties with corrosion on metallic surfaces and equipment upkeep (Cheyne, 2010). Fouling caused rust to occur in addition to endangering surfaces' protective paint coatings (Imbesi et al., 2012). The leaching effects of biocidal AF coatings made marine water tainted and required constant care. Maintenance expenses and corrosion concerns were made worse by the coating film reduction (Eduok et al., 2017). The global market, which is worth billions of dollars a year, is heavily impacted by biocidal coatings and fouling issues (Tamayo et al., 2016). Modern research is focusing on elastomeric, cost-effective, and environment-friendly fire-resistant coatings particularly silicon-based composites for ship hull coatings as a solution to these biofouling problems. These marine AF composites are a cost-effective alternative to poisonous and leaching materials. Moreover, the examination of naturally occurring superhydrophobic surfaces has catalyzed the development of innovative biomimetic and superhydrophobic AF nanosurfaces featuring controlled topological structures (Elbourne et al., 2017).

5.4 Strategic approaches to antifouling techniques

The economic and ecological issues associated with fouling have made AF strategy techniques a focus for scientists and engineers. With the use of technological equipment and chemical approaches, this coordinated effort seeks to develop novel AF strategies. The financial ramifications of fouling highlight how urgent it is to come up with workable plans that will lessen damages. Scientists and professionals are working hard to investigate chemical techniques and engineered devices as practical ways to stop unwanted organisms from settling in an area. Two main strategies for fouling avoidance have been identified: coating techniques and noncoating strategies (Legg et al., 2015).

5.4.1 Noncoating approaches

A number of noncoating approaches, such as electrical, irradiation, and sonochemical procedures, were developed in the past to prevent fouling (Anderson et al., 2003; Awais & Bhuiyan, 2019). Installed within the hull, ultrasonic transducers produce pulses that disrupt active cell processes, especially in the early phases of fouling. Effectiveness necessitates constant operation, with the exception of fast vessel movement, when transmission is affected by the structure and hull design. Certain sandwich core structures and other hull designs absorb a large amount of ultrasonic energy, which reduces their effectiveness. While ultrasonic vibration methods were found to be both expensive and insufficient for preventing ship hull damage (Akinfiev et al., 2007), surface cleaning using water jet technology or mechanical scrubbing was considered crucial. In general, noncoating methods were more costly, less effective, and unfeasible; they were especially useful for small boats (Umoren & Solomon, 2019; Xie et al., 2019). These ultrasonic vibration methods turned out to be insufficient and unreasonably expensive.

5.4.2 Antifouling coatings: a promising and eco-friendly approach

Coatings that prevent fouling have been used extensively as a successful method. Biocidal AF coatings were used in the past; wax and tar were used more than 2000 years ago to prevent fouling on marine ships. As shown in Table 5.1 (Almeida et al., 2007; Callow & Callow, 2002; Carman et al., 2006; Ferrari & Benedetti, 2015; Magin et al., 2010; Marmur, 2004; Peng et al., 2007; Tian, Jiang, et al., 2019; Xie et al., 2019), AF methods

Table 5.1 A wide range survey of fouling-prevention methods and antifouling (AF) advances.

Timeline	Description of AF product	References
Oldest	Tar, asphalt, and wax	Almeida et al. (2007)
700 BCE	Carthaginians & Phoenicians used pitch, sheathing with copper and lead, and tallow	Selim et al. (2017b), Almeida et al. (2007)
500 BCE	Phoenicians developed arsenic and sulfur in oil coatings	Selim et al. (2017b), Xie et al. (2019)
300 BCE–45	Greeks and Romans used tar, wax, and sheeting with lead with nails of copper	Dafforn et al. (2011), Kiil et al. (2001)
10	Seal tar was used by Vikings	Xie et al. (2019), Almeida et al. (2007)
45–125	Plutarch used pitch, algae scrapings	Xie et al. (2019)
1300–1500	Pitch mixed with oils, pitch, and tallow was used by Columbus's vessel	Xie et al. (2019), Almeida et al. (2007)
1618–1625	Arsenic ore, copper, and iron dust	Xie et al. (2019)
1625	First coating patent by William Beale	Xie et al. (2019)
18th century	Wood sheathing on a pitch layer, pitch, fat	Selim et al. (2017b)
1758 BCE	Copper sheathing by the English (Frigate HMS Alarm)	Almeida et al. (2007)
	Copper sheathing with zinc alloy	Almeida et al. (2007)
Iron ships		
1800–1900s	Sir Humphrey Davy reported that copper dissolution in seawater prevented fouling. So, copper, arsenic, and mercury were incorporated into coatings	Selim et al. (2017b), Xie et al. (2019)
1847	Application of insulating primer under the AF layer	Almeida et al. (2007)
1860	Hot plastic paints (metallic soap composition such as copper sulfate)	Selim et al. (2017b)
1863	AF paint by using tar	Xie et al. (2019), Almeida et al. (2007)

(*Continued*)

Table 5.1 (Continued)

Timeline	Description of AF product	References
Late 19th century	Shellac primer and shellac AF coating with different toxicants	Selim et al. (2017b), Almeida et al. (2007)
1926	Cold plastic paints, including coal tar + colophony and synthetic resins	Almeida et al. (2007)
1950–1960	Development of the first organometallic paints (tri-organotins (R)3-Sn in acrylic ester-based coatings)	Selim et al. (2017b)
1976	TBT-SPC technology, 1976 patent, allowed control of biocide release rates	Selim et al. (2017b), Xie et al. (2019), Dafforn et al. (2011), Kiil et al. (2001)
1977	First FR coating patent	Selim et al. (2017b)
1980s	– Development of TBT-SPC coatings allowed control of biocide release rates. – TBT linked to shell abnormalities in oysters and imposex in dog whelks.	Selim et al. (2017b), Xie et al. (2019)
1987–1990	TBT coatings prohibited on vessels	Selim et al. (2017b), Xie et al. (2019)
1990s	Copper release rate restrictions introduced in Denmark and considered elsewhere, e.g., California, United States	Selim et al. (2017b), Almeida et al. (2007)
2000s	Research into environment-friendly AF alternatives increases	Xie et al. (2019)
2001	International Maritime Organization (IMO) adopts "AFS Convention" to eliminate TBT from AF coatings from vessels through: 2003—prohibition of further application of TBT. 2008—prohibition of active TBT presence.	Almeida et al. (2007)
2001	FR coatings based on silicone and fluoropolymer matrixes	Selim et al. (2017b)

(*Continued*)

Table 5.1 (Continued)

Timeline	Description of AF product	References
2002	A group designed engineered polydimethylsiloxane (PDMS)-based microtopographies composed of pillars or ridges with various heights.	Callow and Callow (2002)
2004	Lotus leaf structure has been studied in detail by Marmur showed two-dimensional roughness in leaf appendixes of several micrometers in size and covered with nano-micro sized wax crystals	Marmur (2004)
2006	Carman et al. demonstrated a bioinspired surface, Sharklet AF	Carman et al. (2006)
2009	Chung and others demonstrated that the Sharklet AF topography inhibited biofilm formation of *Staphylococcus aureus* over a period of 21 days.	Peng et al. (2007)
Since 2009	The change in wettability of a surface due to micro-topographical roughness is also likely to be a contributing factor to AF properties.	Magin et al. (2010)
2011	Superhydrophobic surface based on silica colloids and a low surface energy fluorinated silane xerogel reduced the fouling adhesion	Ferrari and Benedetti (2015)
2010–18	Development of inorganic-organic hybrid nanocomposite for self-cleaning and FR coatings (different nanofillers, polymers, and silicone copolymers) were used.	Tian, Jiang, et al. (2019), Selim et al. (2016a), Selim et al. (2019), Roy and Bhowmick (2010), Howell et al. (2014), Nayak et al. (2013), Murase and Fujibayashi (1997)

(*Continued*)

Table 5.1 (Continued)

Timeline	Description of AF product	References
2017–19	Various series of silicone homo (co)polymer/hybrid nanofiller composites as a self-cleaning and FR coatings termed as ternary and quaternary nanocomposites.	Selim et al., (2017b, 2016a), Selim et al. (2019), Selim et al. (2019), Howell et al. (2014), Nayak et al. (2013), Selim et al. (2016b)

have undergone significant development over the course of history. Many historical civilizations, including the Carthaginians, Phoenicians, Greeks, Romans, and Plutarch, have addressed the problem of maritime fouling (Almeida et al., 2007; Xie et al., 2019). Paints that are biocidal to prevent fouling have become widely used since the advent of iron ships and the ensuing corrosion. Developed in the late 1970s, a TBT copolymer served as a self-polishing coating (Almeida et al., 2007; Xie et al., 2019). This early method was effective, but it had several disadvantages, such as fouling toxicity from the use of toxicants like biocides. In Fig. 5.3A, a leaching process utilizing a copolymer of TBT-acrylate and methylmethacrylate is illustrated. The presence of toxic chemicals released from TBT into the saltwater has been found to have adverse effects on microorganisms (Detty et al., 2014). The advantages of this specific coating design include a streamlined hydrodynamic profile during sailing, reduced fuel consumption, and consistent release rates of biocides over time. The robust biocidal properties of TBT-based coatings are widely acknowledged for their effectiveness in AF applications. But because of their strong biocidal properties and detrimental impacts on nontarget organisms, TBT-based coatings were outlawed by the International Maritime Organization in 2008 (Dafforn et al., 2011; Kiil et al., 2001). The development of tin-free material coatings using alternative hazardous biocides, such as Cu^{2+}, was started in response to the approval of tin-based fouling prevention coatings and their accompanying negative effects (Nir & Reches, 2016). Nevertheless, obstacles arising from the deleterious impacts and rates of release impeded the widespread implementation of these substitutes. The fact that many fouling strains could tolerate these coatings was another disadvantage. As a result, "booster" biocides like diuron and Irgarol 1051 were added to copper AF paint formulations (Chambers et al., 2006). Because of the detrimental effects, these biocides have on photosynthetic organisms'

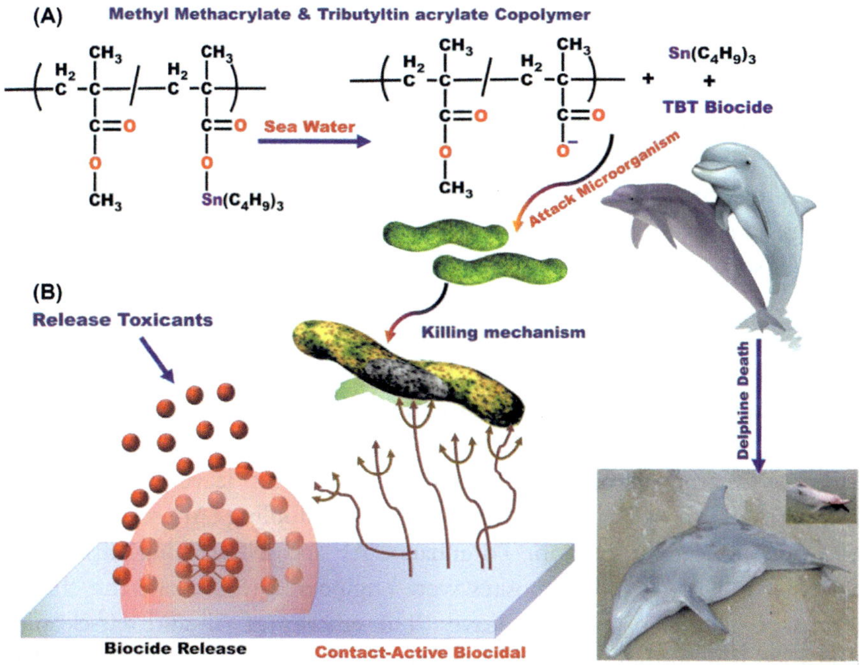

Figure 5.3 (A) The release of biocides from a commonly used copolymer, methylmethacrylate, and tributyltin acrylate into seawater through leaching. (B) The mechanism through which antifouling coatings with biocidal properties exert a toxic effect, preventing the adhesion of fouling organisms. *Reproduced with permission Selim, M. S., Shenashen, M. A., El-Safty, S. A., Sakai, M., Higazy, S. A., Selim, M. M., Isago, H., & Elmarakbi, A. (2017b).* Progress in Materials Science, *87, 1–32, Copyright 2017, Elsevier.*

growth rate, some countries outlawed their use. For example, Denmark outlawed both chemicals, although Australia and the Netherlands only outlawed Irgarol 1051 and diuron, respectively (Sapozhnikova et al., 2013). On the other hand, natural marine substances have become environmentally acceptable substitutes for biocidal AF coatings. These naturally occurring marine chemicals were successfully incorporated into AF building blocks to stop fouling attachments (Li & Ning, 2019; Yebra et al., 2004). Observing marine species use these substances to reduce fouling served as the inspiration for this approach. These included fatty acids, acerogenins, heterocyclic compounds, amino acids, and halogenated chemicals (Yebra et al., 2004). These natural chemicals' primary AF building blocks comprised growth inhibition, attachment prevention, upgrading of negative chemotaxis, fouling repellence, and organism death (Fig. 5.3B). Although these compounds provided environment-friendly and efficient solutions, their use in high-performance

AF systems was limited because of several important factors (Acevedo et al., 2013): the difficulty of releasing these compounds in a controlled manner, the cost and duration of registration procedures, the difficulties of large-scale manufacturing, and the difficulty of incorporating natural biocides into the active site within the coating matrix. Hence, there is a rapidly increasing demand for eco-friendly AF coatings, specifically silicone fouling release (FR) coatings, to steer toward an environmentally conscious AF future. These silicone FR surfaces establish a nonadhesive coating characterized by low surface free energy and absence of leaching properties. The most favorable alternatives that align with environmental considerations are the foundational elements of silicone FR (Table 5.1). Progress has been made in the development of FR paints, particularly those leveraging silicone matrices such as Sylgard 184 and RTV11. In 2004 an innovative approach emerged from scanning electron microscopy examinations of lotus leaves, inspiring the conceptualization of Sharklet AF self-cleaning antifouling (AF) surfaces a biomimetic self-cleaning solution. To enhance AF and self-cleaning attributes, a variety of polymer nanocomposites were engineered to emulate the characteristics of shark skin and lotus leaves. The efficacy of AF and self-cleaning properties was further boosted through the creation of hybrid nanofiller/composites, copolymers, and nanocomposites.

5.5 Marine antifouling through biomimetic surface microtopographies

Many marine animals have inherent AF characteristics, which are thought to be granted by the way their skin patterns affect surface characteristics like surface energy, wettability, and textural roughness (Bai et al., 2013; Kirschner & Brennan, 2012; Zhao et al., 2020). The main benefit of imitating these naturally occurring AF microstructures is that they reduce the risk to marine ecosystems by not requiring the release of biocides. As a result, research on the creation of biomimetic microstructure coatings has become increasingly important and has received a lot of attention lately (Liu & Li, 2012). Reduced contact area between fouling organisms and the surface is one explanation put up for the AF effect of rough microstructures. Studies reveal that fouling organism colonization is intricately impacted by surface topographies, with variables including species, morphological configurations, and dimensions (Cao et al., 2010; Decker et al., 2014). Notably, the surface pattern exhibits higher AF efficacy when the size of the surface texture matches or is smaller than that of the fouling organism.

On the other hand, fouler may settle and take up residence inside the structure if the surface texture is larger than the fouling organism's size (Cao et al., 2010; Schumacher et al., 2007b; Xie et al., 2019). The number of attached fouler increases and adhesion strength diminishes when the structural size is an order of magnitude less than the fouling organism (Cao et al., 2010). Scardino and de Nys (2011) reviewed biomimicking AF surfaces that are modeled after the skin of marine mammals, echinoderms, gorgonians, and sharks. Crucially, inspiration does not just come from aquatic life terrestrial species can also serve as useful models. Several physical fabrication techniques, including photolithography, electron-beam lithography, and ion-beam lithography, were reviewed by Scardino and de Nys (Scardino & de Nys, 2011). They discussed biomimicking AF surfaces modeled after the skin of marine mammals, echinoderms, gorgonians, and sharks. Importantly, the inspiration for such surfaces is not limited to aquatic life; terrestrial species can also provide valuable models. Another set of techniques, including soft lithography, hot embossing, and picosecond laser texturing was reviewed by Richards et al. (2020) in a thorough review. These techniques can be used to replicate biological surface microtopographies. Soft mold replication is the most popular and straightforward technique used in research to replicate biological microstructures on artificial coated surfaces. Fixing the biological specimen on a plate, adding a liquid elastomer precursor and curing agent, and then separating the elastomer sheet to create a negative reproduction of the biological sample are the steps in the process. The negative replica then functions as a mold, and the precursor and curing agent are poured, followed by curing and separation, to create the positive reproduction of the specimen (Bai et al., 2013; Bixler & Bhushan, 2014; Chen et al., 2015b; Liu & Li, 2012).

5.5.1 Mimicking aquatic organisms

The remarkable qualities of shark skin, like AF and drag reduction, are well known. The goal of several investigations has been to imitate in AF coatings the complex surface microstructure of shark skin. The surface of shark skin is not smooth, as is commonly believed; rather, it is made up of microscopic scales called dermal denticles. The alternating arrangement of micro riblets and grooves in these diamond-shaped dermal denticles forms an interlocking structure that produces a low-drag surface (Fig. 5.4A)

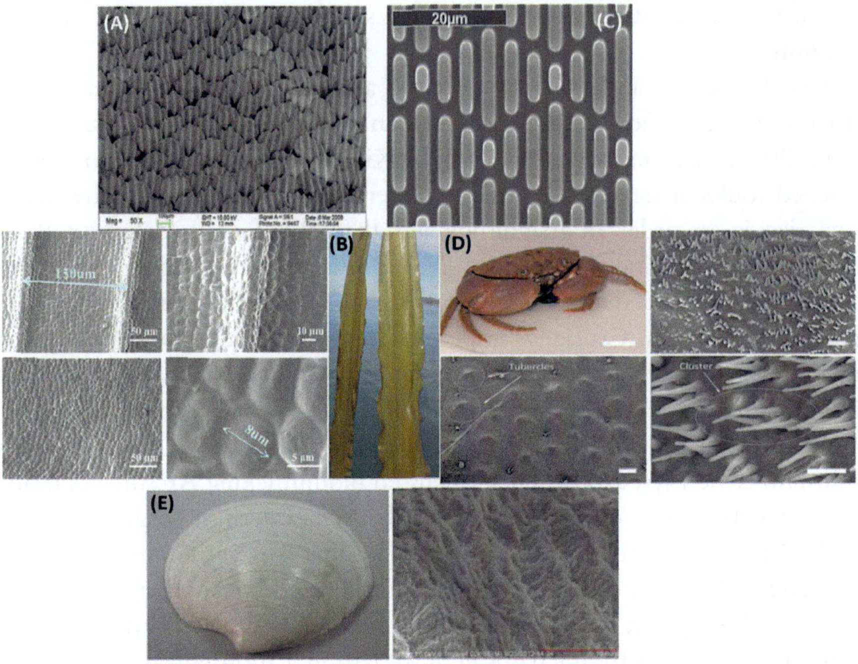

Figure 5.4 (A) Microscopic features on the surface of Shark skin. (B) Image capturing *Laminaria japonica* and its surface microtopography. (C) Surface microtopography of Sharklet antifouling coating. (D) Image featuring a marine crab (*Myomenippe hardwickii*) and the microtopography on its shell surface. (E) Picture showcasing *Dosinia japonica* and the microtopography on its shell surface. *Reproduced with permission (A) and (E) from Bai et al. (2013), Copyright 2012, Elsevier; (B) from Zhao et al. (2020), Copyright 2020, Elsevier; (C) from Schumacher et al. (2007b), Copyright 2007, Taylor & Francis; (D) from Brzozowska et al. (2014), Copyright 2014, American Chemical Society.*

(Bai et al., 2013; Bixler & Bhushan, 2014; Li & Guo, 2019). Bixler and Bhushan (2014) claim that shark skin has hydrophilic qualities. A biomimetic surface AF coating called "Sharklet" has been created and commercially manufactured based on these concepts. It features grooves and ribs that are each 2 μm wide. The riblets' lengths exhibit periodic variations (4, 8, 12, 16, 12, 8 μm) as illustrated in Fig. 5.4C (Carman et al. (2006); Schumacher et al., 2007b). KOH-etched silicon molds and reactive ion etched molds were used to construct a unique surface with a height gradient on the riblets, drawing on a prior investigation of shark skin microtopography (Munther et al., 2018). *Escherichia coli* (*E. coli*) adherence was shown to be reduced by this novel surface; specifically reactive ion etching (RIE)-etched replicas outperformed KOH-etched replicas, reducing adhesion by up to 75% as opposed to 55.69% (Munther et al., 2018). Research on catsharks, more especially *Scyliorhinus canicula*, revealed that surfaces with more compactly packed and smaller dermal denticles were better at preventing fouling (Sullivan & Regan, 2011). To create superhydrophobic surfaces with microgroove and micropit patterns, Sun et al. (2018) used a picosecond laser on stainless steel. Following 5 weeks of submersion in saltwater, the microgroove pattern performed marginally better than the control group, with a biofouling reduction of about 50%. Liu and Li (2012) combined the microstructures of lotus leaves and shark skin to create a superhydrophobic surface. Feld et al. (2019) carried out in-depth examinations of the surface microstructures of three species of slowly swimming sharks, presenting new objectives for biomimicking research as well as insightful information about the functional mechanisms of shark skin. In terms of AF, some marine organisms such as crabs, seaweeds, and mollusk shells perform better than their more mobile relatives despite their generally static character (Brzozowska et al., 2014; Chen et al., 2015b; Greco et al., 2013). Examining the surfaces of *Dosinia japonica* (Fig. 5.4E), *Gafrarium pectinatum*, and *Mimachlamys nobilis*, it was found that the latter two species' surfaces had scales that are less than 1 μm in size and are thought to be useful in avoiding diatom adhesion. Remarkably, *M. nobilis* had the least effective AF performance, whereas *D. japonica* demonstrated the strongest performance (Bai et al., 2013). After researching seaweed surfaces, Chapman et al. (2014) created a biomimicking technique based on Guiry's wrack (Fucus guiryi) and sugar kelp (*Saccharina latissima*) that successfully decreased the adhesion of biomacromolecules and fouling organisms. Taking inspiration from the surface microtopography observed on *Laminaria japonica* (Fig. 5.5B), Zhao et al. (2020) employed the layer-by-layer self-assembly process on a microstructured PDMS replica to fabricate a (GHPEI/ALG) film. The microstructure of this film enhanced its surface antibacterial properties, leading to synergistic effects with other elements. Simultaneously, a gel-like layer of sodium alginate was formed, substantially increasing the surface hydrophilicity and effectively preventing the adhesion of Nitzschia closterium. The surface pattern of crab shells was observed, exhibiting agnails with average diameters and lengths of 1.5 and 4 μm, respectively (Chen et al., 2015b). Algal cell counts were reduced by more than 65% in AF experiments with positive and negative crab shell mimics. Due to their compound eye structure, the eyes of the green crab *Carcinus maenas* have been identified as a potential source of AF solutions for marine sensors (Greco et al., 2013). A microstructured surface inspired by the shell of the marine crab

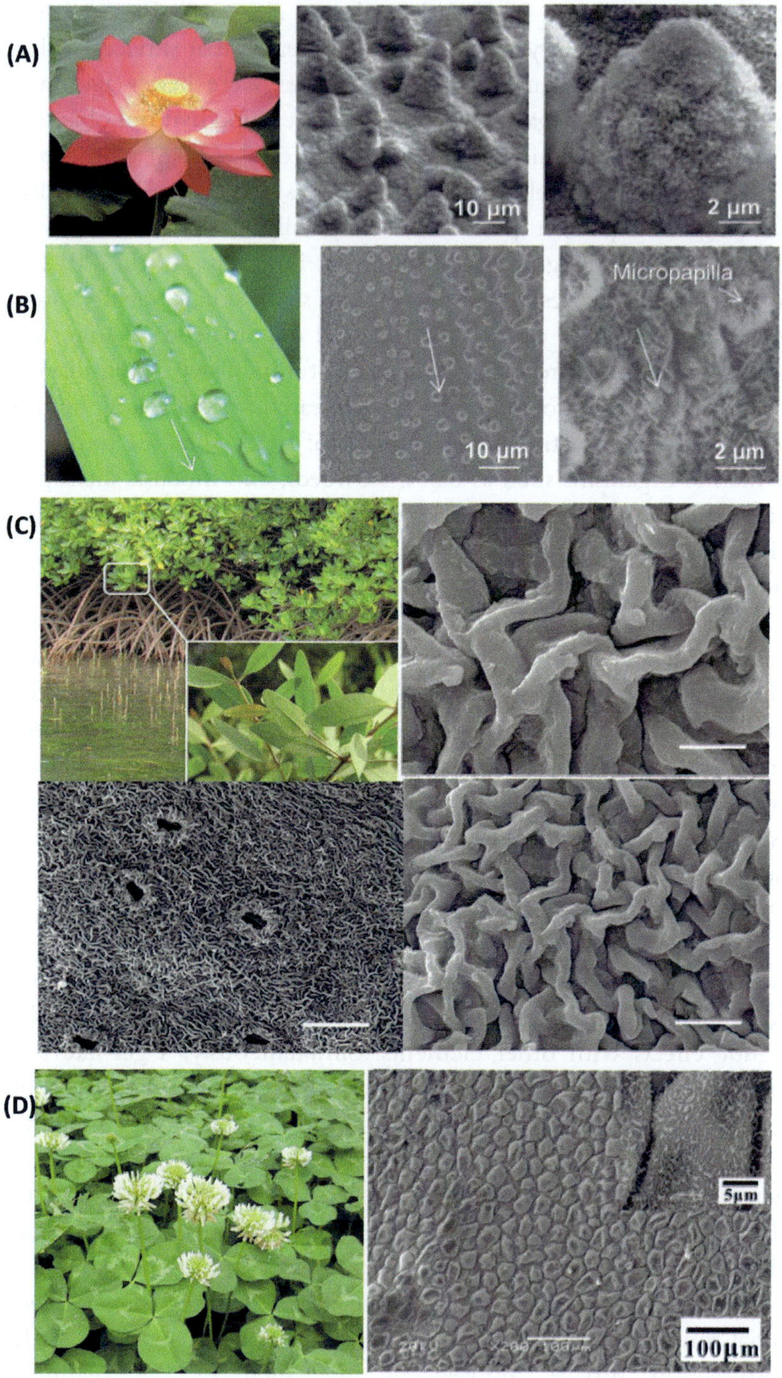

(Continued)

Myomenippe hardwickii (Fig. 5.5D) was merged with chemical modification technology by Brzozowska et al. (2014). Sulfobetaine brushes outperformed layer by layer in laboratory tests that demonstrated the combined chemical alteration and microtopography surfaces' ability to limit biofouling. While a perfluorododecyltrichlorosilane coated and patterned PDMS surface showed distinct AF and FR potency for at least six weeks in field tests, the mechanical strength of the modified surfaces proved insufficient for prolonged field use.

5.5.2 Mimicking the texture of plant leaves

Lotus is well known for having a superhydrophobic surface and for washing itself (Bixler & Bhushan, 2014; Chen et al., 2015b; Li & Guo, 2019). Lotus shows an ability to maintain cleanliness even while growing in lakebeds coated with muck. The surface structure of lotus leaves has been the subject of further research because of this occurrence. Research has demonstrated that the surface of lotus leaves has a waxy layer covering a hierarchical structure, which confers superhydrophobic and self-cleaning capabilities known as the "lotus effect" (Bixler & Bhushan, 2014; Chen et al., 2015b; Selim et al., 2017a) (Fig. 5.5A). This microtopography is formed by randomly organized micropapillae on the surface, with average heights and diameters of around 8 and 7 μm, respectively, and average intervals of 10 μm (Chen et al., 2015b). A substantially greater water contact angle than that of a smooth surface is produced when this structure comes into contact with water because it traps air and creates a cushion layer between the water and the surface (Chen et al., 2015b; Li & Guo, 2019).

Studies showed that copies of lotus leaves, both positive and negative, decreased closterium adhesion by about 73%. Repellency against *Navicula* was higher in negative copies (74% and 54%) compared to positive replicas (Chen et al., 2015b). The beneficial water-repellent and self-cleaning qualities of rice (*Oryza sativa*) leaves have also been revealed by recent investigations (Bixler & Bhushan, 2014). Similar to lotus leaves, rice leaves have

Figure 5.5 A: Image and microtopography on the surface of lotus (*Nelumbo nucifera*) leaves. (B) Photograph and surface microtopography of rice (*Oryza sativa*) leaves. (C) Picture and surface microtopography of mangrove tree (Sonneratia apetala) leaves. (D) Photograph and surface microtopography of clover (Trifolium) leaves. *Reproduced with permission (A) and (B) from Bixler and Bhushan (2014), Copyright 2014, Royal Society of Chemistry; (C) from Fu et al. (2018), Copyright 2018, The Royal Society; (D) from Wan et al. (2012), Copyright 2012, American Chemical Society.*

intricate hierarchical structures on their surfaces, with waxy micropapillae and sinusoidal grooves (Fig. 5.5B). Rice leaves have a water contact angle of 164 degrees, which suggests superhydrophobicity. Because of their small size, the micropapillae proved difficult to copy using urethane polymer; however, covering the replica with hydrophobic silica nanoparticles enhanced self-cleaning and decreased adhesive force. Despite the pressure of sea fouling, the mangrove tree (*Sonneratia apetala*) demonstrates expected fouling-proof ability. The topology of *S. apetala* leaves is ridge-like, with erratically spaced ridges that are roughly 5 μm in height and 1 μm in thickness, separated by 5 μm (Fig. 5.5C). In tests, an artificial surface made of graphite paper showed a comparable capacity to separate tubeworms from the PDMS replica of mangrove tree leaves. The AF process of *S. apetala* leaves is facilitated by low wettability, self-cleanability, and the release of oleanolic acid antifoulant (Feng et al., 2016). Certain terrestrial plants with relatively dry environments also have hydrophobic surfaces on their leaves. Four different plant leaf types were examined by Wan et al. (2012) for their surface microstructures: *Trifolium* (Fig. 5.5D), Herba solani nigri, Forsythia suspensa, and *Parthenocissus tricuspidata.* Four different chemical modifications were applied to duplicated surfaces: PSPMA, PMETAC, PMAA, and PSBMA. The findings suggested that incorporating PSPMA molecular brushes with both negatively and positively replicated clover leaves demonstrated effective antiadhesion and FR characteristics against microalgae such as Chlorella and Nannochloropsis maritima. Furthermore, Tian et al. (Tian, Zhang, et al., 2019) synthesized an electroplated Zn-Fe coating modified with tetradecanoic acid that had an Echinopsis multiplex-like microstructure surface, leading to superhydrophobicity. When the coating was applied to carbon steel, stainless steel, and copper, it showed a wide water contact angle (>160 degrees) and a very low surface energy (1.33 mJ/m^2). These advantageous characteristics point to possible uses in marine AF, while the possibility of antibiofouling has not been studied. Overall, self-cleaning characteristics found in plant leaves provide important information for biomimetic microtopography AF coatings. Certain species that live in swampy or humid environments may have more hydrophobic leaves, which makes them interesting subjects for biomimetic research.

5.5.3 Mimicking the texture of insect wing surfaces

Insects may have extremely thin wings, but they are often exposed to harsh surroundings. These wings show resistance against organic pollutants found in nature, like pollen and hydrocarbons. Insect wings exhibit excellent hydrophobicity when they come into contact with water during a downpour. Scientists have been inspired by these findings to develop surfaces that resemble the nanostructure of insect wings. Dragonflies and cicadas were chosen as bionic templates in a study conducted by Gangadoo et al. (2016). The wing surface structures of two cicada species, namely *Psaltoda claripennis* (Fig. 5.6A) and *Tamasa tristigma* (Fig. 5.6B), as well as one dragonfly species primarily *Rhyothemis graphiptera* (Fig. 5.6C), were examined. The wing sample replicas were created on an epoxy matrix, and their AF properties were then examined. Images captured by micrographs showed that the surface of cicada wings was covered in neat rows of cones, each about 200 nm in height and distance from the others. The surface topography of dragonfly wings was also made up of randomly dispersed nanopillars, each measuring around 200 nm in height (Fig. 5.6A–C). In a thorough 7-day test, the dragonfly wing nanostructure outperformed commercial AF coatings, the blank epoxy sample, and cicada replica epoxy in terms of AF capabilities. Unlike the microstructures of dragonfly and cicadas wings, butterfly wings have a large number of microscales. Bixler et al. claimed that superhydrophobicity, self-cleaning qualities, and a drag-reducing performance that combines the benefits of lotus leaves and shark skin were demonstrated by butterfly wings, particularly those of the blue *Morpho didius* species (Bixler & Bhushan, 2012, 2014). The matched shingle-shaped scales with microgrooves defined the surface microstructure of butterfly wings (Fig. 5.6D) (Bixler & Bhushan, 2014). The duplicated butterfly wing sample had a contact angle of 160 degrees, showing that it was as self-cleaning and water repellent as rice leaves. The microstructure under investigation shows potential for use in AF surfaces.

5.5.4 Innovative coatings: fouling release and self-cleaning

Fouling-release surfaces possess regulated mechanisms that prevent fouling attachments and lower the adhesion strength of fouling coatings. The development of nontoxic FR nanocomposites marks the beginning of a new movement in the transportation sector toward resilient and environmentally acceptable self-cleaning coatings for ship bottoms. The many benefits of these FR surfaces are as follows: low friction, an ultrasmooth surface, improved molecular mobility, decreased free energy, micro/nanoroughness, tin-free composition, extended durability, and nontoxicity and nonleaching properties (Sankar et al., 2015; Wan et al., 2012). These FR

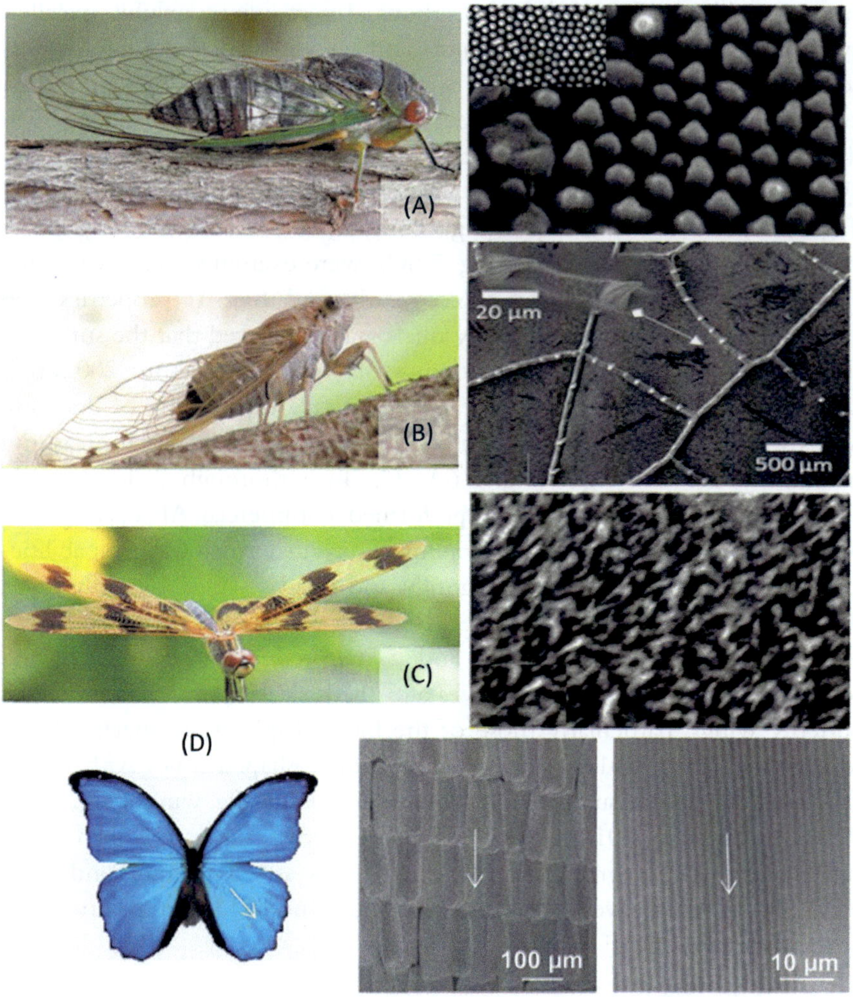

Figure 5.6 Images and surface microtopographies of (A) cicada (*Psaltoda claripennis*), (B) cicada (*Tamasa tristigma*), (C) dragonfly (*Rhyothemis graphiptera*) wings, respectively. (D) Image and surface microtopography of butterfly (Blue Morpho didius) wings. *Reproduced with permission (A)–(C) from Gangadoo et al. (2016) Copyright 2016, Royal Society of Chemistry; (D) from Bixler and Bhushan (2012) Copyright 2012, Royal Society of Chemistry.*

characteristics enable higher ship speed and fewer cargo days by lowering fuel consumption and maintenance expenses (Wynne et al., 2000).

The use of inorganic nano-additives has become necessary to improve the mechanical and FR properties of a wide range of silicone paints, even though silicone paints already have good FR qualities (Chakradhar et al., 2011; Sankar et al., 2015). In addition to lowering surface free energy, inorganic–organic surfaces are essential for enhancing superhydrophobic and AF properties (Chapman & Regan, 2012). Effective superhydrophobic FR nanocomposite surfaces have been identified in PDMS coatings enhanced with various nanofillers, including Fe_3O_4 nanospheres, $TiO_2@SiO_2$ core–shell, Cu_2O nanocubes, and Al_2O_3 nanorods (El-Safty et al., 2012, 2015; Hassen et al., 2018; Selim et al., 2017b, 2018, 2020; Shenashen et al., 2017).

Graphene materials are appropriate for a variety of applications because to their exceptional qualities, which include biocompatibility, cost-effectiveness, corrosion resistance, and eco-friendly security (El-Safty et al., 2015; Emran et al., 2019; Selim et al., 2018; Shenashen et al., 2016, 2017). Nanocomposite coatings based on silicone and graphene provide FR self-cleaning systems that are both economically and mechanically durable (Xue et al., 2008). As reinforcing FR nanofillers, graphene oxide (GO)/metal oxide hybrids provide superhydrophobic and micro/nano-rough self-cleaning surfaces—all essential elements of effective AF coatings (Howell et al., 2014; Nayak et al., 2013; Selim et al., 2015a, 2016a, 2017c). Certain materials have requirements for cleaning their surfaces from debris and water, such as superhydrophobic and superhydrophilic surfaces. For example, solar light irradiation-enhanced photo-induced catalysts can produce superhydrophilic surfaces with contact angles of less than 10 degrees for impurity breakdown. Under photo-induced lighting, these superhydrophilic materials may undergo mechanistic self-cleaning that involves releasing/removing pollutants from surfaces, lowering the contact angle on surfaces, and dissolving the structure of adsorbed toxicant species (El-Safty et al., 2015; Emran et al., 2019; Selim et al., 2018; Shenashen et al., 2016, 2017). On the other hand, water droplet rolling can produce thin slide films as protective layers that improve the early-stage adherence of pollutants, which is how superhydrophobic materials achieve their self-cleaning mechanics (Selim et al., 2015b, 2017b). These extremely water-repellent, superhydrophobic surfaces efficiently thwart fouling settlement and deteriorate surface-fouling adhesion bonds (Durand et al., 2011).

5.6 Challenges and outlook for the future

The persistent challenge of marine fouling necessitates continuous research into novel remedies. AF marine coatings could be greatly advanced by the introduction of biomimetic microtopography, which is modeled after the complex patterns found in nature. A challenge facing this developing technology is assuring the long-term stability and longevity of biomimetic microtopography coatings in severe marine conditions, where mechanical forces, UV radiation, and saltwater exposure may eventually reduce their efficiency. Complex microtopographic shapes are difficult to replicate commercially and need sophisticated manufacturing methods that may increase production costs. Another challenge underscoring the critical importance of scalability is the transition from laboratory-scale demonstrations to large-scale commercial production. It is yet unclear how biomimetic coatings on marine structures interact with other layers, especially those intended to prevent corrosion. The future of biomimetic microtopography coatings is bright, notwithstanding these obstacles. Technological developments in materials and nanotechnology offer prospects for improving their characteristics, and it is possible to create multifunctional coatings with attributes like enhanced hydrophobicity or self-healing. Enhancement through the integration of natural molecules through bioinspired chemistry is another possibility. To guarantee efficacy and set standards, however, extensive field testing and validation in actual maritime habitats are necessary. Widespread acceptance depends on addressing financial issues and creating production procedures that are economical. Finally, given the significant potential advantages of biomimetic microtopography AF marine coatings, this is an area that begs for further investigation. This calls for interdisciplinary cooperation, technological advancement, and a dedication to sustainable practices as the field of study develops.

5.7 Conclusions

Efficacious and ecologically sustainable AF solutions are desperately needed in navigation, detection, engineering, and aquaculture because to the increasing human activity on the sea. In addition to offering workable remedies for marine biofouling, nature also provides important design cues for nontoxic AF coatings. As a result, maritime AF companies are paying more attention to biomimetic coatings. This chapter scrutinizes the prevalent application of biomimetic AF techniques, which seek to mimic the structure, function, and topography of living organisms. Comprehensive data are provided, along with pros and cons of biomimetic surface microtopographies. Only a small number of marine AF coatings have been successfully used in practice, despite intensive study into the subject. This presents a significant obstacle to industrialized manufacture. Difficulties include costly and complex production procedures combined with inadequate endurance and durability in marine conditions. Comprehensive knowledge of the mechanisms underlying biofouling settlement is still needed. We argue that merging successful biomimetic AF tactics could lead to the creation of novel methods with remarkable stability and repellency.

References

Abarzua, S., & Jakubowski, S. (1995). Biotechnological investigation for the prevention of biofouling. I. Biological and biochemical principles for the prevention of biofouling. *Marine Ecology Progress Series*, *123*, 301–312.

Acevedo, M. S., Puentes, C., Carreño, K., León, J. G., Stupak, M., García, M., Pérez, M., & Blustein, G. (2013). *International Biodeterioration & Biodegradation*, *83*, 97–104.

Akinfiev, T., Janushevskis, A., & Lavendelis, E. (2007). *Transport & Engineering*, *6*(24), 133–145.

Almeida, E., Diamantino, T. C., & de Sousa, O. (2007). *Progress in Organic Coatings*, *59*, 2–20.

Amador, G. J., & Hu, D. L. (2015). *The Journal of Experimental Biology*, *218*, 3164.

Anderson, C., Atlar, M., Callow, M., Candries, M., Milne, A., & Townsin, R. L. (2003). *Journal of Marine Design and Operations*, *B4*, 11–23.

Aslam, M., Ahmad, R., & Kim, J. (2018). *Separation and Purification Technology*, *206*, 297–315.

Awais, M., & Bhuiyan, A. A. (2019). *International Journal of Heat and Mass Transfer*, *41*, 580–603.

Bai, X. Q., Xie, G. T., Fan, H., Peng, Z. X., Yuan, C. Q., & Yan, X. P. (2013). Study on biomimetic preparation of shell surface microstructure for ship antifouling. *Wear*, *306*, 285–295.

Bitton, G. (2002). *Encyclopedia of Environmental Microbiology*. New York: Wiley.

Bixler, G. D., & Bhushan, B. (2012). *Philosophical Transactions: Mathematical, Physical and Engineering Sciences*, *370*, 2381.

Bixler, G. D., & Bhushan, B. (2014). Rice- and butterfly-wing effect inspired self-cleaning and low drag micro/nanopatterned surfaces in water, oil, and air flow. *Nanoscale*, *6*, 76–96.

Bloecher, N., & Floerl, O. (2020). Efficacy testing of novel antifouling coatings for pen nets in aquaculture: How good are alternatives to traditional copper coatings? *Aquaculture (Amsterdam, Netherlands)*, *519*734936.

Brzozowska, A. M., Parra-Velandia, F. J., Quintana, R., Zhu, X. Y., Lee, S. S. C., Chin-Sing, L., Janczewski, D., Teo, S. L. M., & Vancso, J. G. (2014). Biomimicking micropatterned surfaces and their effect on marine biofouling. *Langmuir: the ACS Journal of Surfaces and Colloids*, *30*, 9165–9175.

Callow, M. E., & Callow, J. A. (2002). *Biologist (Columbus, Ohio)*, *49*(1), 10.

Cao, X., Pettitt, M. E., Wode, F., Arpa Sancet, M. P., Fu, J., Ji, J., Callow, M. E., Callow, J. A., Rosenhahn, A., & Grunze, M. (2010). Interaction of zoospores of the green alga Ulva with bioinspired micro- and nanostructured surfaces prepared by polyelectrolyte layer-by-layer self-assembly. *Advanced Functional Materials*, *20*, 1984–1993.

Carman, M. L., Estes, T. G., Feinberg, A. W., Schumacher, J. F., Wilkerson, W., Wilson, L. H., Callow, M. E., Callow, J. A., & Brennan, A. B. (2006). Engineered antifouling microtopographies - correlating wettability with cell attachment. *Biofouling*, *22*, 11–21.

Carteaua, D., Vallèe-Rèhela, K., Linossier, I., Quiniou, F., Davy, R., Compère, C., Delbury, M., & Faÿ, F. (2014). *Progress in Organic Coatings*, 77(2), 485–493.

Chakradhar, R. P. S., Kumara, V. D., Raob, J. L., & Bharathibai, B. (2011). *Applied Surface Science*, *257*, 8569–8575.

Chambers, L. D., Stokes, K. R., Walsh, F. C., & Wood, R. J. K. (2006). *Surface and Coatings Technology*, *201*, 3642–3652.

Chapman, J., Hellio, C., Sullivan, T., Brown, R., Russell, S., Kiterringham, E., Le Nor, L., & Regan, F. (2014). Bioinspired synthetic macroalgae: Examples from nature for antifouling applications. *International Biodeterioration and Biodegradation*, *86*, 6–13.

Chapman, J., & Regan, F. (2012). *Advanced Engineering Materials*, *14*(4), B175–B184.

Chen, Z. F., Zhao, W. J., Xu, J. H., Mo, M. T., Peng, S. S., Zeng, Z. X., Wu, X. D., & Xue, Q. J. (2015b). Designing environmentally benign modified silica resin coatings with biomimetic textures for antibiofouling. *RSC Advances*, *5*, 36874–36881.

Clemente, C. J., Bullock, J. M., Beale, A., & Federle, W. (2010). *The Journal of Experimental Biology*, *213*, 635.

Compere, C., Bellon-Fontaine, M. N., Bertrand, P., Costa, D., Marcus, P., & Poleunis, C. (2001). *Biofouling*, *17*, 129–145.

Dafforn, K. A., Lewis, J. A., & Johnston, E. L. (2011). *Marine Pollution Bulletin*, *62*, 453–465.

Decker, J. T., Sheats, J. T., & Brennan, A. B. (2014). Engineered antifouling microtopographies: Surface pattern effects on cell distribution. *Langmuir: the ACS Journal of Surfaces and Colloids*, *30*, 15212–15218.

Demirel, Y. K., Uzun, D., Zhang, Y., & Turan, O. (2018). In A. I. Ölçer, M. Kitada, D. Dalaklis, & F. Ballini (Eds.), *Trends and Challenges in Maritime Energy Management* (p. 325). Cham, Switzerland: Springer International Publishing.

Detty, M. R., Ciriminna, R., Bright, F. V., & Pagliaro, M. (2014). *Accounts of Chemical Research*, *47*(2), 678–687.

Durand, N., Mariot, D., Améduri, B., Boutevin, B., & Ganachaud, F. (2011). *Langmuir: the ACS Journal of Surfaces and Colloids*, *27*(7), 4057–4067.

Eduok, U., Faye, O., & Szpunar, J. (2017). *Progress in Organic Coatings*, *111*, 124–163.

Elbourne, A., Crawford, R. J., & Ivanova, E. P. (2017). *Journal of Colloid and Interface Science*, *508*, 603–616.

El-Safty, S. A., Sakai, M., Selim, M., & Hendi, A. A. (2015). *ACS Applied Materials & Interfaces*, 7(24), 13217–13231.

El-Safty, S. A., Shenashen, M. A., Ismael, M., & Khairy, M. (2012). *Advanced Functional Materials*, *22*, 3013–3021.

Emran, M. Y., El-Safty, S. A., Shenashen, M. A., & Minowa, T. (2019). *Sensors & Actuators, B: Chemical*, *284*, 456–467.

Feld, K., Kolborg, A. N., Nyborg, C. M., Salewski, M., Steffensen, J. F., & Berg-Sorensen, K. (2019). Dermal denticles of three slowly swimming shark species: Microscopy and flow visualization. *Biomimetics*, *4*, 38.

Feng, D. Q., Wang, W., Wang, X., Qiu, Y., & Ke, C. H. (2016). Low barnacle fouling on leaves of the mangrove plant Sonneratia apetala and possible anti-barnacle defense strategies. *Marine Ecology Progress Series*, *544*, 169–182.

Feng, X. J., & Jiang, L. (2006). *Advanced Materials*, *18*, 3063.

Ferrari, M., & Benedetti, A. (2015). *Advances in Colloid and Interface Science*, *222*, 291–304.

Flemming, H.-C., Murthy, P. S., Venkatesan, R., & Cooksey, K. (2009). *Marine and Industrial Biofouling*. Berlin, Germany: Springer.

Fu, J. M., Zhang, H., Guo, Z. B., Feng, D. Q., Thiyagarajan, V., & Yao, H. M. (2018). Combat biofouling with microscopic ridge-like surface morphology: a bioinspired study. *Journal of the Royal Society, Interface/the Royal Society*, *15*20170823.

Gangadoo, S., Chandra, S., Power, A., Hellio, C., Watson, G. S., Watson, J. A., Green, D. W., & Chapman, J. (2016). Biomimetics for early stage biofouling prevention: Templates from insect cuticles. *Journal of Materials Chemistry B*, *4*, 5747–5754.

Greco, G., Lanero, T. S., Torrassa, S., Young, R., Vassalli, M., Cavaliere, A., Rolandi, R., Pelucchi, E., Faimali, M., & Davenport, J. (2013). Microtopography of the eye surface of the crab *Carcinus maenas*: An atomic force microscope study suggesting a possible antifouling potential. *Journal of the Royal Society, Interface/the Royal Society*, *10*20130122.

Hakim, M. L., Nugroho, B., Nurrohman, M. N., Suastika, I. K., & Utama, I. K. A. P. (2019). *IOP Conference Series: Earth and Environmental Science*, *339*012037.

Hansen, W. R., & Autumn, K. (2005). *Proceedings of the National Academy of Sciences of the United States of America*, *102*, 385.

Hassen, D., Shenashen, M. A., El-Safty, A. R., Elmarakbi, A., & El-Safty, S. A. (2018). *Scientific Reports*, *8*, 3740.

Hellio, C., Maréchal, J. P., Da Gama, B. A. P., Pereira, R. C., & Clare, A. S. (2009). In C. Hellio, & D. Yebra (Eds.), *Advances in Marine Antifouling Coatings and Technologies* (p. 572). Cambridge: Woodhead Publishing.

Hoa, N. D., & El-Safty, S. A. (2011). *Chemistry: A European Journal*, *17*(46), 12896–12901.

Howell, C., Vu, T. L., Lin, J. J., Kolle, S., Juthani, N., Watson, E., Weaver, J. C., Alvarenga, J., & Aizenberg, J. (2014). *ACS Applied Materials & Interfaces*, *6*(15), 13299–13307.

Cheyne, I. (2010). Regulation of marine antifouling in international and EC law. In S. Dürr, & J. C. Thomason (Eds.), *Biofouling* (pp. 306–318). Chichester: Wiley-Blackwell.

Imbesi, P. M., Gohad, N. V., Eller, M. J., Orihuela, B., Rittschof, D., Schweikert, E. A., Mount, A. S., & Wooley, K. L. (2012). *ACS Nano*, *6*(2), 1503–1512.

Ivanova, E. P., Hasan, J., Webb, H. K., Gervinskas, G., Juodkazis, S., Truong, V. K., Wu, A. H., Lamb, R. N., Baulin, V. A., Watson, G. S., Watson, J. A., Mainwaring, D. E., & Crawford, R. J. (2013). *Nature Communications*, *4*, 2838.

Jain, A., & Bhosle, N. B. (2009). Biochemical composition of the marine conditioning film: Implications for bacterial adhesion. *Biofouling*, *25*, 13–19.

Kelleher, S. M., Habimana, O., Lawler, J., O'reilly, B., Daniels, S., Casey, E., & Cowley, A. (2016). *ACS Applied Materials & Interfaces*, *8*, 14966.

Kiil, S., Weinell, C. E., Pedersen, M. S., & Dam-Johansen, K. (2001). *Industrial & Engineering Chemistry Research*, *40*(18), 3906–3920.

Kirschner, C. M., & Brennan, A. B. (2012). Bio-inspired antifouling strategies. *Annual Review of Materials Research*, *42*, 211–229.

Lami, R. (2019). In G. Tommonaro (Ed.), *Quorum Sensing* (p. 55). San Diego, CA: Academic.

Lee, W., Ahn, C. H., Hong, S., Kim, S., Lee, S., Baek, Y., & Yoon, J. (2010). Evaluation of surface properties of reverse osmosis membranes on the initial biofouling stages under no filtration condition. *Journal of Membrane Science*, *351*, 112–122.

Legg, M., Yücel, M. K., Garcia de Carellan, I., Kappatos, V., Selcuk, C., & Gan, T. H. (2015). *Ocean Engineering*, *103*, 237–247.

Li, Y., & Ning, C. (2019). *Bioactive Materials*, *4*, 189–195.

Li, Z. H., & Guo, Z. G. (2019). Bioinspired surfaces with wettability for antifouling application. *Nanoscale*, *11*, 22636–22663.

Liu, M., Wang, S., Wei, Z., Song, Y., & Lei, J. (2009). *Advanced Materials*, *21*, 665.

Liu, Y. H., & Li, G. J. (2012). A new method for producing "lotus effect" on a biomimetic shark skin. *Journal of Colloid and Interface Science*, *388*, 235–242.

Magin, C. M., Cooper, S. P., & Brennan, A. B. (2010). *Materials Today*, *13*(4), 36–44.

Maréchal, J.-P., & Hellio, C. (2009). *International Journal of Molecular Sciences, 10*(11), 4623–4637.

Marmur, A. (2004). *Langmuir: the ACS Journal of Surfaces and Colloids, 20*, 3517–3519.

Munther, M., Palma, T., Angerona, I. A., Salari, S., Ghassemi, H., Vasefi, M., Beheshti, A., & Davami, K. (2018). Microfabricated biomimetic placoid scale-inspired surfaces for antifouling applications. *Applied Surface Science, 453*, 166–172.

Murase, H., & Fujibayashi, T. (1997). *Progress in Organic Coatings, 31*, 97–104.

Nayak, B. K., Caffrey, P. O., Speck, C. R., & Gupta, M. C. (2013). *Applied Surface Science, 266*, 27–32.

Nir, S., & Reches, M. (2016). *Current Opinion in Biotechnology, 39*, 48–55.

Okamura, H., Aoyama, I., Liu, D., Maguire, R. J., Pacepavicius, G. J., & Lau, Y. L. (2000). *Water Research, 34*, 3523.

Omae, I. (2003). *Applied Organometallic Chemistry, 17*, 81.

Owen, R., Knap, A., Toaspern, M., & Carbery, K. (2002). *Marine Pollution Bulletin, 44*, 623.

Peng, P., Voelcker, N. H., Kumar, S., & Griesser, H. J. (2007). *Biointerphases, 2*(2), 95–104.

Ralston, E., & Swain, G. (2011). *Marine Technology Society Journal, 45*, 216.

Richards, C., Slaimi, A., O'Connor, N. E., Barrett, A., Kwiatkowska, S., & Regan, F. (2020). Bioinspired surface texture modification as a viable feature of future aquatic antifouling strategies: a review. *International Journal of Molecular Sciences*, 21.

Roy, N., & Bhowmick, A. K. (2010). *Polymer, 51*(22), 5172–5185.

Salta, M., Wharton, J. A., Stoodley, P., Dennington, S. P., Goodes, L. R., Werwinski, S., Mart, U., Wood, R. J., & Stokes, K. R. (2010). *Philosophical Transactions of the Royal Society A, 368*, 4729.

Sankar, G. G., Sathya, S., Murthy, P. S., Das, A., Pandiyan, R., Venugopalan, V. B., & Doble, M. (2015). *International Biodeterioration and Biodegradation, 104*, 307–314.

Sapozhnikova, Y., Wirth, E., Schiff, K., & Fulton, M. (2013). *Marine Pollution Bulletin, 69* (1– 2), 189–194.

Scardino, A. J., & de Nys, R. (2011). Mini review: Biomimetic models and bioinspired surfaces for fouling control. *Biofouling, 27*, 73–86.

Schultz, M. P. (2007). *Biofouling, 23*, 331–341.

Schultz, M. P., Bendick, J. A., Holm, E. R., & Hertel, W. M. (2010). *Biofouling, 27*(1), 87–98.

Schumacher, J. F., Carman, M. L., Estes, T. G., Feinberg, A. W., Wilson, L. H., Callow, M. E., Callow, J. A., Finlay, J. A., & Brennan, A. B. (2007b). Engineered antifouling microtopographies - effect of feature size, geometry, and roughness on settlement of zoospores of the green alga Ulva. *Biofouling, 23*, 55–62.

Selim, M. S., Elmarakbi, A., Azzam, A. M., Shenashen, M. A., ELSaeed, A. M., & El-Safty, S. A. (2018). *Progress in Organic Coatings, 116*, 21–34.

Selim, M. S., El-Safty, S. A., Azzam, A. M., Shenashen, M. A., El-Sockary, M. A., & Abo Elenien, O. M. (2019). *ChemistrySelect, 4*, 3395–3407.

Selim, M. S., El-Safty, S. A., El-Sockary, M. A., Hashem, A. I., Abo Elenien, O. M., EL-Saeed, A. M., & Fatthallah, N. A. (2015a). *RSC Advances, 5*(78), 63175–63185.

Selim, M. S., El-Safty, S. A., El-Sockary, M. A., Hashem, A. I., Abo Elenien, O. M., EL-Saeed, A. M., & Fatthallah, N. A. (2015b). *RSC Advances, 5*(26), 19933–19943.

Selim, M. S., El-Safty, S. A., El-Sockary, M. A., Hashem, A. I., Abo Elenien, O. M., EL-Saeed, A. M., & Fatthallah, N. A. (2016a). *Materials & Design, 101*, 218–225.

Selim, M. S., El-Safty, S. A., ElSockary, M. A., Hashem, A. I., Abo Elenien, O. M., EL-Saeed, A. M., & Fatthallah, N. A. (2016b). *Data in Brief, 8*, 1357–1364.

Selim, M. S., Mo, P. J., Zhang, Y. P., Hao, Z., & Wen, H. (2020). *Ceramics International*. Available from https://doi.org/10.1016/j.ceramint.2019.12.183. (In press.

Selim, M. S., Shenashen, M. A., Elmarakbi, A., Fatthallah, N. A., Hasegawa, S.-i, & El- Safty, S. A. (2017a). Synthesis of ultrahydrophobic and thermally stable inorganic–organic nanocomposites for self-cleaning foul release coatings. *Chemical Engineering Journal, 320*, 653–666.

Selim, M. S., Shenashen, M. A., El-Safty, S. A., Sakai, M., Higazy, S. A., Selim, M. M., Isago, H., & Elmarakbi, A. (2017b). *Progress in Materials Science, 87*, 1–32.

Selim, M. S., Shenashen, M. A., Hasegawa, S., Fatthallah, N. A., Elmarakbi, A., & El-Safty, S. A. (2017c). *Chemical Engineering Journal, 320*, 653–666.

Selim, M. S., Yang, H., Wang, F. Q., Fatthallah, N. A., Li, X., Li, Y., & Huang, Y. (2019). *Journal of Coatings Technology and Research*, 1–16.

Shenashen, M. A., Akhtar, N., Selim, M. M., Morsy, W. M., Yamaguchi, H., Kawada, S., Alhamid, A. A., Ohashi, N., Ichinose, I., Alamoudi, A. S., & El-Safty, S. A. (2017). *Chemistry, an Asian Journal, 12*(15), 1952–1964.

Shenashen, M. A., Hassen, D., El-Safty, S. A., Akhtar, N., Chatterjee, A., & Elmarakbi, A. (2016). *Advanced Materials Interfaces, 3*(24), 1600743.

Silverman, H. G., & Roberto, F. F. (2007). Understanding marine mussel adhesion. *Marine Biotechnology, 9*, 661–681.

Soroldoni, S., Castro, Í. B., Abreu, F., Duarte, F. A., Choueri, R. B., Möller, O. O., Fillmann, G., & Pinho, G. L. L. (2018). *Water Research, 137*, 47–56.

Sullivan, T., & Regan, F. (2011). The characterization, replication and testing of dermal denticles of Scyliorhinus canicula for physical mechanisms of biofouling prevention. *Bioinspiration & Biomimetics, 6*046001.

Sun, K., Yang, H., Xue, W., He, A., Zhu, D. H., Liu, W. W., Adeyemi, K., & Cao, Y. (2018). Antibiofouling superhydrophobic surface fabricated by picosecond laser texturing of stainless steel. *Applied Surface Science, 436*, 263–267.

Tamayo, L., Azócar, M., Kogan, M., Riveros, A., & Páez, M. (2016). *Materials Science and Engineering C, 69*, 1391–1409.

Tian, G. Y., Zhang, M., Zhao, Y., Li, J. X., Wang, H. F., Zhang, X. Y., & Yan, H. (2019). High corrosion protection performance of a novel nonfluorinated biomimetic superhydrophobic ZnFe coating with Echinopsis multiplex-like structure. *ACS Applied Materials & Interfaces, 11*, 38205–38217.

Tian, S., Jiang, D., Pu, J., Sun, X., Li, Z., Wu, B., Zheng, W., Liu, W., & Liu, Z. (2019). *Chemical Engineering Journal, 370*, 1–9.

Umoren, S. A., & Solomon, M. M. (2019). *Progress in Materials Science, 104*, 380–450.

Van Hullebusch, E. D., Zandvoort, M. H., & Lens, P. N. L. (2003). *Reviews in Environmental Science and Bio/Technology, 2*(1), 9–33.

Wahl, M. (1989). *Marine Ecology Progress Series, 58*, 175.

Wan, F., Pei, X. W., Yu, B., Ye, Q., Zhou, F., & Xue, Q. J. (2012). Grafting polymer brushes on biomimetic structural surfaces for anti-algae fouling and foul release. *ACS Applied Materials & Interfaces, 4*, 4557–4565.

Wynne, K. J., Swain, G. W., Fox, R. B., Bullock, S., & Uilk, J. (2000). *Biofouling, 16*, 277–288.

Xie, Q. Y., Pan, J. S., Ma, C. F., & Zhang, G. Z. (2019). Dynamic surface antifouling: Mechanism and systems. *Soft Matter, 15*, 1087–1107.

Xue, C. H., Jia, S. T., Zhang, J., Tian, L. Q., Chen, H. Z., & Wang, M. (2008). *Science and Technology of Advanced Materials, 9*(3)035008.

Xue, L., Lu, X., Wei, H., Long, P., Xu, J., & Zheng, Y. (2014). *Journal of Colloid and Interface Science, 421*, 178–183.

Xue, Z., Wang, S., Lin, L., Chen, L., Liu, M., Feng, L., & Jiang, L. (2011). *Advanced Materials*, *23*, 4270.

Yebra, D. M., Kiil, S., & Dam-Johansen, K. (2004). *Progress in Organic Coatings*, *50*, 75–104.

Zhang, P., Lin, L., Zang, D., Guo, X., & Liu, M. (2017). *Small (Weinheim an der Bergstrasse, Germany)*, *13*1503334.

Zhao, L. M., Chen, R. R., Lou, L. J., Jing, X. Y., Liu, Q., Liu, J. Y., Yu, J., Liu, P. L., & Wang, J. (2020). Layer-by-layer-assembled antifouling films with surface microtopography inspired by *Laminaria japonica*. *Applied Surface Science*, *511*145564.

CHAPTER 6

Mimicking nature: advancements in self-cleaning coatings

Ruby Aslam, Qihui Wang, Chongkang Zhao, Qi Zhang and Zhitao Yan
School of Civil Engineering and Architecture, Chongqing University of Science and Technology, Chongqing, P.R. China

6.1 Introduction

Biomimetic coatings draw inspiration from the natural world, aiming to replicate self-cleaning mechanisms (Katiyar et al., 2021; Wang et al., 2020). One fascinating example is the lotus leaf's water-repellent surface structure, which has inspired scientists to create biomimetic coatings with similar properties (Yamamoto et al., 2015). Similarly, shark skin's texture, which reduces drag and prevents fouling, has served as a model for developing coatings with similar effects (Jo et al., 2021; Latthe et al., 2014). In a rapidly evolving world where innovation and sustainability intersect, the pursuit of intelligent, self-sustaining materials has gained significant momentum. These pioneering self-cleaning biomimetic coatings are at the forefront, marking a new era in surface engineering. Guided by nature's brilliance, they have the potential to revolutionize numerous industries, including architecture, automotive, and healthcare (Sharma et al., 2023/2023).

Self-cleaning biomimetic coatings have expanded beyond laboratories, finding practical use across various industries (Yang et al., 2020). In the realm of architecture, these coatings enhance building esthetics while repelling dirt and pollutants, safeguarding against corrosion. This dual function reduces maintenance needs and extends structural longevity, promoting sustainable urban design. In the automotive sector, these coatings transform vehicles into symbols of efficiency and convenience by minimizing dirt adhesion and protecting against environmental corrosion. This minimizes the need for frequent cleaning and maintenance, safeguarding automotive components. Additionally, these coatings have made their

Smart Biomimetic Coatings
DOI: https://doi.org/10.1016/B978-0-443-21738-8.00006-0

mark in textiles, preserving clothing. In healthcare, they offer superior hygiene and corrosion protection for medical instruments. Solar panels benefit from enhanced energy efficiency, with economic and environmental advantages (Qin & Lu, 2023; Sarkın et al., 2020). The marine industry sees reduced maintenance costs as boat hulls remain clean from fouling and corrosion (Chen et al., 2021/2021). Food packaging, consumer electronics, aerospace, and water treatment systems can all harness the extraordinary properties of self-cleaning biomimetic coatings, particularly their anticorrosion capabilities (Thuy et al., 2021).

This chapter embarks on a fascinating journey into the world of self-cleaning biomimetic coatings. The chapter will delve deep into the science behind them, explore their diverse applications, and consider the far-reaching implications of this remarkable technology. This chapter uncover the ingenious strategies inspired by nature, discover the innovative materials and processes propelling this field, and examine how these coatings are set to revolutionize the daily livesthis chapter will explore the self-cleaning biomimetic coatings, where the lines between science, engineering, and nature blur to create a cleaner, more efficient, and sustainable future.

6.2 Biomimetic coatings: an introduction

Growing interest has been shown in biomimetic structures that are simulated after numerous natural components, such as plant leaves, animal feathers, and insect cuticles (Chánová & Rypáček, 2013; Naik & Singamaneni, 2017). Among these, the superhydrophobicity of lotus leaves has received substantial research for producing surfaces with hierarchically organized dual-roughness structures that repel water and can also clean themselves. Lotus leaves have finely branched, hydrophobic epicuticular wax nanostructures covering the micropapillae (Kim et al., 2018). Additionally, antireflection coatings have been created to lessen surface reflection and capture incoming light as a result of the microstructure cornea of some nocturnal moths (Zhang et al., 2016). Hierarchical micro/nanostructures can produce surface characteristics that are multipurpose and combine self-cleaning and antireflection, making them appropriate for flat panel displays, automotive dashboards, and optical equipment (Zhang et al., n.d.).

Biomimetic coatings aim to mimic the unique properties of natural surfaces, including their texture, chemical composition, and surface energy. Scientists analyze natural surfaces to identify the features responsible for their self-cleaning properties. These features serve as a foundation for designing new materials with similar attributes. Biomimetic coatings can be crafted from various materials, such as polymers, ceramics, and metals. Fine-tuning their properties is achievable by adjusting the material's composition, structure, or processing conditions. These coatings find utility across diverse applications. These are discussed in the following sections.

6.2.1 Antifouling coatings for ships

Marine pollution results from the buildup of marine organisms like bacteria, microalgae, diatoms, and invertebrates on underwater structures, disrupting their proper functioning (Chambers et al., 2014; Selim et al., 2017). Biofilms are primarily responsible for this form of pollution in the marine environment (Chen et al., 2021). Biomimetic coatings offer a solution for crafting antifouling coatings on ships, effectively reducing drag, enhancing fuel efficiency, and thereby mitigating biological pollution. Extensive reports detail the application of biomimetic coatings to combat fouling in ships and various marine equipment (Chang et al., 2022; Lin et al., 2023; Wu et al., 2023/2023).

6.2.2 Antiicing coatings for aircraft

Biomimetic coatings can be used to create antiicing coatings for aircraft, which can reduce the risk of ice buildup on the wings and improve safety (Jiang et al., 2022/2022; Zeng et al., 2021/2021; Zhou et al., 2023).

6.2.3 Waterproof coatings for fabrics

Biomimetic coatings can be used to create waterproof coatings for fabrics, which can improve their durability and performance (Abbas et al., 2018; Hasan et al., n.d.).

6.2.4 Medical implants

Biomimetic coatings can be used to create medical implants that are more compatible with the body and less likely to be rejected (Bhaduri, 2017).

6.2.5 Environmental applications

Biomimetic coatings can be used in a variety of environmental applications, such as water treatment or air purification (Mittal, 2023). They can be used to create membranes for water filtration, which can improve the efficiency and effectiveness of the filtration process.

6.2.6 Solar panels

Biomimetic coatings can be used to create self-cleaning surfaces for solar panels, which can improve their efficiency and reduce maintenance costs (Omar 1 & Bakar, 2022; Qin & Lu, 2023).

6.2.7 Food packaging

Biomimetic coatings can be used to create food packaging that is more resistant to bacteria and other contaminants, which can improve food safety and reduce waste (Thuy et al., 2021; Ruzia et al., 2022).

6.2.8 Energy storage

Biomimetic coatings can be used to create materials for energy storage, such as batteries or supercapacitors (Biomimetic, 2022).

6.2.9 Sensors

Biomimetic coatings can be used to create sensors that are more sensitive and selective, which can improve their accuracy and reliability (Ye et al., 2022).

6.2.10 Robotics

Biomimetic coatings can be used to create materials for robotics that are more flexible, durable, or responsive to their environment (Antony et al., 2022; Dong et al., 2022).

6.3 Benefits of using biomimetic coatings for self-cleaning

A group of materials known as "self-cleaning surfaces" have the innate ability to eradicate any dirt or bacteria from their surfaces in a number of different ways. For many applications in society, such as solar energy (Strauss et al., 2015), antifogging (Shang & Zhou, 2016), self-healing (Chen et al., 2016), water–oil separation (Ge et al., 2014; Liu et al., 2012), water purification surfaces (Xu et al., 2015), and smart devices (Jeong et al., 2009; Lee et al., 2007; Lee et al., 2010), robust self-cleaning surfaces are highly wanted material systems.

6.4 Self-cleaning effect

Scientists are working extensively on developing adaptable self-cleaning surfaces, taking inspiration from nature. They frequently take cues from many natural wonders, like water striders, gecko feet, and lotus leaves. In the natural world, surfaces like butterfly wings, cabbage leaves, and Indian cress plants are excellent examples of superhydrophobic surfaces (Webb et al., 2014). The "lotus effect" and its extreme hydrophobicity are most clearly illustrated by the hydrophobic self-cleaning abilities of Nelumbo nucifera lotus plant leaves (Liu et al., 2015; Zhai et al., 2004). Other natural surfaces, such as rice leaves and insect wings, illustrated by butterflies, also display the coveted "lotus effect" (Bhushan & Jung, 2011). It is not just restricted to lotus leaves. These surfaces trap air holes within their micro/nanostructures to achieve superhydrophobicity. For example, rice leaves display anisotropic texturing with minimal contact angle hysteresis ($<< 10°$), characterized by microroughness along the leaf and a variety of micro- and nanosurface features. The core of rice leaves features waxy nano-bumps with longitudinal grooves and transverse sinusoidal structures, while their tips are adorned with eggbeater structures sporting four cohered hairs. Ridge terminations on these surfaces exhibit hydrophilic properties, promoting air retention underwater and bestowing superhydrophobicity (Gundersen et al., 2017). Similarly, butterfly wings derive their superhydrophobicity from micro- and nanostructured surfaces, with microgrooves creating a rough surface that minimizes adhesion. Self-cleaning properties on rice leaves and butterfly wings emerge from the combined influence of anisotropic flow directions along their orientations, vacancies, rigidity, and interfaces (Zheng et al., 2007). These natural superhydrophobic surfaces collectively serve as a wellspring of inspiration for developing self-cleaning surfaces and antifouling features, emulating the effectiveness of their natural counterparts (Bixler & Bhushan, 2012; Shenashen et al., 2017).

The phenomenon of self-cleaning is closely related to the surface contact angle, which forms at the interface between the solid surface, liquid, and vapor. Typically, a contact angle less than 90° indicates a hydrophilic surface, while angles exceeding 90° classify a surface as hydrophobic. Moreover, a surface with a water contact angle near zero is termed ultra (super)hydrophilic (Bhushan et al., 2010), whereas an angle exceeding 150° is typically categorized as ultra (super)hydrophobic (Jeevahan et al., 2018). These distinctions arise from the surfaces' low free energy and their micro-/nanobinary rough topography (Ma & Hill, 2006).

6.5 Types of self-cleaning coatings and their mechanism of action

Self-cleaning coatings fall into two primary categories: hydrophobic and hydrophilic. Hydrophobic coatings repel dust and dirt, causing particles to slide off or roll away from their surfaces. On the other hand, hydrophilic coatings utilize photocatalysis under U.V. radiation to reduce pollutants and dust on their surfaces. It is important to emphasize that the water contact angle is a crucial factor in achieving effective self-cleaning and robust antipollution measures (He, 2016).

Hydrophobic surfaces can be further classified into hydrophobic and superhydrophobic surfaces, primarily based on how droplets interact with them. Surface wettability plays a vital role in the development of efficient self-cleaning coatings. As mentioned earlier, the self-cleaning ability of a hydrophobic surface is demonstrated by how water droplets clean dust particles. In Fig. 6.1, you can see the differences in the sliding and rolling movements of droplets during the self-cleaning process (Chen et al., 2016). For example, on a superhydrophobic surface, spherical droplets remove dust and dirt by rolling, while on a hydrophobic surface, semi-spherical droplets eliminate contaminants through sliding motions.

In a study conducted by Parkin and Palgrave, it was noted that the rolling motion of droplets is more effective for surface cleaning compared to the sliding motion (Parkin & Palgrave, 2005). As a result, for a hydrophobic surface to achieve efficient self-cleaning, it should have a highly favorable static wettability contact angle and a minimal roll-off angle.

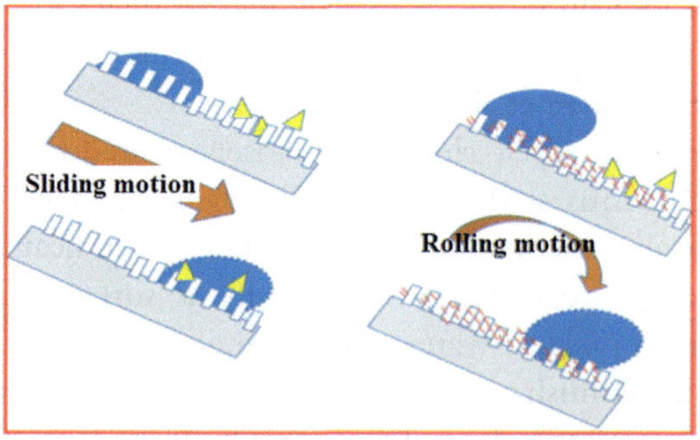

Figure 6.1 ***The sliding and rolling motion of droplets during the self-cleaning process (Chen et al., 2016).***

Johnson et al. played a pivotal role in advancing superhydrophobic surfaces on real glass surfaces. They accomplished this by combining theoretical wettability models, including the Young model, the Wenzel model, and the Cassie–Baxter state, with insights from the natural structure of the lotus plant (Johnson & Dettre, 1964). They proposed a direct connection between the drop's energy, the vibrational energy of the drops, and the height of the energy barrier. When the drop's periphery encounters constriction during motion, it requires less energy to overcome the height barrier. This constriction of the drop's periphery is influenced by the advancing angle curve (θ_A) and receding angle curve (θ_R), which dictate the dynamic movement of drops on the energy barrier. The hysteresis contact angle (θ_H) describes the dynamic motion of a liquid droplet at the triple-interface contact line and is defined as the difference between θ_A and θ_R, as expressed in the following (Wang et al., 2020):

$$\theta_H = \theta_A - \theta_R$$

θ_A corresponds to the liquid's expansion, while θ_R indicates the liquid's contraction. The micro and nanotextures on hydrophobic surfaces impede the liquid's expansion, significantly increasing the contact angle of the liquid droplet. This results in liquid droplets on superhydrophobic surfaces rolling off more quickly. In contrast, hydrophilic surfaces inhibit the liquid's contraction, leading to a reduction in the contact angle of the liquid droplet. Additionally, it is crucial to develop self-cleaning coatings with low van Der Waals forces, which reduce adhesion to dust. This enables dust to be expelled through external forces, not solely relying on water droplets.

The self-cleaning mechanism of superhydrophilic coatings can be activated with or without UV light. Photocatalysts like TiO_2 or other semiconductor materials establish a photocatalytic mechanism on the superhydrophilic surface, reducing dirt particles upon exposure to sufficient UV light. In Fig. 6.2, the photocatalysis process in action for the self-cleaning mechanism has been shown (Chen & Poon, 2009).

Superhydrophilic coatings achieve the spreading of water droplets into a thin film of water, primarily due to the presence of polar functional groups found in superhydrophilic polymers, which include hydroxyl, carboxyl, and carbonyl chains. These polar functional groups have a strong affinity for water, leading to complete wetting of the solid surface, resulting in a water contact angle typically ranging from 0 to 20 degrees (Chen et al., 2016). In the process of photocatalysis, water droplets generate

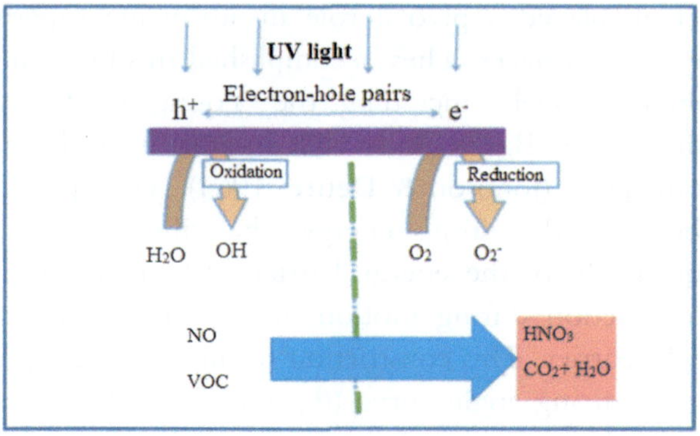

Figure 6.2 ***Photocatalysis process for a self-cleaning mechanism (Chen et al., 2016).***

OH^- anions, which subsequently oxidize into OH radicals. Concurrently, O_2 species transform into $O_2^{\bullet-}$ radicals. These electron–hole radicals play a crucial role in photocatalytic oxidation, effectively reducing organic contaminants and micropollutants. Although titanium dioxide is a common choice for photocatalyst materials, it has a relatively high band gap energy, approximately 3.2 eV, which limits its absorption to only UV radiation. To extend its responsiveness to visible light, various impurities such as polyaniline, nitrogen, iron, tungsten, and silicon dioxide have been introduced as dopants into titanium dioxide materials.

6.6 Self-cleaning applications of biomimetic coatings: a literature review

The first self-cleaning coating was introduced by Paz et al. (1995) specifically designed for windows and windshield applications. Utilizing TNB/FAS nanobelts, Lai et al. (2012) employed a one-step electrophoretic deposition process to create a cross-aligned superhydrophobic film. This film exhibited high transparency of 80% on an indium tin oxide (ITO)-coated glass substrate. By precisely controlling the deposition time, they demonstrated the ability to shift between a "sticky" hydrophobic state (characterized by a high contact angle and strong adhesion) and a "sliding" superhydrophobic state (marked by a high contact angle with weak adhesion). Notably, this coating showcased remarkable chemical stability across a broad range of pH solutions and effectively exhibited self-cleaning properties.

In another notable advancement, Park et al. (2013) engineered large-scale multifunctional transparent ITO nanorod films with extreme wetting states, either superhydrophobic or superhydrophilic. These films exhibited high transmittance, low resistivity for antistatic properties, and resistance to fogging. The achievement of these properties was made possible through the process of radio frequency (RF)-magnetron sputtering deposition. When the ITO nanorod film was prepared at 500°C for 60 minutes and coated with fluoroalkylsilane, it exhibited exceptional transparency (averaging 85% transmittance at 500 nm) and maintained stable superhydrophobic characteristics (a high-water contact angle of 172.11, an almost zero sliding angle, and self-cleaning capabilities). Consequently, the large-scale multifunctional transparent ITO nanorod films presented in this study are poised to expand the possibilities in the field of novel optoelectrical applications.

Furthermore, Park et al. (2014) developed photoanodes with antifogging and antireflection properties by applying a coating of hydrophilic SiO_2 nanoparticles. Yang et al. (2012) created a porous surface utilizing a PDDA-PFO/SiO_2 coating, permitting water to pass through while causing oil to remain on the surface, making it oil-repellent. Chen et al. (2016) investigated a novel slippery surface mechanism by analyzing the peristome surface of *Nepenthes alata*, which holds promise for potential applications in developing artificial fluid transport systems. The effect of SiO_2-TiO_2-PDMS coating on superhydrophobicity and self-cleaning performance of building walls was investigated by various characterization methods (Li et al., 2022). Fig. 6.3 shows the results for the surface of coated and uncoated walls contaminated with Fe_2O_3. It can be found in Fig. 6.3A that the surface of the uncoated wall was easily adhered by Fe_2O_3 powder, and the contaminants were difficult to be washed away by water. In contrast, Fig. 6.3B shows that the coated walls could be easily cleaned out with deionized water even if particulate contaminants were adhered to the surface.

Lee and Fearing (2008) introduced the initial gecko-inspired dry self-cleaning adhesive, employing a high-aspect-ratio fibrillar polypropylene (PP) array. The fabricated fibrillar adhesive displayed a 33% recovery of shear adhesion on clean samples after 30 simulated steps on a dry, clean, and rigid surface. Subsequently, Gillies et al. (Gillies et al., 2013) designed a dry self-cleaning fibrillar structure comprising both hard and soft PP. They observed that hard fibers could recover 96%−115% of shear adhesion even after fouling with small and large particles, with some even

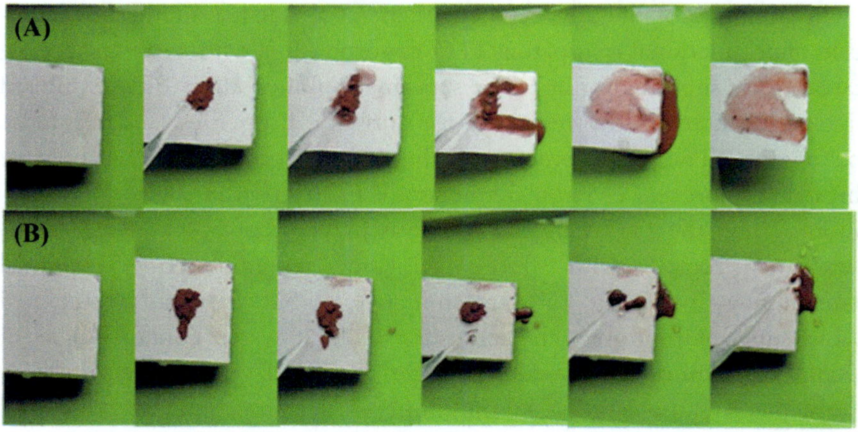

Figure 6.3 ***Optical images of particulate contaminants on the surface of building wall samples before and after spraying. (A) Particle pollutants contaminate the uncoated wall surface and (B) particle pollutants contaminate the coating with* n *(PDMS):*n *(TEOS) = 1: 5 (Xia et al., 2023)*** *. From Xia, X., Liu, J., Liu, Y., Lei, Z., Han, Y., Zheng, Z., & Yin, J. (2023). Preparation and characterization of biomimetic SiO_2-TiO_2-PDMS composite hydrophobic coating with self-cleaning properties for wall protection applications.* Coatings, 13*(2), 224. https://doi.org/10.3390/coatings13020224.*

performing better than before fouling. However, soft fibers exhibited only a 55% recovery when fouled with large particles because these particles had a tendency to embed themselves within the soft polymers, impeding further self-cleaning. Furthermore, Mengüç et al. (2014) created vertically aligned elastomer microfibers and evaluated the self-cleaning properties of this biomimetic material postcontamination. They noted that, during a load-drag-unload dry contacting self-cleaning process, large particles tended to roll off during the drag phase. If particles were smaller than the adjacent fiber distances, they might become embedded between the fibers. However, when particles were much smaller than the fibers, they could stay on the surfaces of the fibers, making removal more challenging.

A superhydrophobic self-cleaning coating was developed for brass surfaces through a multistep process involving electrochemical etching, brushing with a PDMS layer, and the deposition of carbon soot particles (Li et al., 2022). Fig. 6.4 provides a schematic representation of the entire preparation process for these superhydrophobic coating samples. The coatings' self-cleaning effectiveness was assessed using chalk dust particles to simulate solid contaminants and a variety of liquids, such as grape juice,

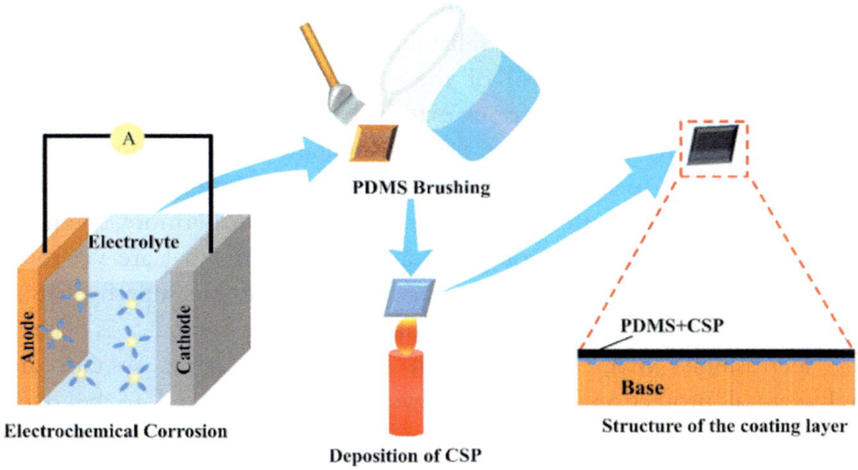

Figure 6.4 ***Schematic diagram of the preparation process of superhydrophobic coatings samples (Li et al., 2022).***
From Li, F., Liu, Y., Zhou, H., & Tian, G. (2022). Preparation and evaluation of PDMS/carbon soot particles superhydrophobic biomimetic composite coating with self-cleaning and durability. Biomimetics, *7(3). https://doi.org/10.3390/biomimetics7030132.*

beer, cola, and blue ink, to mimic liquid contaminants. Remarkably, the coating maintained its superhydrophobic properties even after undergoing physical and chemical damage tests.

In a separate study, a ZnO electrosprayed coating with antibacterial and self-cleaning attributes was documented (Valenzuela et al., 2019/2019). ZnO-functionalized materials displayed an even external surface composed of microspheres with diameters falling within the range of 100–300 nanometers. These ZnO coatings also exhibited the ability to prevent bacterial colonization and biofilm formation on surfaces.

6.7 Future developments and outlook

This chapter provides a concise overview of the current landscape of self-cleaning materials and delves into a detailed analysis of the mechanisms underlying their self-cleaning properties. The latter part of this review explores the extensive range of potential applications for these fascinating materials. The future trajectory of self-cleaning surfaces is expected to involve the integration of various cutting-edge functionalities such as antireflection, water repellency, self-healing, antifogging, micromanipulation, and antistickiness. On the engineering front, advancements in the fabrication process are poised to enhance the cost-effectiveness, flexibility, sustainability, durability, and reliability of these intelligent surfaces. Looking forward, the control of these smart surfaces will be achieved through the application of various external stimuli, including mechanical, thermal, electrical, and magnetic fields. Simultaneously, ongoing research will explore ways to introduce additional novel and intriguing properties into self-cleaning structures to expand their utility. Furthermore, the natural world offers a multitude of multifunctional systems that are yet to be discovered. Moreover, the demand for superhydrophobic/superhydrophilic and self-cleaning surfaces with enhanced corrosion resistance is becoming increasingly vital, particularly in premium transport systems and architectural protection. However, several challenges need to be overcome before these technologies can be effectively applied on a commercial scale. Many of the techniques reported thus far are not yet ready for large-scale production in real-world applications. The primary hurdles include the complex nature of micro/nanostructured hierarchical designs and the costs associated with acquiring low surface energy materials necessary for surface modification.

Another critical concern pertains to the long-term durability of these surfaces under real-world service conditions, which is a significant aspect that requires thorough consideration for widespread adoption. Therefore a deeper understanding of the mechanisms at play in natural systems is essential for the replication of these properties in the next generation of multifunctional self-cleaning surfaces. Consequently, a sustained and rigorous study of diverse biological surfaces found in nature and the development of futuristic multifunctional surfaces with unprecedented properties are on the horizon.

Acknowledgments

This work is fully supported by the National Natural Science Foundation of China (Grant No. 52178458); National Science Foundation of Chongqing Science and Technology Commission (Grant No. CSTB2022NSCQ-MSX0363 and CSTB2023NSCQ-LZX0051).

References

Abbas, Mudassar, Iftikhar, Hina, Malik, Mumtaz, & Nazir, Ahsan (2018). Surface coatings of TiO_2 nanoparticles onto the designed fabrics for enhanced self-cleaning properties. *Coatings*, *8*(1). Available from https://doi.org/10.3390/coatings8010035.

Antony, Sherin, Anju, T. R., & Thomas, Bejoy (2022). *Nature-inspired biomimetic polymeric materials and their applications* (pp. 1–31). Springer Science and Business Media LLC. Available from 10.1007/978-981-16-6603-2_50-1.

Bhaduri, Sarit B. (2017). Biomimetic coating technology for orthopedic implants. *Current Opinion in Chemical Engineering*, *3*, 49–55.

Bhushan, B., & Jung, Y. C. (2011). Natural and biomimetic artificial surfaces for superhydrophobicity, self-cleaning, low adhesion, and drag reduction. *Progress in Materials Science*, *56*(1), 1–108. Available from https://doi.org/10.1016/j.pmatsci.2010.040.003, https://www.journals.elsevier.com/progress-in-materials-science.

Bhushan, Bharat, Jung, Yong Chae, & Nosonovsky, Michael (2010). *Lotus effect: Surfaces with roughness-induced superhydrophobicity, self-cleaning, and low adhesion* (pp. 1437–1524). Springer Nature. Available from 10.1007/978-3-642-02525-9_42.

Biomimetic. (2022). Polymer-based composite coating inhibits zinc dendrite growth for high-performance zinc-ion batteries. *ACS Applied Materials & Interfaces*, 10384–10393.

Bixler, G. D., & Bhushan, B. (2012). Bioinspired rice leaf and butterfly wing surface structures combining shark skin and lotus effects. *Soft Matter*, *8*(44), 11271–11284. Available from https://doi.org/10.1039/c2sm26655e.

Chambers, L. D., Wharton, J. A., Wood, R. J. K., Walsh, F. C., & Stokes, K. R. (2014). Techniques for the measurement of natural product incorporation into an antifouling coating. *Progress in Organic Coatings*, 77(2), 473–484. Available from https://doi.org/10.1016/j.porgcoat.2013.110.013.

Chang, Xueting, Li, Mingyu, Tang, Sikai, Shi, Liang, Chen, Xiaoqiu, Niu, Shicong, Zhu, Xiaojie, Wang, Dongsheng, & Sun, Shibin (2022). Superhydrophobic micro-nano structured PTFE/WO_3 coating on low-temperature steel with outstanding anti-pollution, anti-icing, and anti-fouling performance. *Surface and Coatings Technology*, *434*. Available from https://doi.org/10.1016/j.surfcoat.2022.128214.

Chen, Huawei, Zhang, Pengfei, Zhang, Liwen, Liu, Hongliang, Jiang, Ying, Zhang, Deyuan, Han, Zhiwu, & Jiang, Lei (2016). Continuous directional water transport on the peristome surface of *Nepenthes alata. Nature*, *532*(7597), 85–89. Available from https://doi.org/10.1038/nature17189.

Chen, J., & Poon, Cs (2009). Photocatalytic construction and building materials: From fundamentals to applications. *Building and Environment*, *44*(9), 1899–1906. Available from https://doi.org/10.1016/j.buildenv.2009.010.002.

Chen, Kunlin, Wu, Yi, Zhou, Shuxue, & Wu, Limin (2016). Recent development of durable and self-healing surfaces with special wettability. *Macromolecular Rapid Communications*, *37*(6), 463–485. Available from https://doi.org/10.1002/marc.201500591.

Chen, Liren, Duan, Yanyi, Cui, Mei, Huang, Renliang, Su, Rongxin, Qi, Wei, & He, Zhimin (2021). The total environment biomimetic surface coatings for marine antifouling: Natural antifoulants, synthetic polymers and surface microtopography. *Science of the Total Environment*, *766*.

Chánová, E. M., & Rypáček, F. (2013). *Biomimetic coatings for biomaterial surfaces. Biomimetic biomaterials: Structure and applications* (pp. 91–126). Czech Republic: Elsevier Ltd. Available from. Available from http://www.sciencedirect.com/science/book/9780857094162, 10.1533/9780857098887.1.91.

Dong, Xiaoxiao, Luo, Xiaohang, Zhao, Hong, Qiao, Chenyu, Li, Jiapeng, Yi, Jianhong, Yang, Li, Oropeza, Francisco J., Hu, Travis Shihao, Xu, Quan, & Zeng, Hongbo (2022). Recent advances in biomimetic soft robotics: fabrication approaches, driven strategies and applications. *Soft Matter*, *18*(40), 7699–7734. Available from https://doi.org/10.1039/d2sm01067d.

Ge, Jin, Ye, Yin-Dong, Yao, Hong-Bin, Zhu, Xi, Wang, Xu, Wu, Liang, Wang, Jin-Long, Ding, Hang, Yong, Ni, He, Ling-Hui, & Yu, Shu-Hong (2014). Pumping through porous hydrophobic/oleophilic materials: An alternative technology for oil spill remediation. *Angewandte Chemie International Edition, 53*(14), 3612–3616. Available from https://doi.org/10.1002/anie.201310151.

Gillies, A. G., Puthoff, J., Cohen, M. J., Autumn, K., & Fearing, R. S. (2013). Dry self-cleaning properties of hard and soft fibrillar structures. *ACS Applied Materials and Interfaces, 5*(13), 6081–6088. Available from https://doi.org/10.1021/am400839n.

Gundersen, H., Leinaas, H. P., & Thaulow, C. (2017). Collembola cuticles and the three-phase line tension. *Journal of Nanotechnology, 8*(1), 1714–1722. Available from https://doi.org/10.3762/bjnano.80.172, http://www.beilstein-journals.org/bjnano/content/pdf/2190-4286-8-172.pdf.

Ruzia, M., Celik, N., & Onses, M.S. (2022). Superhydrophobic coatings for food packaging applications: A review. Food Packaging and Shelf Life, 32 (2022), 100823.

Hasan, Z., Rahaman, M.D., & Islam, J.M. M. (n.d.). Self-cleaning textiles: Structure, fabrication and applications. In: Fundamentals of natural fibres and textiles. A volume in the textile institute book series book 2021.

He, J. (2016). Self-cleaning coatings: Structure, fabrication and application. *Royal Society of Chemistry*.

Jeevahan, Jeya, Chandrasekaran, M., Britto Joseph, G., Durairaj, R. B., & Mageshwaran, G. (2018). Superhydrophobic surfaces: A review on fundamentals, applications, and challenges. *Journal of Coatings Technology and Research, 15*(2), 231–250. Available from https://doi.org/10.1007/s11998-017-0011-x.

Jeong, H. E., Lee, J. K., Kim, H. N., Moon, S. H., & Suh, K. Y. (2009). A nontransferring dry adhesive with hierarchical polymer nanohairs. *Proceedings of the National Academy of Sciences of the United States of America, 106*(14), 5639–5644. Available from https://doi.org/10.1073/pnas.0900323106SouthKorea, http://www.pnas.org/content/106/14/5639.full.pdf.

Jiang, Shanshan, Diao, Yunhe, & Yang, Huige (2022). Historical perspective recent advances of bio-inspired anti-icing surfaces. *Advances in Colloid and Interface Science, 308*.

Jo, W., Kang, H. S., Choi, J., Jung, J., Hyun, J., Kwon, J., Kim, I., Lee, H., & Kim, H. T. (2021). Light-designed shark skin-mimetic surfaces. *Nano Letters, 21*(13), 5500–5507. Available from https://doi.org/10.1021/acs.nanolett.1c00436, http://pubs.acs.org/journal/nalefd.

Johnson, R. E., & Dettre, R. H. (1964). Contact angle hysteresis. III. Study of an idealized heterogeneous surface. *Journal of Physical Chemistry, 68*(7), 1744–1750. Available from https://doi.org/10.1021/j100789a012.

Katiyar, N. K., Goel, G., Hawi, S., & Goel, S. (2021). Nature-inspired materials: Emerging trends and prospects. *NPG Asia Materials, 13*(1). Available from https://doi.org/10.1038/s41427-021-00322-y, http://www.nature.com/am/index.html.

Kim, Woochan, Kim, Daun, Park, Sunho, Lee, Dohyeon, Hyun, Hoon, & Kim, Jangho (2018). Engineering lotus leaf-inspired micro- and nanostructures for the manipulation of functional engineering platforms. *Journal of Industrial and Engineering Chemistry, 61*, 39–52. Available from https://doi.org/10.1016/j.jiec.2017.110.045.

Lai, Yuekun, Tang, Yuxin, Gong, Jiaojiao, Gong, Dangguo, Chi, Lifeng, Lin, Changjian, & Chen, Zhong (2012). Transparent superhydrophobic/superhydrophilic TiO_2-based coatings for self-cleaning and anti-fogging. *Journal of Materials Chemistry, 22*(15). Available from https://doi.org/10.1039/c2jm16298a.

Latthe, Sanjay, Terashima, Chiaki, Nakata, Kazuya, & Fujishima, Akira (2014). Superhydrophobic surfaces developed by mimicking hierarchical surface morphology of lotus leaf. *Molecules (Basel, Switzerland), 19*(4), 4256–4283. Available from https://doi.org/10.3390/molecules19044256.

Lee, H., Lee, B. P., & Messersmith, P. B. (2007). A reversible wet/dry adhesive inspired by mussels and geckos. *Nature, 448*(7151), 338–341. Available from https://doi.org/10.1038/nature05968, http://www.nature.com/nature/index.html.

Lee, J., & Fearing, R. S. (2008). Contact self-cleaning of synthetic gecko adhesive from polymer microfibers. *Langmuir: The ACS Journal of Surfaces and Colloids, 24*(19), 10587–10591. Available from https://doi.org/10.1021/la8021485.

Lee, S. G., Lee, D. Y., Lim, H. S., Lee, D. H., Lee, S., & Cho, K. (2010). Switchable transparency and wetting of elastomeric smart windows. *Advanced Materials, 22*(44), 5013–5017. Available from https://doi.org/10.1002/adma.201002320.

Li, Fengqin, Liu, Yong, Zhou, Honggen, & Tian, Guizhong (2022). Preparation and evaluation of PDMS/carbon soot particles superhydrophobic biomimetic composite coating with self-cleaning and durability. *Biomimetics*, 7(3). Available from https://doi.org/10.3390/biomimetics7030132.

Lin, Shujie, Bi, Huichao, Weinell, Claus Erik, Azizaddini, Seyednezamaddin, & Dam-Johansen, Kim (2023). Systematic cleaning and evaluation of exposed fouling control coating systems using a novel laboratory scale automated underwater cleaning system. *Progress in Organic Coatings, 182.* Available from https://doi.org/10.1016/j.porgcoat.2023.107712.

Liu, Mingjie, Xue, Zhongxin, Liu, Huan, & Jiang, Lei (2012). Surface wetting in liquid-liquid-solid triphase systems: Solid-phase-independent transition at the liquid-liquid interface by lewis acid-base interactions. *Angewandte Chemie International Edition, 51*(33), 8348–8351. Available from https://doi.org/10.1002/anie.201202293.

Liu, Y., Li, S., Zhang, J., Liu, J., Han, Z., & Ren, L. (2015). Corrosion inhibition of biomimetic super-hydrophobic electrodeposition coatings on copper substrate. *Corrosion Science, 94*, 190–196. Available from https://doi.org/10.1016/j.corsci.2015.020.009, https://www.journals.elsevier.com/corrosion-science.

Ma, Minglin, & Hill, Randal M. (2006). Superhydrophobic surfaces. *Current Opinion in Colloid & Interface Science, 11*(4), 193–202. Available from https://doi.org/10.1016/j.cocis.2006.060.002.

Mengüç, Y., Rohrig, M., Abusomwan, U., Holscher, H., & Sitti. (2014). Staying sticky: Contact self-cleaning of gecko-inspired adhesives. *Journal of the Royal Society, Interface/the Royal Society, 11.*

Mittal, Tanu (2023). Self-cleaning smart photocatalytic coatings for water treatment. *Materials Today: Proceedings, 78*, 891–894. Available from https://doi.org/10.1016/j.matpr.2022.120.094.

Naik, Rajesh R., & Singamaneni, Srikanth (2017). Introduction: Bioinspired and biomimetic materials. *Chemical Reviews, 117*(20), 12581–12583. Available from https://doi.org/10.1021/acs.chemrev.7b00552.

Omar 1, Azimah, & Bakar, Ab. Halim Abu (2022). Application of transparent self-cleaning coating for photovoltaic panel: A review. *Current Opinion in Chemical Engineering, 2.*

Park, H. K., Yoon, S. W., Chung, W. W., Min, B. K., & Do, Y. R. (2013). *Journal of Materials Chemistry A, 1.*

Park, J. T., Kim, J. H., & Lee, D. (2014). Excellent anti-fogging dye-sensitized solar cells based on superhydrophilic nanoparticle coatings. *Nanoscale, 6*(13), 7362–7368. Available from https://doi.org/10.1039/c4nr00919c, http://www.rsc.org/publishing/journals/NR/Index.asp.

Parkin, I. P., & Palgrave, R. G. (2005). Self-cleaning coatings. *Journal of Materials Chemistry, 15*(17), 1689–1695. Available from https://doi.org/10.1039/b412803f.

Paz, Y., Luo, Z., Rabenberg, L., & Heller, A. (1995). Photooxidative self-cleaning transparent titanium dioxide films on glass. *Journal of Materials Research, 10*(11), 2842–2848. Available from https://doi.org/10.1557/jmr.1995.2842.

Qin, Jing, & Lu, Hao (2023). A review of self-cleaning coatings for solar photovoltaic systems: Theory, materials, preparation, and applications. *Environmental Science and Pollution Research*, *30*(40), 91591–91616. Available from https://doi.org/10.1007/s11356-023-28550-5.

Sarkın, Ali Samet, Ekren, Nazmi, & Sağlam, Şafak (2020). A review of anti-reflection and self-cleaning coatings on photovoltaic panels. *Solar Energy*, *199*, 63–73. Available from https://doi.org/10.1016/j.solener.2020.010.084.

Selim, M. S., Shenashen, M. A., El-Safty, S. A., Higazy, S. A., Selim, M. M., Isago, H., & Elmarakbi, A. (2017). Recent progress in marine foul-release polymeric nanocomposite coatings. *Progress in Materials Science*, *87*, 1–32. Available from https://doi.org/10.1016/j.pmatsci.2017.020.001.

Shang, Qianqian, & Zhou, Yonghong (2016). Fabrication of transparent superhydrophobic porous silica coating for self-cleaning and anti-fogging. *Ceramics International*, *42*(7), 8706–8712. Available from https://doi.org/10.1016/j.ceramint.2016.020.105.

Sharma, T., Sultan, M.T. B.H., Shahar, F.S., èukaszewicz, A., Józwik, J., Md, A.U., Shah, R.G., & Grzejda, R. (2023). *From nature to the skies: Exploring bio-inspired polymer coatings for aerospace advancements*.

Shenashen, M. A., Hassen, D., El-Safty, S. A., Isago, H., Elmarakbi, A., & Yamaguchi, H. (2017). Axially oriented tubercle vein and X-crossed sheet of N-Co_3O_4@C hierarchical mesoarchitectures as potential heterogeneous catalysts for methanol oxidation reaction. *Chemical Engineering Journal*, *313*, 83–98. Available from https://doi.org/10.1016/j.cej.2016.120.003, http://www.elsevier.com/inca/publications/store/6/0/1/2/7/3/index.htt.

Strauss, J. A., Soave, P. A., Ribeiro, R. S., & Horowitz, F. (2015). Absorber and self-cleaning surfaces on modified polymer plates for solar harvesting in the humid (sub) tropics. *Solar Energy*, *122*, 579–586. Available from https://doi.org/10.1016/j.solener.2015.090.020.

Thuy, Vu. Thi Tuyet, Hao, Lam Tan, Jeon, Hyeonyeol, Koo, Jun Mo, Park, Jaeduk, Lee, Eun Seong, Hwang, Sung Yeon, Choi, Sejin, Park, Jeyoung, & Oh, Dongyeop X. (2021). Sustainable, self-cleaning, transparent, and moisture/oxygen-barrier coating films for food packaging. *Green Chemistry*, *23*(7), 2658–2667. Available from https://doi.org/10.1039/d0gc03647a.

Valenzuela, L., Iglesias, A., Faraldos, M., & Bahamonde, A. (2019). Antimicrobial surfaces with selfcleaning properties functionalized by photocatalytic ZnO electrosprayed coatings. *Journal of Hazardous Materials*, *369*.

Wang, Y., Naleway, S. E., & Wang, B. (2020). Biological and bioinspired materials: Structure leading to functional and mechanical performance. *Bioactive Materials*, *5*(4), 745–757. Available from https://doi.org/10.1016/j.bioactmat.2020.060.003, http://www.keaipublishing.com/en/journals/bioactive-materials/.

Webb, H. K., Crawford, R. J., & Ivanova, E. P. (2014). Wettability of natural superhydrophobic surfaces. *Advances in Colloid and Interface Science*, *210*, 58–64. Available from https://doi.org/10.1016/j.cis.2014.010.020.

Wu, Xiao, Yang, Chao, Wu, Lingli, Zhang, Chuchu, Cui, Gan, & Xin, Yanping (2023). Self-repairing and anti-fouling performance of anticorrosive coating in marine environment. *Polymer Testing*, *124*.

Xia, Xiaojing, Liu, Jue, Liu, Yang, Lei, Zijie, Han, Yutong, Zheng, Zeping, & Yin, Jian (2023). Preparation and characterization of biomimetic SiO_2-TiO_2-PDMS composite hydrophobic coating with self-cleaning properties for wall protection applications. *Coatings*, *13*(2). Available from https://doi.org/10.3390/coatings13020224.

Xu, Q., Xu, H., Chen, J., Lv, Y., Dong, C., & Sreeprasad, T. S. (2015). Graphene and graphene oxide: Advanced membranes for gas separation and water purification.

Inorganic Chemistry Frontiers, *2*(5), 417–424. Available from https://doi.org/10.1039/c4qi00230j, http://pubs.rsc.org/en/journals/journal/qi.

Yamamoto, M., Nishikawa, N., Mayama, H., Nonomura, Y., Yokojima, S., Nakamura, S., & Uchida, K. (2015). Theoretical explanation of the lotus effect: Superhydrophobic property changes by removal of nanostructures from the surface of a lotus leaf. *Langmuir: the ACS Journal of Surfaces and Colloids*, *31*(26), 7355–7363. Available from https://doi.org/10.1021/acs.langmuir.5b00670, http://pubs.acs.org/journal/langd5.

Yang, J., Zhang, Z., Xu, X., Zhu, X., Men, X., & Zhou, X. (2012). Superhydrophilic-superoleophobic coatings. *Journal of Materials Chemistry*, *22*(7), 2834–2837. Available from https://doi.org/10.1039/c2jm15987b.

Yang, Yushan, Shen, Huajie, & Qiu, Jian (2020). Fabrication of biomimetic robust self-cleaning superhydrophobic wood with canna-leaf-like micro/nanostructure through morph-genetic method improved water-, UV-, and corrosion resistance properties. *Journal of Molecular Structure*, *1219*. Available from https://doi.org/10.1016/j.molstruc.2020.128616.

Ye, X., Li, Y., Zhang, Y., & Wang, P. (2022). A comprehensive review: Recent developments of biomimetic sensors. *Journal of Bionic Engineering*, *19*(4), 853–876. Available from https://doi.org/10.1007/s42235-022-00181-5, https://rd.springer.com/journal/42235.

Zeng, Dan, Li, Yong, Huan, Dajun, Liu, Hongquan, Luo, Hongyun, Cui, Yingxue, Zhu, Chunling, & Wang, Jingxin (2021). Physicochemical and Engineering Aspects Robust epoxy-modified superhydrophobic coating for aircraft anti-icing systems. *Colloids and Surfaces A*, *628*.

Zhai, L., Cebeci, F. C., Cohen, R. E., & Rubner, M. F. (2004). Stable superhydrophobic coatings from polyelectrolyte multilayers. *Nano Letters*, *4*(7), 1349–1353. Available from https://doi.org/10.1021/nl049463j.

Zhang, L., Uzoma, P.C., Xiaoyang, C., Penkov, O.V., & Hu,H. (n.d.). Bio-inspired hierarchical micro/nanostructured surfaces for superhydrophobic and anti-ice applications. *Frontiers in Bioengineering and Biotechnology*, *10*.

Zhang, Mingqian, Feng, Shile, Wang, Lei, & Zheng, Yongmei (2016). Lotus effect in wetting and self-cleaning. *Biotribology*, *5*, 31–43. Available from https://doi.org/10.1016/j.biotri.2015.080.002.

Zheng, Y., Gao, X., & Jiang, L. (2007). Directional adhesion of superhydrophobic butterfly wings. *Soft Matter*, *3*(2), 178–182. Available from https://doi.org/10.1039/b612667g.

Zhou, Haonan, Xu, Qingmeng, Zhao, Jing, Luo, Hongjie, Huang, Xiao, & Huang, Jizhong (2023). Biomimetic super slippery surface with excellent and durable anti-icing property for immovable heritage conservation. *Progress in Organic Coatings*, *184*. Available from https://doi.org/10.1016/j.porgcoat.2023.107818.

CHAPTER 7

Biomimetic coatings for bone regeneration

Jeenat Aslam[1] and Hilal Ahmad Parray[2]
[1]Department of Chemistry, College of Science, Taibah University, Yanbu, Al-Madina, Saudi Arabia
[2]Department of Pathology, University of Texas, Dallas, TX, United States

7.1 Introduction

Bone tissue engineering (BTE) is an important field in craniofacial and orthopedic surgery (Antoniac, Paltanea et al., 2022; Cavalu, Antoniac, et al., 2020; Iulian et al., 2018). Biomimetic scaffolds are essential for repairing flaws brought on by osteoporosis, osteoarthritis, Paget's disease, and osteogenesis imperfecta as well as defects brought on by prosthetic implants (Cavalu, Antoniac, et al., 2020; Cavalu, Fritea, et al., 2020). Inflammation, regeneration, and remodeling are all part of the complex process of bone rebuilding, and they are all controlled by different biological and physical processes. Mesenchymal stem cells normally differentiate into osteoblasts, and hematopoietic stem cells are directly linked to the creation of osteoclasts. Stem cells, in conjunction with growth hormones or cytokines, are essential to this process (Fierro et al., 2017). Smaller bone defects tend to heal on their own, while bigger lesions frequently need additional treatments (Antoniac, Miculescu et al., 2022; Quan et al., 2022). Based on the magnitude of the defect and the loss of cortical circumference, Schemitsch (2017) created a classification scheme for bone defects. When extracted through invasive methods, autografts or allografts carry a risk of infection, disease transfer, and possible graft rejection (Savin et al., 2017; Xue et al., 2022). Typically, autologous vascularized fibular graft, allograft, and iliac crest bone are used. Another strategy is to use bone transport fixators; however, these have been connected to longer healing durations and more discomfort. Although donor site morbidity effects and restricted supply provide obstacles, autografts are still regarded as the gold standard in orthopedics (Fernandez-Yague et al., 2015). Allografts raise issues with graft vascularization and immunogenic reactions, and grafting methods are costly. Treatment problems for bone abnormalities are expected due to the growing demand for grafts worldwide (Bud et al., 1908; Manjua et al., 2021; Romanec et al., 2018).

Smart Biomimetic Coatings
DOI: https://doi.org/10.1016/B978-0-443-21738-8.00007-2

Bone regeneration is an intricate and dynamic process important for upholding the structural integrity and function of the skeletal system (Ansari, 2019). A fine balance between bone formation and resorption is required for this process, which is regulated by a number of signaling pathways, growth factors, and cellular interactions. Bone abnormalities, which cause pain, disability, and a reduced quality of life, can arise from the disruption of this balance, which can be caused by trauma, disease, or aging (Pajarinen et al., 2019). By mimicking the natural milieu of bone tissue, biomimetic coatings have become a viable tactic to promote bone regeneration in recent years. These coatings are specialized surfaces or materials that mimic the extracellular matrix (ECM) naturally found in bone tissue and are intended for use in bone regeneration (Wang et al., 2017). Moreover, coatings improve cell adhesion, proliferation, and differentiation by imitating the structural and compositional characteristics of the ECM, which facilitates efficient bone regeneration (Jiang et al., 2021).

Biomimetic coatings, which typically include elements like collagen, hydroxyapatite, and growth hormones, produce an environment that is compatible with biology. These coatings, which are frequently used in orthopedic and dental implants as well as to repair abnormalities in the bone, enhance osseointegration and hasten bone healing. As a result, biomimetic coatings offer a potential solution to the problems related to bone regeneration in clinical and medical contexts (Shih & Varghese, 2019). This chapter explores the theories, practices, and developments around the use of biomimetic coatings to promote bone regeneration.

7.2 Architectures in bone tissue engineering

Bone scaffolds, designated as artificial platforms for defect support and repair, are crucial in cases of organ or tissue damage, necessitating a three-dimensional (3D) structure. Biocompatibility, mechanical qualities, biodegradability, pore size and interconnectivity, osteoinductivity, porosity, stability, antimicrobial effects, osteoconductivity, osteointegration, and osteogenesis are important characteristics and design elements (Fig. 7.1) (Prasadh & Wong, 2018). The porosity range of 200–350 μm has been suggested by recent research for bone tissue regeneration (Babaie & Bhaduri, 2018; Raut et al., 2020), and this is necessary for 3D scaffolds to be considered optimal implants since it allows for tissue growth, signaling, cellular ingress, and vascularization. Two-dimensional structures function as scaffolds in cases of minor bone deficiencies, improving the biomaterial

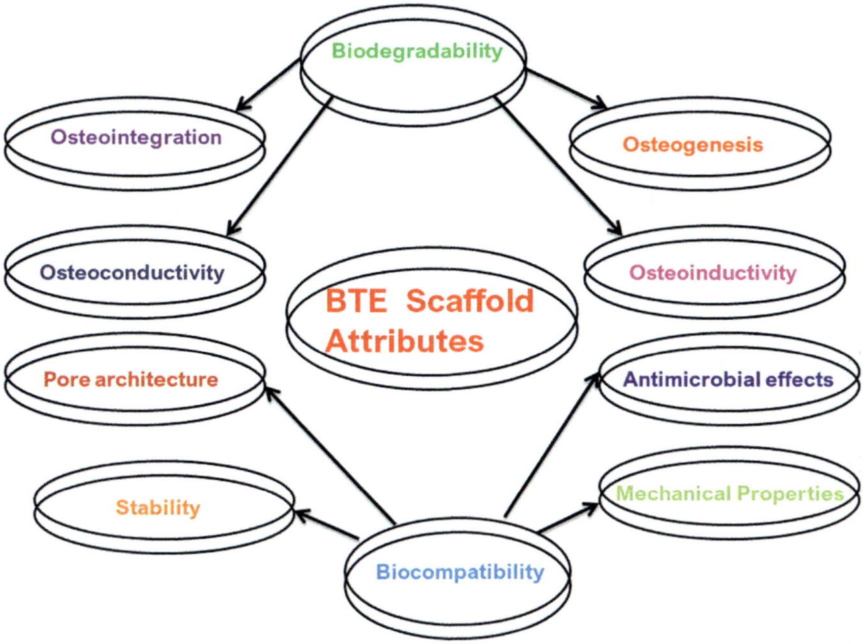

Figure 7.1 Vital BTE features in scaffold development for tissue regeneration. *BTE*, Bone tissue engineering.

interaction between the implant and the cell (Streza et al., 2023). Scaffolds are anticipated to create a biomechanical medium for tissue regeneration by fostering an environment that is favorable for cell adhesion, proliferation, and differentiation after implantation. They allow for the encapsulation of cells for later release and interaction with growth factors, and they aid in the diffusion of oxygen and nutrients (Mohan et al., 2022). In addition to its usefulness for drug and cell delivery, scaffolds can help restore normal functionality in cases of organ failure or disease. Porous structures that resemble bone are crucial for blood flow, nutrition delivery, and the interaction of osteogenic cells with bioactive substances in BTE. These processes help to promote mineralization and angiogenesis in the transplanted graft. Scaffold topological features and chemical makeup have a significant impact on their surface qualities, which are essential for cell adhesion and proliferation. For osteoblast adhesion and differentiation, surface roughness is thought to be essential, and for a successful and healthy bone grafting procedure, the scaffold's mechanical characteristics should resemble those of real bone. The success of the regenerative process is determined by pore distribution, exposed surface area, material porosity, cell penetration rate within the scaffold volume, and ECM architecture. The implant must support bone ingrowth until the new bone becomes self-sustaining (Abbasian et al., 2019; Jazayeri et al., 2018; Liu et al., 2019).

7.3 Biomaterials used for bone tissue engineering

Biomedical scaffolds with different components have been the focus of recent studies (Pupilli et al., 2022). Unfortunately, these implants are usually expensive, which has led to research into scaffolds that do not contain "biologics," which have some significant benefits. These scaffolds are specifically designed to draw in and recruit neighboring tissue cells, which promotes improved production of new bone. The addition of appropriate bioactive substances may help attract cells that have osteogenic properties (Campodoni et al., 2021; Pupilli et al., 2022). As a result, mineralized matrices from all over the implant structure greatly accelerate the healing process (Maia et al., 2022). Angiogenesis is another important mechanism that helps the growing tissue meets its needs (Russo et al., 2013). The forefront of tissue engineering research over the last few decades has focused on developing bone tissue scaffolds as a safer and more effective alternative. Current methods, illustrated in Fig. 7.2, involve using natural (e.g., starch-based polymers, chitosan, collagen, alginate, organic calcium phosphate) or synthetic materials (e.g., polyethylene glycol, polycaprolactone, poly(lactic-*co*-glycolic acid), urethanes, inorganic calcium phosphates, calcium carbonate) alone or in combination

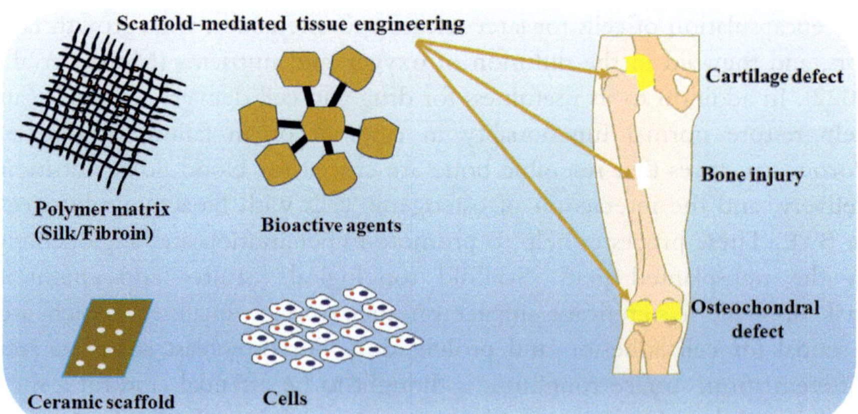

Figure 7.2 Diagram illustrating tissue regeneration through scaffold-based tissue engineering approaches.

(Li et al., 2014). Fabrication techniques for these materials include 3D printing, solvent casting, freeze-drying, gas foaming, and electrospinning (Thavornyutikarn et al., 2014; Zhou et al., 2020).

In BTE, bioactive materials like bioglass and ceramics based on calcium phosphate are frequently used. By means of an ion-exchange reaction with natural tissue, these materials promote the development of an active apatite layer on the scaffold (Mazzoni et al., 2021). Bioactive ceramic scaffolds have characteristics similar to human bone, such as osteoconductivity, corrosion resistance, and biocompatibility, but they also have the disadvantage of being brittle and porous, which increases the chance of fracture (Pupilli et al., 2022). In BTE, hydroxyapatite, calcium phosphates, and β-tricalcium phosphate are the most often used ceramics. Bioactive glasses are another important class of materials; these glasses are usually made of SiO_2, P_2O_5, and B_2O_3. The formation of a calcium phosphate layer is facilitated by the migration of phosphate and calcium ions, which is facilitated by the silanol groups produced by the dissolution of SiO_2 (Daskalakis et al., 2022). When B_2O_3 is partially substituted for SiO_2 in some bioactive glasses, borosilicate or borate glasses with a regulated rate of biodegradation are produced. Na_2O and CaO, two phosphate glasses, show a quicker rate of scaffold breakdown. Although bioactive glasses have regulated osteoconduction and resorbability, their mechanical characteristics are not the same as those of real bone; therefore it is necessary to carefully adjust the rate of ion release and disintegration to avoid toxicity. A problem with bioactive glass in 3D porous scaffolds is that it crystallizes during the sintering process (Xiao et al., 2016). As a result, these materials can be used as scaffolds at low-load defect areas or in composite structures that include bioactive ceramics or polymers (Fucile et al., 2020).

Polymers, which come from either synthetic or natural sources, are one of the materials that are frequently used in the construction of scaffolds. Based on the final result, intrinsic nature, and processing circumstances, the main characteristics of polymeric implants are classified. The chemical composition and structure determine several intrinsic qualities, such as density, solubility, crystallinity, transition temperature, mechanical properties, transparency, and electromagnetic behavior (Gloria et al., 2010). Important processing parameters that show how the material behaves during production are viscosity, melt strength, and melt flow index. The characteristics of the finished product include features related to appearance, how it behaves in the environment, and how it degrades (George et al., 2020). One important feature of polymeric scaffolds is their biodegradability, which indicates a slow disintegration process. Ring-opening polymerization materials and stepwise polycondensation materials are the two primary types of biodegradable polymers. The first group includes proteins and polysaccharides (John & Thomas, 2008), whereas the second group includes aliphatic and aromatic polyesters. The human body contains numerous natural polymers that are broken down by enzymes including lysosomes and amylases. Synthetic polymer breakdown frequently occurs through hydrolytic reactions, with erosion and hydrolysis being two of the most prominent nonbiological degradation mechanisms. Molecular weight and crystallinity grade have an impact on the mechanical characteristics of polymers and are closely related to the material's degradation process (Goonoo & Bhaw-Luximon, 2020; Pilia et al., 2013). To successfully treat biodegradable polymers and rebuild load-bearing tissues like bone, sufficient mechanical strength must be maintained. When new implants are introduced to the market, rheological parameters such as Young's modulus, flexural modulus, maximum strain, and tensile/compressive strength are regularly measured (Donnaloja et al., 2020). Advantages of synthetic polymeric implants include regulated production conditions that allow for customization of the material's mechanical characteristics, porosity, and rate of degradation for a range of medical uses (Echeverria Molina et al., 2021; Ye et al., 2022). Their structure is homogeneous and they can be made in vast quantities. Although they are scarce, natural polymers interact with cells more effectively (Samal et al., 2015). Unlike synthetic polymers, their primary disadvantage is the lack of control over their properties, and their toxicity needs to be carefully considered (Hartley et al., 2022). Electromagnetic forces can be used to modify magnetic nanoparticles (MNPs) in situ and integrate them into scaffolds (Petretta et al., 2021; Russo et al., 2016). At major bone defect sites, this manipulation in a magnetic field may lead to increased osteogenesis and angiogenesis (Goranov et al., 2020). Several studies in the literature have shown that scaffolds reinforced with MNPs promote osteoblast development and proliferation by turning on particular signaling pathways, whether a magnetic field is present or not (Fan et al., 2020; Xia et al., 2018). Furthermore, the application of techniques such as magnetic hyperthermia or photothermal therapy to the treatment of bone malignancies becomes possible.

7.4 Biomimetic scaffold fabrication approaches

Researchers have focused their efforts on developing biomimetic surfaces to mineralize scaffolds and direct the osteogenic differentiation of stem cells, in addition to employing ceramic materials in scaffold construction.

A nanocrystalline anisotropic fibril is formed in the normal bone structure by the deposition of carbonated apatite on collagen I fibrils (Weiner & Addadi, 1997). The deposition process of carbonated apatite is regulated by a range of anionic proteins found in the bone matrix, which function as both initiators and inhibitors (Boskey & Robey, 2013). Researchers have concentrated on adding anionic groups to the polymeric network by taking cues from nature. Six distinct functional groups ($-CH_3$, $-PO_4H_2$, $-COOH$, $-CONH_2$, $-OH$, and $-NH_2$) on self-assembled monolayers of alkane thiols were studied by Tanahashi et al. They discovered that the most potent groups for causing mineralization were $-PO_4H_2$ and $-COOH$, with negatively charged species showing higher efficacy. In contrast, there was no mineralization of the neutral methyl group. Since positively charged species showed less mineralization than their negatively charged counterparts, the production of apatite is considered to be the result of calcium ion-induced complexation (Tanahashi & Matsuda, 1997). Benoit et al. tethered various groups in a PEG hydrogel system to show this effect in a 3D setting. The increased release of osteopontin (OPN) with an increasing concentration of the phosphate group indicated that the additional phosphate group regulated stem cells toward an osteoblastic lineage (Benoit et al., 2008). In a similar vein, Deepthi et al. used plasma treatment to alter the polymer surface. Nitrogen and argon gases were plasma treated on electrospun scaffolds to add new functional groups onto the membrane. Increased alkaline phosphate activity and biomineralization seen by alizarin red staining (Sankar et al., 2014) are indications that this alteration favorably affected osteogenic development. Kim et al. have demonstrated the osteogenic favorability of sulfated groups in a study. Higher quantities of chondroitin sulfate (CS) promoted osteogenic development and enhanced mineralization, as shown by CS/PEG hydrogels. Furthermore, in a cranial lesion model, PEG hydrogels containing 10% CS incorporation demonstrated improved bone growth (Kim et al., 2017). Taken as a whole, these investigations highlight how surface functionalization affects stem cell behavior and confirm that it positively regulates osteogenic differentiation.

7.5 Developing an intelligent framework for bone tissue regeneration

The global demand for bone grafts is substantially high, driven by the growing need for functional bone graft materials to address congenital or acquired bone defects, developmental issues, trauma, and the presence of tumors (Giannoudis et al., 2005). The integration of a bone transplant predominantly proceeds through the interdigitation process (Morone et al., 1998), a multistep cascade, including the buildup of inflammatory cells toward the graft site as the initial response (Claes et al., 2012). The host mesenchymal cells then differentiate into chondroblasts and osteoblasts by chemotaxis toward the graft. By modifying the osteoblasts onto the 3D framework of the graft, the biomaterial's composition and arrangement eventually direct bone formation through cell attachment and morphology (Bueno & Glowacki, 2009). The process of bone formation is intricate and involves multiple components, including the differentiation and proliferation of osteoprogenitor cells, the creation of collagen, the regulation of mineralization, and the expression of functional proteins like osteocalcin and alkaline phosphatase (Szulc et al., 2005). Due to the distinct properties of bone in various skeleton regions, such as vascularization, mineral density, porosity, and growth potential, the long-term survival and regeneration of a bone implant is difficult. There is a strong need to produce biomimetic materials that improve osteoblast adherence to the biomaterial surface, facilitating bone bonding and osteoinduction, given the difficulties in harvesting autografts and the poor osteoinductive powers of many synthetic materials (Betz, 2002). In addition to providing structural support during the process, the ideal bone graft should include all the components required for integration and the new bone creation cascade. The most crucial essential feature for the perfect bone transplant is osseointegration, which is defined as the direct structural and functional link between the surface of a load-carrying implant and living bone (Mavrogenis et al., 2009). Branemark first proposed the idea of osseointegration in 1982, highlighting the critical part that implant–host tissue interaction plays in the potential for fracture healing (Branemark, 1983). There are several ways to define osseointegration: anatomically, clinically, histologically, and ultrastructurally. However, for the purposes of this discussion, the clinical definition is more pertinent. According to Branemark, osseointegration refers to the direct anatomical and functional bond between a load-bearing implant's surface and organized, live bone. At a newly implanted site, fracture repair is contingent upon a well-defined series of cellular reactions, including the foreign body reaction (Barrère et al., 2006; Branemark, 1983). The interaction between the implant and the host tissue is the main factor influencing the remodeling phase. Techniques for the functional design of interfaces with specialized binding sites for BTE applications can be developed. In vivo performance would be improved by biofunctional substrates with active surfaces that might trigger biomimetic mineralization while also enabling selective binding. Molecular modeling of such organic–inorganic interfaces, with improved efficiency, should take into account interactions specific to a certain biotype as well as geometric, stereochemical, and electrostatic constraints. When it comes to bone implants, surface functions that enable biomimetic mineralization are preferred because of the significant amount of naturally occurring inorganic content. Table 7.1 presents the biomimetic techniques and substrates that have been explored in detail, together with important data that has been acquired.

7.6 Bioinspired mineralization in mimicking nature

A material is said to be "biocompatible" if it causes the proper host tissue reactions. Surface modification is recognized as an effective way to control cellular interactions without changing the material's basic bulk functional characteristics, particularly in certain situations (Castner & Ratner, 2002). Through clever physicochemical or biochemical changes of polymers, desired biological reaction functions can be achieved (Schweizer & Taubert, 2007). Biomimetic mineralization is the technique of artificially simulating biomineralization conditions in a laboratory environment, usually accomplished with the use of organic templates like lipid membranes, cell walls, or macromolecular frameworks. The biological moieties and the biomineral precursors interact specifically or selectively to achieve this. Over the last several decades, a great deal of research has been done on methods that promote the development of biomimetic hydroxyapatite (Guentsch et al., 2012; Nudelman et al., 2012).

7.6.1 Calcium phosphate coatings

The complex processes of hard tissue development, remineralization, and disintegration entail several calcium phosphate stages (LeGeros, 1991). Metastable intermediates are formed by a number of biological mineralization processes and then change into more thermodynamically stable phases (Cazalbou et al., 2004). According to kinetic studies, precursor phases of calcium phosphate, such as dicalcium phosphate dihydrate and octacalcium phosphate, are formed and eventually change into stable hydroxyapatite (Christoffersen & Christoffersen, 1981). The kinds of mineralization (normal or pathological) and pH are two elements that

Table 7.1 Exploring biomimetic strategies for biomineralization and osseointegration: key insights and gathered information.

	Innovative substrates and approaches for biomineralization, osseointegration, and osteogenesis	Key insights	References
1	Synthetic hydroxyapatite (HA) and its composites	• Electrostatic interaction of the HAP surface with the calcium and the phosphate ions	Kim et al. (2004)
2	Bioglass and bioglass-calcium phosphate composites	• Carbonate apatite layer formation • Good osteointegration both in vitro and in vivo	Granja et al. (2001)
3	U HMWPE, biodegradable starch/ethylene Vinyl alcohol blend, PU foams	• Formation of continuous and adherent Ca-P • Layer on the surface • Needle-like crystals formed *cauliflower* like morphology	Reis et al. (1997)
4	Surface functionalization by phosphorylation • Bamboo (Li et al., 1997) • Chitosan (Sailaja, Mohanty et al., 2009; Sailaja, Sreenivasan et al., 2009) • Poly(HEMA-co-MMA) (Varma et al., 1999) • PVA (Sailaja, Mohanty et al., 2009; Sailaja, Sreenivasan et al., 2009) • Regenerated cellulose (Granja et al., 2001)	• Increased number of nuclear sites and apatite formation • Nucleation and porous HAP coating • Direct bone bonding and elicited new bone formation • Promotes in vitro biomineralization and in vitro cell adhesion • Increased surface roughness and leads to better binding of Calcium ions	Li et al. (1997), Sailaja, Mohanty et al. (2009), Sailaja, Sreenivasan et al. (2009), Varma et al. (1999), Granja et al. (2001)
5	• Surface modification Polyethersulphone • PMMA (ATP coupling) electrospun PCL—gelatin	• Promotes nucleation and growth of calcium phosphate • Uniform apatite layer formation upto 20 μm thickness	Tanahashi and Matsuda (1997), Tovani et al. (2020), Varma et al. (2003), Li et al. (2008)

6	RGD and BMP-integrated polymer matrices	• Structural integrity modulation and aligned biomineralization • Enhance bone specific marker protein expression and thereby mineralization	Goonoo & Bhaw-Luximon (2020), Li et al. (1997)
6	Biodegradable polymer composites • Viscose cellulose sponge • Starch/ethylene vinyl alcohol blend (SEVA-C) • Gelatin—poly(acrylic acid) matrix • poly(lactide-co-glycolide)	• Compatible for tissue in-growth • Attractive as scaffold for bone tissue engineering • Promotes cell adhesion • Feasibility of orientation by stretching	Bigi et al. (2004), Oliveira et al. (2002)
7	• Titanium metal • Polished and gritted titanium (Ti6Al4V)	• NaOH and heat treatment generates amorphous sodium titanate on the metal and induces bone-like apatite layer	Kim et al. (2004), Nancollas (1992)
8	Stem cell–based approaches	• In vivo osteogenesis • Promising source for bone tissue engineering	Granja et al. (2001), Kokubo et al. (1990), Märtson et al. (1998)

Source: From Sailaja G. S., Mohanty, T. V. Kumary, M. P. Valappil, R. Parameshwaran, H. K. Varma, S, Ramesh, P. Vellappally, A., Varma, H. K. (2009). Biomimetic approaches with smart interfaces for bone regeneration. *Journal of Biomedical Science*, *15*, 1–9. (Original work published 2009).

affect the nature of the phases that develop (Nancollas, 1992). Furthermore, the rate of mineralization and demineralization is strongly influenced by extralattice ions or foreign molecules present in the system. It was proposed by Kim et al. that the creation of calcium-poor amorphous calcium phosphate during the early soaking phase leads to the formation of bone-like apatite or calcium-rich amorphous calcium phosphate in the in vitro environment (Kim et al., 2004).The parameters involved in synthesis and postsynthesis can have an adverse effect on the functional characteristics of biomimetic apatites (Vandecandelaere et al., 2012). To strategically design bioceramic materials that perform optimally and minimize unwanted biological effects, such as prolonged macroplage activation, it is imperative to understand the interactions between molecules and cells on bioceramic surfaces (Dee & Bizios, 1996). Organoapatites, which are composed entirely of amino acids such as poly (L-lysine), poly(L-sodium glutamate), poly(sodium acrylate), or poly(L-lysine), have been shown to exhibit bone apposition in canine and cortical bone after 35 weeks of implantation (Shirkhanzadeh & Liu, 1994).Many studies have concentrated on surface modification approaches to enable the biomimetic mineralization of calcium phosphate, since bone is an organic–inorganic hybrid tissue with 58% mineralized hydroxyapatite. Graft copolymerization, chemical derivatization, ionizing radiation, plasma gas discharge, photochemical grafting, and chemical modification are some of the methods used (Li, 2003; Ozawa & Yao, 2002; Reis et al., 1997; Tanahashi & Matsuda, 1997; Tovani et al., 2020). Surface phosphorylation has been found to be one of these techniques that works well for surface functionalization (Li et al., 1997; Sailaja, Mohanty et al., 2009; Sailaja, Sreenivasan et al., 2009; Varma et al., 1999). Direct phosphorylation was shown by Varma et al. to produce a calcium phosphate coating on chitosan, but PMMA needed surface functionalization by ATP molecule coupling to produce HAP coating (Varma et al., 2003). Significant apatite coating and improved cytocompatibility were seen in vitro in surface-phosphorylated poly(vinyl alcohol) (PVA) (Sailaja, Mohanty et al., 2009; Sailaja, Sreenivasan et al., 2009). Li et al. (1997) phosphorylated bamboo using sodium hydroxide-phosphoric acid rather than urea-phosphoric acid, and Granja et al. (2001) phosphorylated regenerated cellulose using phosphoric acid and triethyl phosphate. An additional technique for surface phosphorylation was demonstrated in a different study using poly(hydroxyl ethyl methacrylate-co-methyl methacrylate), which encouraged calcium phosphate to develop biomimetically (Varma et al., 1999).

It has been shown that the functionalized material can stimulate the production of new bone and direct bone bonding (Sailaja, Mohanty et al., 2009; Sailaja, Sreenivasan et al., 2009).

7.6.2 Bioglass coating

The application of a bioactive glass coating, another recognized method for establishing a calcium phosphate coating, is primarily driven by the increase in the ionic product of apatite in the surrounding body fluid. The dissolution of Ca^{2+} ions from the bioactive glass, which is already supersaturated with regard to apatite, is what is responsible for this increase. Kokubo has explained the mechanics of this process in a number of groundbreaking studies (Kokubo et al., 1990). Several studies confirm that bioglass plays an important function in encouraging the development of apatite that resembles bone. The hydrated silica that forms on the surface of bioactive glasses causes a large number of apatite nuclei to be created on their surfaces.

7.6.3 Facilitating biomineralization with bioactive molecules

The immobilization of biomacromolecules on organic substrates using spacer groups, both temporarily and permanently, is recognized as a bioinspired approach that provides greater steric freedom, leading to improved specific activity. Hydroxyapatite is nucleated and grows in a site-directed or template-directed manner when exposed to surface functional groups such as $-COOH$, $-PO_4$, $-NH_2$, and $-OH$. Under physiological or simulated physiological settings, biomaterial substrates with surface-functionalized reactive anionic groups such as $-OH$, $-NH_2$, $-COOH$, and $-PO_4$ can interact with mineral precursor ions and promote the nucleation of the calcium phosphate phase. Surface functionalization confers attributes such hydrophilicity, improved cytocompatibility, and biomolecular recognition in addition to bioinspired mineralization. On functionalized self-assembled monolayers on a gold surface, the growth rate of apatite crystals is $PO_4 > COOH > CONH_2 > OH > NH_2 > CH_3$(Tanahashi & Matsuda, 1997). Nucleation of inorganic crystals on organic surfaces is driven by a decrease in activation energy. Compared to convex or planar surfaces, concave surfaces acquire an enhanced spatial charge concentration of functional groups, which is thought to be caused by surface charge-concentrated pockets that speed up the nucleation of crystals (Mann, 2002; Xin et al., 2005). A highly phosphorylated phosphoserine molecule and cysteine amino acids form the architecture of an Arg–Gly–Asp (RGD) ended self-assembled surfactant that has been shown to specifically govern nucleation and hydroxyapatite development, as well as improve cell adhesion. RGD units improved cell adhesion, while this architecture encouraged HAP nucleation (Hartgerink et al., 2001). Lu et al. demonstrated mineralization of rabbit skeletal muscle and increased bone marker expression with the aid of bone morphogenetic proteins (BMP) BMP-7 delivered from a PLGA matrix (Lu et al., 2003).

7.7 Biomimetic coatings

Technological developments in the last several years have made it possible to place calcium phosphate layers on a substrate at physiological temperatures (Nandakumar et al., 2010; Takahashi et al., 2008), instead of the previously necessary grossly unphysiological temperatures above 1000°C. In addition, hydroxyapatite and tri- or tetracalcium phosphate, which are created at extremely high temperatures, have a structure more akin to bone mineral than the crystals created by this technique, known as carbonated apatite (Klein et al., 1994).

7.7.1 Bioactive agent-induced functionalization in biomimetic coatings

The biomimetic coating technique possesses a unique advantage in that it can be rendered osteoinductive through the coprecipitation of an osteogenic agent, incorporating it into the crystalline latticework of the coating (Liu et al., 2003). Previously, these compounds could only be faintly adsorbed onto a premade biomimetic calcium phosphate coating due to their proteinaceous nature and susceptibility to deactivation at high temperatures (Murphy et al., 2000). In these situations, the superficially adsorbed depot of an osteogenic agent is released quickly and runs out in a matter of hours when exposed to a physiological environment. Due to the drug's quick release, there is a brief increase in local concentration, which may compromise osteogenic activity (Liu et al., 2005; Murphy et al., 2000). On the other hand, over a few weeks (Wernike et al., 2010), a coating-incorporated depot of this drug is progressively released (Liu et al., 2005), through a cell-mediated process. In animal models, these circumstances allow for the efficient induction and maintenance of osteogenic activity at both ectopic and orthotopic sites (Liu et al., 2005; Murphy et al., 2000).

7.7.2 Enhancing bone substitutes through biomimetic coatings employing deposition techniques

Kokubo et al. (1990) introduced the idea of biomimetic mineralization, which is the deposition of a layer of calcium phosphate that decreases fibrous encapsulation (Nagano et al., 1996), encourages bone marrow stromal cells to differentiate into osteoblasts (Ohgushi & Caplan, 1999), and facilitates the ingrowth of osseous tissue, allowing direct contact with implanted materials (Hong et al., 2020). This coating method can be used on a variety of materials, such as organic polymers, metals, and bioceramics (Kravanja & Finšgar, 2022). The original biomimetic method, however, is only applicable to surfaces that operate as mineralization nucleation sites due to the presence of active chemical groups (Song et al., 2005). Methyl groups (CH_3) are thought to be unfavorable for the process of biomimetic mineralization (Yin et al., 2004), but chemical groups such as dihydrogen phosphate (H_2PO_4) or carboxylic acid (COOH) have demonstrated great conduciveness to the process (Tanahashi & Matsuda, 1997). The absence of active chemical groups on the surfaces of many bone substitutes, particularly polymeric materials, has led to efforts to covalently attach functional anionic ones (Filmon et al., 2002). These changes run the danger of jeopardizing the material's biological and physicochemical characteristics, though. Biomimetic mineralization is also influenced by 3D structure and surface shape (Oliveira et al., 2007). An improved biphasic biomimetic coating method comprising two fundamental phases was created to overcome these obstacles (Liu et al., 2006). This method effectively applied biomimetically not just titanium implants (Koju et al., 2017), but also four polymeric bone substitutes (Wu et al., 2008), deproteinized bovine bone (Fujioka-Kobayashi et al., 2022), and each with distinct physicochemical properties, all without the need for extra surface modification. The surface chemistry, surface geometry, and 3D structures of the underlying materials had no bearing on the morphological or physicochemical characteristics of the coatings (Liu et al., 2005). The amorphous seeding layer is responsible for the consistent outcomes. This biphasic biomimetic coating method is a promising strategy for BTE because it can potentially mineralize a wider range of bone substitutes without the need for additional surface modification. Mineralizing deep surfaces with complex structures is a difficulty for current coating processes when applied to 3D scaffolds that require interconnective porosity. Li et al. (2007) describe an indirect coating technique in which apatite is coated on paraffin spheres, which are subsequently molded into foam, forming apatite layers on the pore surfaces within the scaffold. However, there is a chance that any leftover solvent could damage the host tissues or transplanted cells (Lee et al., 2004). A different method for preparing coatings uses a dynamic perfusion methodology (Oliveira et al., 2007), which has been shown to be successful in creating distinct apatite layers inside scaffold interiors under flow perfusion circumstances.

7.8 Conclusion and future prospective

In conclusion, biomimetic coatings hold great promise in regenerative medicine, advancing osteoconductivity and bioactivity in diverse implants. These coatings, which imitate calcium phosphate layers and are applied to a variety of materials, including metals and polymers, are inspired by the process of natural bone production and improve osseointegration. The effectiveness of cellular differentiation is increased by active functional groups and the regulated release of osteoinductive chemicals. Even with advancements, problems still exist. Clinical translation depends on prolonged release, increased protein incorporation, and coating method optimization. Exciting research opportunities include investigating novel biomaterials, tailoring coatings for particular anatomical areas, and tackling 3D scaffold difficulties.

Precision in biomimetic coatings is guided by developments in surface functionalization and molecular modeling. The incorporation of growth factors into these coatings opens up opportunities for intricate tissue regeneration. To advance biomimetic coatings and make them truly transformational treatments for bone deformities and fractures, interdisciplinary cooperation will be essential to pushing the bounds of these coatings.

References

Abbasian, M., Massoumi, B., Mohammad-Rezaei, R., Samadian, H., & Jaymand, M. (2019). Scaffolding polymeric biomaterials: Are naturally occurring biological macromolecules more appropriate for tissue engineering? *International Journal of Biological Macromolecules*, *134*, 673–694. Available from https://doi.org/10.1016/j.ijbiomac.2019.04.197, 01418130.

Ansari, M. (2019). Bone tissue regeneration: Biology, strategies and interface studies. *Progress in Biomaterials*, *8*(4), 223–237. Available from https://doi.org/10.1007/s40204-019-00125-z, http://www.springer.com/journal/40204.

Antoniac, I., Miculescu, M., Păltânea, V. M., Stere, A., Quan, P. H., Păltânea, G., Robu, A., & Earar, K. (2022). Magnesium-based alloys used in orthopedic surgery. *Materials.*, *15*(3), 1148.

Antoniac, I., Paltanea, V. M., Paltanea, G., Antoniac, A., Nemoianu, I. V., Petrescu, M. I., Dura, H., & Bodog, A. D. (2022). Additive manufactured magnesium-based scaffolds for tissue engineering. *Materials*, 8693.

Babaie, E., & Bhaduri, S. B. (2018). Fabrication aspects of porous biomaterials in orthopedic applications: A review. american chemical society, United States. *ACS Biomaterials Science and Engineering*, *4*(1), 1–39. Available from https://doi.org/10.1021/acsbiomaterials.7b00615, http://pubs.acs.org/journal/abseba.

Barrère, F., van Blitterswijk, C. A., & de Groot, K. (2006). Bone regeneration: Molecular and cellular interactions with calcium phosphate ceramics. *International Journal of Nanomedicine*, *1*(3), 317–332. Available from http://www.dovepress.com/getfile.php?fileID = 200.Netherlands.

Benoit, D. S. W., Schwartz, M. P., Durney, A. R., & Anseth, K. S. (2008). Small functional groups for controlled differentiation of hydrogel-encapsulated human mesenchymal stem cells. *Nature Materials*, 7(10), 816–823. Available from https://doi.org/10.1038/nmat2269, http://www.nature.com/nmat/.

Betz, R. R. (2002). Limitations of autograft and allograft: New synthetic solutions. *Orthopedics*, *25*(5), s561–s570.

Bigi, A., Bracci, B., Cojazzi, G., Panzavolta, S., & Rubini, K. (2004). In vitro mineralization of gelatin-polyacrylic acid complex matrices. *Journal of Biomaterials Science, Polymer Edition*, *15*(3), 243–254. Available from https://doi.org/10.1163/156856204322977166.

Boskey, A. L., & Robey, P. G. (2013). *The regulatory role of matrix proteins in mineralization of bone. Marcus and Feldman's osteoporosis* (pp. 235–255). United States: Elsevier Inc. Available from http://www.sciencedirect.com/science/book/9780124158535.

Branemark, P. I. (1983). Osseointegration and its experimental background. *The Journal of Prosthetic Dentistry*, *50*(3), 399–410. Available from https://doi.org/10.1016/S0022-3913(83)80101-2, 00223913.

Bud, E. S., Bocanet, V. I., Muntean, M. H., Vlasa, A., Bucur, S. M., Păcurar, M., Dragomir, B. R., Olteanu, C. D., & Bud, A. (1908). Accuracy of three-dimensional (3D) printed dental digital models generated with three types of resin polymers by extra-oral optical scanning. *Journal of Clinical Medicine*, *10*.

Bueno, E. M., & Glowacki, J. (2009). Cell-free and cell-based approaches for bone regeneration. *Nature Reviews Rheumatology*, *5*(12), 685–697. Available from https://doi.org/10.1038/nrrheum.2009.228.

Campodoni, E., Velez, M., Fragogeorgi, E., Morales, I., De La Presa, P., Stanicki, D., Dozio, S. M., Xanthopoulos, S., Bouziotis, P., Dermisiadou, E., Rouchota, M., Loudos, G., Marín, P., Laurent, S., Boutry, S., Panseri, S., Montesi, M., Tampieri, A., & Sandri, M. (2021). Magnetic and radio-labeled bio-hybrid scaffolds to promote and track in vivo the progress of bone regeneration. *Biomaterials Science*, *9*(22), 7575–7590. Available from https://doi.org/10.1039/d1bm00858g, 20474849, http://pubs.rsc.org/en/journals/journal/bm.

Castner, D. G., & Ratner, B. D. (2002). Biomedical surface science: Foundations to frontiers. *Surface Science*, *500*(1–3), 28–60. Available from https://doi.org/10.1016/S0039-6028(01)01587-4, 00396028.

Cavalu, S., Antoniac, I. V., Mohan, A., Bodog, F., Doicin, C., Mates, I., Ulmeanu, M., Murzac, R., & Semenescu, A. (2020). Nanoparticles and nanostructured surface fabrication for innovative cranial and maxillofacial surgery. *Materials*, *13*(23). Available from https://doi.org/10.3390/ma13235391, 1996-1944.

Cavalu, S., Fritea, L., Brocks, M., Barbaro, K., Murvai, G., Costea, T. O., Antoniac, I., Verona, C., Romani, M., Latini, A., Zilli, R., & Rau, J. V. (2020). Novel Hybrid Composites based on PVA/SeTiO_2 nanoparticles and natural hydroxyapatite for orthopedic applications: Correlations between structural, morphological and biocompatibility properties. *Materials*, *13* (9). Available from https://doi.org/10.3390/ma13092077, 1996-1944.

Cazalbou, S., Combes, C., Eichert, D., & Rey, C. (2004). Adaptative physico-chemistry of bio-related calcium phosphates. *Journal of Materials Chemistry*, *14*(14), 2148–2153. Available from https://doi.org/10.1039/b401318b.

Christoffersen, J., & Christoffersen, M. R. (1981). Kinetics of dissolution of calcium hydroxyapatite. IV. The effect of some biologically important inhibitors. *Journal of Crystal Growth*, *53*(1), 42–54. Available from https://doi.org/10.1016/0022-0248(81)90054-3.

Claes, L., Recknagel, S., & Ignatius, A. (2012). Fracture healing under healthy and inflammatory conditions. *Nature Reviews Rheumatology*, *8*(3), 133–143. Available from https://doi.org/10.1038/nrrheum.2012.1.

Daskalakis, E., Huang, B., Vyas, C., Acar, A. A., Fallah, A., Cooper, G., Weightman, A., Koc, B., Blunn, G., & Bartolo, P. (2022). Novel 3D bioglass scaffolds for bone tissue regeneration. *Polymers*, *14*, 445.

Dee, K. C., & Bizios, R. (1996). Mini-review: Proactive biomaterials and bone tissue engineering. *Biotechnology and Bioengineering*, *50*(4), 438–442. Available from https://doi.org/10.1002/(SICI)1097-0290(19960520), 50:4 < 438::AID-BIT11 > 3.0.CO;2-F.

Donnaloja, F., Jacchetti, E., Soncini, M., & Raimondi, M. T. (2020). Natural and synthetic polymers for bone scaffolds optimization. *Polymers*, *12*(4). Available from https://doi.org/10.3390/polym12040905, 2073–4360.

Echeverria Molina, M. I., Malollari, K. G., & Komvopoulos, K. (2021). Design challenges in polymeric scaffolds for tissue engineering. *Frontiers in Bioengineering and Biotechnology*, *9*.

Fan, D., Wang, Q., Zhu, T., Wang, H., Liu, B., Wang, Y., Liu, Z., Liu, X., Fan, D., & Wang, X. (2020). Recent advances of magnetic nanomaterials in bone tissue repair. *Frontiers in Chemistry*, *8*. Available from https://doi.org/10.3389/fchem.2020.00745, 2296–2646.

Fernandez-Yague, M. A., Abbah, S. A., McNamara, L., Zeugolis, D. I., Pandit, A., & Biggs, M. J. (2015). Biomimetic approaches in bone tissue engineering: Integrating biological and physicomechanical strategies. *Advanced Drug Delivery Reviews*, *84*, 1–29. Available from https://doi.org/10.1016/j.addr.2014.09.005, 18728294, http://www.elsevier.com/locate/drugdeliv.

Fierro, F. A., Nolta, J. A., & Adamopoulos, I. E. (2017). Concise review: Stem cells in osteoimmunology. *Stem Cells*, *35*(6), 1461–1467. Available from https://doi.org/10.1002/stem.2625, 15494918, http://onlinelibrary.wiley.com/journal/10.1002/(ISSN)1549-4918.

Filmon, R., Grizon, F., Baslé, M. F., & Chappard, D. (2002). Effects of negatively charged groups (carboxymethyl) on the calcification of poly(2-hydroxyethyl methacrylate). *Biomaterials*, *23*(14), 3053–3059. Available from https://doi.org/10.1016/s0142-9612(02)00069-8, 01429612.

Fucile, P., Onofrio, I., Papallo, I., Gallicchio, V., Rega, A., D'Antò, V., Improta, G., de Santis, R., Gloria, A., & Russo, T. (2020). Strategies for the design of additively manufactured nanocomposite scaffolds for hard tissue regeneration. *Acta IMEKO*, *9*(4), 53–59. Available from https://doi.org/10.21014/acta_imeko.v9i4.739, https://acta.imeko.org/index.php/acta-imeko/article/view/IMEKO-ACTA-09%20%282020%29-04-07/pdf.

Fujioka-Kobayashi, M., Katagiri, H., Lang, N. P., Imber, J. C., Schaller, B., & Saulacic, N. (2022). Addition of synthetic biomaterials to deproteinized bovine bone mineral (DBBM) for bone augmentation—A preclinical in vivo study. *International journal of molecular sciences* (18).

George, A. M., Reddy Peddireddy, S. P., Thakur, G., & Rodrigues, F. C. (2020). *Biopolymer-based scaffolds* (pp. 717–749). Elsevier BV. Available from 10.1016/b978-0-12-816897-4.00029-1.

Giannoudis, P. V., Dinopoulos, H., & Tsiridis, E. (2005). Bone substitutes: An update. *Injury*, *36*(3), S20–S27. Available from https://doi.org/10.1016/j.injury.2005.07.029.

Gloria, A., De Santis, R., & Ambrosio, L. (2010). Polymer-based composite scaffolds for tissue engineering. *Journal of Applied Biomaterials and Biomechanics*, *8*(2), 57–67. Available from http://www.jabb.biz/public/JABB/Article/Attach.action?cmd = Download&uid = 8F1D6B98-1616-4DB7-B06C-2D19F45D3088.Italy.

Goonoo, N., & Bhaw-Luximon, A. (2020). *Nanomaterials combination for wound healing and skin regeneration. Advanced 3D-Printed Systems and Nanosystems for Drug Delivery and Tissue Engineering* (pp. 159–217). Mauritius: Elsevier. Available from https://www.sciencedirect.com/book/9780128184714, 10.1016/B978-0-12-818471-4.00007–8.

Goranov, V., Shelyakova, T., De Santis, R., Haranava, Y., Makhaniok, A., Gloria, A., Tampieri, A., Russo, A., Kon, E., Marcacci, M., Ambrosio, L., & Dediu, V. A. (2020). 3D patterning of cells in magnetic scaffolds for tissue engineering. *Scientific Reports*, *10*(1). Available from https://doi.org/10.1038/s41598-020-58738-5.

Granja, P. L., Pouységu, L., Deffieux, D., Daudé, G., De Jéso, B., Labrugère, C., Baquey, C., & Barbosa, M. A. (2001). Cellulose phosphates as biomaterials. II. Surface chemical modification of regenerated cellulose hydrogels. *Journal of Applied Polymer Science*, *82*(13), 3354–3365. Available from https://doi.org/10.1002/app.2194.

Guentsch, A., Seidler, K., Nietzsche, S., Hefti, A. F., Preshaw, P. M., Watts, D. C., Jandt, K. D., & Sigusch, B. W. (2012). Biomimetic mineralization: Long-term observations in patients with dentin sensitivity. *Dental Materials*, *28*(4), 457–464. Available from https://doi.org/10.1016/j.dental.2012.01.003, 01095641.

Hartgerink, J. D., Beniash, E., & Stupp, S. I. (2001). Self-assembly and mineralization of peptide-amphiphile nanofibers. *Science (New York, N.Y.)*, *294*(5547), 1684–1688. Available from https://doi.org/10.1126/science.1063187.

Hartley, E., Moon, H., & Neves, A. (2022). Biodegradable synthetic polymers for tissue engineering: A mini-review. *Reinvention: a Journal of Undergraduate Research*, 48–70.

Hong, J. Y., Ko, S. Y., Lee, W., Chang, Y. Y., Kim, S. H., & Yun, J. H. (2020). Enhancement of bone ingrowth into a porous titanium structure to improve osseointegration of dental implants: A pilot study in the canine model. *Materials*, *13*(14). Available from https://doi.org/10.3390/ma13143061, 19961944, https://res.mdpi.com/d_attachment/materials/materials-13-03061/article_deploy/materials-13-03061.pdf.

Iulian, A., Dan, L., Camelia, T., Claudia, M., & Sebastian, G. (2018). *Synthetic materials for osteochondral tissue engineering, Advances in experimental medicine and biology* (1058). Romania: Springer New York LLC. Available from http://www.springer.com/series/5584, 10.1007/978-3-319-76711-6_2.

Jazayeri, H. E., Rodriguez-Romero, M., Razavi, M., Tahriri, M., Ganjawalla, K., Rasoulianboroujeni, M., Malekoshoaraie, M. H., Khoshroo, K., & Tayebi, L. (2018). The cross-disciplinary emergence of 3D printed bioceramic scaffolds in orthopedic bioengineering. *Ceramics International*, *44*(1), 1–9. Available from https://doi.org/10.1016/j.ceramint.2017.09.095, 02728842.

Jiang, S., Wang, M., & He, J. (2021). A review of biomimetic scaffolds for bone regeneration: Toward a cell-free strategy. *Bioengineering and Translational Medicine*, *6*(2). Available from https://doi.org/10.1002/btm2.10206, 23806761, http://onlinelibrary.wiley.com/journal/10.1002/(ISSN)2380-6761.

John, M., & Thomas, S. (2008). Biofibres and biocomposites. *Carbohydrate Polymers*, *71*(3), 343–364. Available from https://doi.org/10.1016/j.carbpol.2007.05.040, 01448617.

Kim, H. D., Lee, E. A., An, Y. H., Kim, S. L., Lee, S. S., Yu, S. J., Jang, H. L., Nam, K. T., Im, S. G., & Hwang, N. S. (2017). Chondroitin sulfate-based biomineralizing surface hydrogels for bone tissue engineering. *ACS Applied Materials and Interfaces*, *9*(26), 21639–21650. Available from https://doi.org/10.1021/acsami.7b04114, 19448252, http://pubs.acs.org/journal/aamick.

Kim, H. M., Himeno, T., Kawashita, M., Kokubo, T., & Nakamura, T. (2004). The mechanism of biomineralization of bone-like apatite on synthetic hydroxyapatite: An in vitro assessment. *Journal of the Royal Society Interface*, *1*(1), 17–22. Available from https://doi.org/10.1098/rsif.2004.0003, 17425662, http://rsif.royalsocietypublishing.org/.

Klein, C. P. A. T., Patka, P., Wolke, J. G. C., de Blieck-Hogervorst, J. M. A., & de Groot, K. (1994). Long-term in vivo study of plasma-sprayed coatings on titanium alloys of tetracalcium phosphate, hydroxyapatite and α-tricalcium phosphate. *Biomaterials*, *15*(2), 146–150. Available from https://doi.org/10.1016/0142-9612(94)90264-x, 01429612.

Koju, N., Sikder, P., Ren, Y., Zhou, H., & Bhaduri, S. B. (2017). Biomimetic coating technology for orthopedic implants. *Current Opinion in Chemical Engineering*, *15*, 49–55. Available from https://doi.org/10.1016/j.coche.2016.11.005, http://www.elsevier.com/wps/find/journaldescription.cws_home/725837/description#description.

Kokubo, T., Ito, S., Huang, Z. T., Hayashi, T., Sakka, S., Kitsugi, T., & Yamamuro, T. (1990). Ca, P-rich layer formed on high-strength bioactive glass-ceramic A-W. *Journal of Biomedical Materials Research*, *24*(3), 331–343. Available from https://doi.org/10.1002/jbm.820240306, 0021–9304.

Kravanja, K. A., & Finšgar, M. (2022). A review of techniques for the application of bioactive coatings on metal-based implants to achieve controlled release of active ingredients. *Materials & Design*, *217*. Available from https://doi.org/10.1016/j.matdes.2022.110653, 02641275.

Lee, S. H., Kim, B. S., Kim, S. H., Kang, S. W., & Kim, Y. H. (2004). Thermally produced biodegradable scaffolds for cartilage tissue engineering. *Macromolecular Bioscience*, *4*(8), 802–810. Available from https://doi.org/10.1002/mabi.200400021.

LeGeros, R. Z. (1991). Calcium phosphates in oral biology and medicine. *Monographs in Oral Science*, *15*, 1–201.

Li, J., Beaussart, A., Chen, Y., & Mak, A. F. T. (2007). Transfer of apatite coating from porogens to scaffolds: Uniform apatite coating within porous poly(DL-lactic-co-glycolic acid) scaffold in vitro. *Journal of Biomedical Materials Research – Part A*, *80*(1), 226–233. Available from https://doi.org/10.1002/jbm.a.31096, 15524965.

Li, J. J., Kaplan, D. L., & Zreiqat, H. (2014). Scaffold-based regeneration of skeletal tissues to meet clinical challenges. *Journal of Materials Chemistry B*, *2*(42), 7272–7306. Available from https://doi.org/10.1039/c4tb01073f, 2050750X, http://pubs.rsc.org/en/journals/journalissues/tb.

Li, P. (2003). Biomimetic nano-apatite coating capable of promoting bone ingrowth. *Journal of Biomedical Materials Research – Part A*, *66*(1), 79–85. Available from https://doi.org/10.1002/jbm.a.10519, 00219304, http://onlinelibrary.wiley.com/journal/10.1002/(ISSN)1552-4965.

Li, S., Liu, Q., De Wijn, J., Wolke, J., Zhou, B., & De Groot, K. (1997). In-vitro apatite formation on phosphorylated bamboo. *Journal of Materials Science: Materials in Medicine*, *8*(9), 543–549. Available from https://doi.org/10.1023/A:1018546730925, 09574530.

Li, X., Xie, J., Yuan, X., & Xia, Y. (2008). Coating electrospun poly(ε-caprolactone) fibers with gelatin and calcium phosphate and their use as biomimetic scaffolds for bone tissue engineering. *Langmuir: the ACS Journal of Surfaces and Colloids*, *24*(24), 14145–14150. Available from https://doi.org/10.1021/la802984a, 0743–7463.

Liu, Y., Degroot, K., & Hunziker, E. (2005). BMP-2 liberated from biomimetic implant coatings induces and sustains direct ossification in an ectopic rat model. *Bone*, *36*(5), 745–757. Available from https://doi.org/10.1016/j.bone.2005.02.005, 87563282.

Liu, Y., Li, J. P., Hunziker, E. B., & de Groot, K. (2006). Incorporation of growth factors into medical devices via biomimetic coatings. *Philosophical Transactions of the Royal Society A: Mathematical, Physical and Engineering Sciences*, *364*(1838), 233–248. Available from https://doi.org/10.1098/rsta.2005.1685, 1364-503X.

Liu, Y., Hunziker, E. B., Layrolle, P., Van Blitterswijk, C., Calvert, P. D., & De Groot, K. (2003). Remineralization of demineralized albumin-calcium phosphate coatings. *Journal of Biomedical Materials Research - Part A*, *67*(4), 1155–1162. Available from https://doi.org/10.1002/jbm.a.20019, 00219304, http://onlinelibrary.wiley.com/journal/10.1002/(ISSN)1552-4965.

Liu, Y., Nelson, T., Chakroff, J., Cromeens, B., Johnson, J., Lannutti, J., & Besner, G. E. (2019). Comparison of polyglycolic acid, polycaprolactone, and collagen as scaffolds for the production of tissue engineered intestine. *Journal of Biomedical Materials Research — Part B Applied Biomaterials*, *107*(3), 750–760. Available from https://doi.org/10.1002/jbm.b.34169, 15524981, http://onlinelibrary.wiley.com/journal/10.1002/(ISSN)1552-4965.

Lu, H. H., Kofron, M. D., El-Amin, S. F., Attawia, M. A., & Laurencin, C. T. (2003). In vitro bone formation using muscle-derived cells: A new paradigm for bone tissue engineering using polymer-bone morphogenetic protein matrices, Academic Press Inc., United States*Biochemical and Biophysical Research Communications*, *305*(4), 882–889. Available from https://doi.org/10.1016/S0006-291X(03)00858-1, 0006291X, http://www.sciencedirect.com/science/journal/0006291X.

Maia, F. R., Bastos, A. R., Oliveira, J. M., Correlo, V. M., & Reis, R. L. (2022). Recent approaches towards bone tissue engineering. *Bone*, *154*, 116256.

Manjua, A. C., Cabral, J. M. S., Portugal, C. A. M., & Ferreira, F. C. (2021). Magnetic stimulation of the angiogenic potential of mesenchymal stromal cells in vascular tissue engineering. *Science and Technology of Advanced Materials*, *22*(1), 461–480. Available from https://doi.org/10.1080/14686996.2021.1927834, http://www.tandfonline.com/loi/tsta20#.V0KNDU1f3cs.

Mann, S. (2002). *Biomineralization: Principles and concepts in bioinorganic materials chemistry*. Oxford Chemistry Masters, Oxford Chemistry Masters.

Märtson, M., Viljanto, J., Hurme, T., & Saukko, P. (1998). Biocompatibility of Cellulose Sponge with Bone. *European Surgical Research*, *30*(6), 426–432. Available from https://doi.org/10.1159/000008609.

Mavrogenis, A. F., Dimitriou, R., Parvizi, J., & Babis, G. C. (2009). Biology of implant osseointegration. *Journal of Musculoskeletal Neuronal Interactions*, *9*(2), 61–71, 11087161. Available from http://www.ismni.org/jmni/pdf/36/01MAVROGENIS.pdf.Greece.

Mazzoni, E., Iaquinta, M. R., Lanzillotti, C., Mazziotta, C., Maritati, M., Montesi, M., Sprio, S., Tampieri, A., Tognon, M., & Martini, F. (2021). Bioactive materials for soft tissue repair. *Frontiers in Bioengineering and Biotechnology*. Available from https://doi.org/10.3389/fbioe.2021.613787.

Mohan, A. G., Ciurea, A. V., Antoniac, I., Paltanea, V. M., Bodog, V., Maghiar, A., Marcut, O., Ghiurau, L., & Bodog, A. (2022). Cranioplasty after two giant intraosseous angiolipomas of the cranium: Case report and literature review. *Healthcare*, *10*(4), 655.

Morone, M. A., Boden, S. D., Hair, G., Martin, G. J., Racine, M., Titus, L., & Hutton, W. C. (1998). Gene expression during autograft lumbar spine fusion and the effect of bone morphogenetic protein 2. *Clinical Orthopaedics and Related Research*, *351*, 252–265. Available from https://doi.org/10.1097/00003086-199806000-00030, https://journals.lww.com/clinorthop/pages/default.aspx.

Murphy, W. L., Kohn, D. H., & Mooney, D. J. (2000). Growth of continuous bonelike mineral within porous poly(lactide-co- glycolide) scaffolds in vitro. *Journal of Biomedical Materials Research*, *50*(1), 50–58. Available from https://doi.org/10.1002/(SICI)1097-4636. (200004)50:1 < 50::AID-JBM8 > 3.0.CO;2-F.

Nagano, M., Kitsugi, T., Nakamura, T., Kokubo, T., & Tanahashi, M. (1996). Bone bonding ability of an apatite-coated polymer produced using a biomimetic method: A mechanical and histological study in vivo. *Journal of Biomedical Materials Research*, *31*(4), 487–494. Available from https://doi.org/10.1002/(SICI)1097-4636. (199608) 31:4 < 487::AID-JBM8 > 3.3.CO;2-M.

Nancollas, G. H. (1992). The involvement of calcium phosphates in biological mineralization and demineralization processes. *Pure and Applied Chemistry*, *64*(11), 1673–1678. Available from https://doi.org/10.1351/pac199264111673.

Nandakumar, A., Yang, L., Habibovic, P., & van Blitterswijk, C. (2010). Calcium phosphate coated electrospun fiber matrices as scaffolds for bone tissue engineering. *Langmuir: The ACS Journal of Surfaces and Colloids*, *26*(10), 7380–7387. Available from https://doi.org/10.1021/la904406b.

Nudelman, F., Bomans, P. H. H., George, A., De With, G., & Sommerdijk, N. A. J. M. (2012). The role of the amorphous phase on the biomimetic mineralization of collagen. *Faraday Discussions*, *159*, 357–370. Available from https://doi.org/10.1039/c2fd20062g, 13645498.

Ohgushi, H., & Caplan, A. I. (1999). Stem cell technology and bioceramics: From cell to gene engineering. *Journal of Biomedical Materials Research*, *48*(6), 913–927. Available from https://doi.org/10.1002/(SICI)1097-4636(1999), 48:6 < 913::AID-JBM22 > 3.0.CO;2-0.

Oliveira, A.L., Alves, C.M., & Reis, R.L. (2002). Cell adhesion and proliferation on biomimetic calcium-phosphate coatings produced by a sodium silicate gel methodology. *Journal of Materials Science: Materials in Medicine*, *12*, 1181–1188. https://doi.org/10.1023/A:1021106525097.

Oliveira, A. L., Malafaya, P. B., Costa, S. A., Sousa, R. A., & Reis, R. L. (2007). Micro-computed tomography (μ -CT) as a potential tool to assess the effect of dynamic coating routes on the formation of biomimetic apatite layers on 3D-plotted biodegradable polymeric scaffolds. *Journal of Materials Science: Materials in Medicine*, *18*(2), 211–223. Available from https://doi.org/10.1007/s10856-006-0683-8.

Ozawa, N., & Yao, T. (2002). Micropattern formation of apatite by combination of a biomimetic process and transcription of resist pattern. *Journal of Biomedical Materials Research*, *62*(4), 579–586. Available from https://doi.org/10.1002/jbm.10281.

Pajarinen, J., Lin, T., Gibon, E., Kohno, Y., Maruyama, M., Nathan, K., Lu, L., Yao, Z., & Goodman, S. B. (2019). Mesenchymal stem cell-macrophage crosstalk and bone healing. *Biomaterials*, *196*, 80–89. Available from https://doi.org/10.1016/j.biomaterials.2017.12.025, http://www.journals.elsevier.com/biomaterials/.

Petretta, M., Gambardella, A., Desando, G., Cavallo, C., Bartolotti, I., Shelyakova, T., Goranov, V., Brucale, M., Dediu, V. A., Fini, M., & Grigolo, B. (2021). Multifunctional 3D-printed magnetic polycaprolactone/hydroxyapatite scaffolds for bone tissue engineering. *Polymers*, *13*(21). Available from https://doi.org/10.3390/polym13213825.

Pilia, M., Guda, T., & Appleford, M. (2013). Development of composite scaffolds for load-bearing segmental bone defects. *BioMed Research International*, *2013*, 1–15. Available from https://doi.org/10.1155/2013/458253.

Prasadh, S., & Wong, R. C. W. (2018). Unraveling the mechanical strength of biomaterials used as a bone scaffold in oral and maxillofacial defects. *Japanese Stomatological Society, Singapore Oral Science International*, *15*(2), 48–55. Available from https://doi.org/10.1016/S1348-8643(18)30005-3, http://www.elsevier.com/wps/find/journaldescription.cws_home/725218/description#description.

Pupilli, F., Ruffini, A., Dapporto, M., Tavoni, M., Tampieri, A., & Sprio, S. (2022). Design strategies and biomimetic approaches for calcium phosphate scaffolds in bone tissue regeneration. *Biomimetics*, 112.

Quan, P. H., Antoniac, I., Miculescu, F., Antoniac, A., Manescu, V., Robu, V., Biţa, A., Miculescu, A.-I., Saceleanu, M., Bodog, A. D., et al. (2022). Fluoride treatment and in vitro corrosion behavior of Mg-Nd-Y-Zn-Zr alloys type. *Materials*. Available from https://doi.org/10.3390/ma15020566.

Raut, H. K., Das, R., Liu, Z., Liu, X., & Ramakrishna, S. (2020). Biocompatibility of biomaterials for tissue regeneration or replacement. *Biotechnology Journal*, *15*(12).

Available from https://doi.org/10.1002/biot.202000160, 18607314, http://onlinelibrary.wiley.com/journal/10.1002/(ISSN)1860-7314.

Reis, R.L., Cunha, A.M., Fernandes, M.H., & Correia R.N. (1997). Treatments to induce the nucleation and growth of apatite-like layers on polymeric surfaces and foams. *Journal of Materials Science: Materials in Medicine*, *12*, 897–905. https://doi.org/10.1023/A:1018514107669.

Romanec, C., Rosu, S., Macovei, G., Scutariu, M. M., Dragomir, B., & Olteanu, N. D. (2018). Morphofunctional features in angle second class malocclusion on dental gypsum models. *Materiale Plastice*, *55*, 686–690. Available from https://doi.org/10.37358/mp.18.4.5101, http://www.revmaterialeplastice.ro/pdf/ROMANEC%204%2018.pdf.

Russo, A., Panseri, S., Shelyakova, T., Sandri, M., Dionigi, C., Ortolani, A., Meikle, S., Lacey, J., Tampieri, A., Dediu, V. et al. (2013). Critical long bone defect treated by magnetic scaffolds and fixed by permanent magnets. In: *Proceedings of the 2nd global congress on nanoengineering for medicine and biology*, Boston, MA, USA.

Russo, A., Bianchi, M., Sartori, M., Parrilli, A., Panseri, S., Ortolani, A., Sandri, M., Boi, M., Salter, D. M., Maltarello, M. C., Giavaresi, G., Fini, M., Dediu, V., Tampieri, A., & Marcacci, M. (2016). Magnetic forces and magnetized biomaterials provide dynamic flux information during bone regeneration. *Journal of Materials Science: Materials in Medicine*, *27*(3), 1–13. Available from https://doi.org/10.1007/s10856-015-5659-0, 15734838, http://www.wkap.nl/journalhome.htm/0957-4530.

Sailaja, G. S., Mohanty, T. V., Kumary, M. P., Valappil, R., Parameshwaran, H. K., Varma, S., Ramesh, P., Vellappally, A., & Varma, H. K. (2009). Biomimetic approaches with smart interfaces for bone regeneration. *Journal of Biomedical Science*, *15*, 1–9.

Sailaja, G. S., Sreenivasan, K., Yokogawa, Y., Kumary, T. V., & Varma, H. K. (2009). Bioinspired mineralization and cell adhesion on surface functionalized poly(vinyl alcohol) films. *Acta Biomaterialia*, *5*(5), 1647–1655. Available from https://doi.org/10.1016/j.actbio.2008.12.005, 17427061.

Samal, S. K., Goranov, V., Dash, M., Russo, A., Shelyakova, T., Graziosi, P., Lungaro, L., Riminucci, A., Uhlarz, M., Bañobre-López, M., Rivas, J., Herrmannsdörfer, T., Rajadas, J., De Smedt, S., Braeckmans, K., Kaplan, D. L., & Dediu, V. A. (2015). Multilayered magnetic gelatin membrane scaffolds. *ACS Applied Materials and Interfaces*, 7(41), 23098–23109. Available from https://doi.org/10.1021/acsami.5b06813, 19448252, http://pubs.acs.org/journal/aamick.

Sankar, D., Shalumon, K. T., Chennazhi, K. P., Menon, D., & Jayakumar, R. (2014). Surface plasma treatment of poly(caprolactone) micro, nano, and multiscale fibrous scaffolds for enhanced osteoconductivity. *Tissue Engineering. Part A*, *20*(11–12), 1689–1702. Available from https://doi.org/10.1089/ten.tea.2013.0569, 1937–3341.

Savin, C., Murariu, A., Gavrila, L., & Balan, A. (2017). Dental material biocompatibility: A cross-sectional study. *International Journal of Medical Dentistry.*, *21*, 94–97.

Schemitsch, E. H. (2017). Size matters: Defining critical in bone defect size!. *Journal of Orthopaedic Trauma*, *31*, S20–S22. Available from https://doi.org/10.1097/BOT.0000000000000978, 15312291, http://journals.lww.com/jorthotrauma.

Schweizer, S., & Taubert, A. (2007). Polymer-controlled, bio-inspired calcium phosphate mineralization from aqueous solution. *Macromolecular Bioscience*, 7(9–10), 1085–1099. Available from https://doi.org/10.1002/mabi.200600283.

Shih, Y. V., & Varghese, S. (2019). Tissue engineered bone mimetics to study bone disorders ex vivo: Role of bioinspired materials. *Biomaterials*, *198*, 107–121. Available from https://doi.org/10.1016/j.biomaterials.2018.06.005, 18785905, http://www.journals.elsevier.com/biomaterials/.

Shirkhanzadeh, M., & Liu, G. Q. (1994). Biocompatible delivery systems for osteoinductive proteins: Immobilization of L-lysine in micro-porous hydroxyapatite coatings. *Materials Letters*, *21*(1), 115–118. Available from https://doi.org/10.1016/0167-577x(94)90134-1, 0167577X.

Song, J., Malathong, V., & Bertozzi, C. R. (2005). Mineralization of synthetic polymer scaffolds: A bottom-up approach for the development of artificial bone. *Journal of the American Chemical Society*, *127*(10), 3366–3372. Available from https://doi.org/10.1021/ja043776z.

Streza, A., Antoniac, A., (Paltanea), V. M., Paltanea, G., Robu, A., Dura, H., Verestiuc, L., Stanica, E., Voicu, S. I., Antoniac, I., Cristea, M. B., Dragomir, B. R., Rau, J. V., & Manolea, M.-M. (2023). Effect of filler types on cellulose-acetate-based composite used as coatings for biodegradable magnesium implants for trauma. *Materials*, *16*(2). Available from https://doi.org/10.3390/ma16020554.

Szulc, P., Garnero, P., Marchand, F., Duboeuf, F., & Delmas, P. D. (2005). Biochemical markers of bone formation reflect endosteal bone loss in elderly men—MINOS study. *Bone*, *36* (1), 13–21. Available from https://doi.org/10.1016/j.bone.2004.09.004, 87563282.

Takahashi, K., Van Den Beucken, J. J. J. P., Wolke, J. G. C., Hayakawa, T., Nishiyama, N., & Jansen, J. A. (2008). Characterization and in vitro evaluation of biphasic calcium pyrophosphate-tricalciumphosphate radio frequency magnetron sputter coatings. *Journal of Biomedical Materials Research – Part A*, *84*(3), 682–690. Available from https://doi.org/10.1002/jbm.a.31341, 15524965.

Tanahashi, M., & Matsuda, T. (1997). Surface functional group dependence on apatite formation on self-assembled monolayers in a simulated body fluid. *Journal of Biomedical Materials Research*, *34*(3), 305–315. Available from https://doi.org/10.1002/(SICI) 1097-4636(19970305), 34:3 < 305::AID-JBM5 > 3.3.CO;2–4.

Thavornyutikarn, B., Chantarapanich, N., Sitthiseripratip, K., Thouas, G. A., & Chen, Q. (2014). Bone tissue engineering scaffolding: computer-aided scaffolding techniques. *Progress in Biomaterials*, *3*(2–4), 61–102. Available from https://doi.org/10.1007/s40204-014-0026-7, 21940517, http://www.springer.com/journal/40204.

Tovani, C. B., Oliveira, T. M., Soares, M. P. R., Nassif, N., Fukada, S. Y., Ciancaglini, P., Gloter, A., & Ramos, A. P. (2020). Strontium Calcium Phosphate Nanotubes as Bioinspired Building Blocks for Bone Regeneration. *ACS Applied Materials and Interfaces*, *12*(39), 43422–43434. Available from https://doi.org/10.1021/acsami.0c12434, 19448252, http://pubs.acs.org/journal/aamick.

Vandecandelaere, N., Rey, C., & Drouet, C. (2012). Biomimetic apatite-based biomaterials: on the critical impact of synthesis and post-synthesis parameters. *Journal of Materials Science: Materials in Medicine*, *23*(11), 2593–2606. Available from https://doi.org/10.1007/s10856-012-4719-y.

Varma, H. K., Sreenivasan, K., Yokogawa, Y., & Hosumi, A. (2003). In vitro calcium phosphate growth over surface modified PMMA film. *Biomaterials*, *24*(2), 297–303. Available from https://doi.org/10.1016/s0142-9612(02)00318-6.

Varma, H. K., Yokogawa, Y., Espinosa, F. F., Kawamoto, Y., Nishizawa, K., Nagata, F., & Kameyama, T. (1999). Porous calcium phosphate coating over phosphorylated chitosan film by a biomimetic method. *Biomaterials*, *20*(9), 879–884. Available from https://doi.org/10.1016/S0142-9612(98)00243-9.

Wang, X., Yu, T., Chen, G., Zou, J., Li, J., & Yan, J. (2017). Preparation and characterization of a chitosan/gelatin/extracellular matrix scaffold and its application in tissue engineering. *Tissue Engineering Part C: Methods*, *23*(3), 169–179. Available from https://doi.org/10.1089/ten.tec.2016.0511.

Weiner, S., & Addadi, L. (1997). Design strategies in mineralized biological materials. *Journal of Materials Chemistry*, 7(5), 689–702. Available from https://doi.org/10.1039/a604512j, 09599428.

Wernike, E., Hofstetter, W., Liu, Y., Wu, G., Sebald, H. J., Wismeijer, D., Hunziker, E. B., Siebenrock, K. A., & Klenke, F. M. (2010). Long-term cell-mediated protein release from calcium phosphate ceramics. *Journal of Biomedical Materials Research – Part A*, *92*(2), 463–474. Available from https://doi.org/10.1002/jbm.a.32411Switzerland, 15524965, http://www3.interscience.wiley.com/cgi-bin/fulltext/121677406/PDFSTART.

Wu, G., Liu, Y., Iizuka, T., & Hunziker, E. B. (2008). *BMP-2-functionalized polymers for bone engineering: the influence of polymer geometry on biomimetic coating with a layer of calcium phosphate and on osteogenic potential. World Biomaterials Congress.* World Biomaterials Congress.

Xia, Y., Sun, J., Zhao, L., Zhang, F., Liang, X. J., Guo, Y., Weir, M. D., Reynolds, M. A., Gu, N., & Xu, H. H. K. (2018). Magnetic field and nano-scaffolds with stem cells to enhance bone regeneration, Elsevier Ltd, China*Biomaterials, 183*, 151–170. Available from http://www.journals.elsevier.com/biomaterials/.

Xiao, W., Zaeem, M. A., Bal, B. S., & Rahaman, M. N. (2016). Creation of bioactive glass (13–93) scaffolds for structural bone repair using a combined finite element modeling and rapid prototyping approach. *Materials Science and Engineering C, 68*, 651–662. Available from https://doi.org/10.1016/j.msec.2016.06.011, 09284931.

Xin, R., Leng, Y., Chen, J., & Zhang, Q. (2005). A comparative study of calcium phosphate formation on bioceramics in vitro and in vivo. *Biomaterials, 26*(33), 6477–6486. Available from https://doi.org/10.1016/j.biomaterials.2005.04.028.

Xue, N., Ding, X., Huang, R., Jiang, R., Huang, H., Pan, X., Min, W., Chen, J., Duan, J.-A., Liu, P., et al. (2022). Bone tissue engineering in the treatment of bone defects. *Pharmaceuticals*. Available from https://doi.org/10.3390/ph15070879.

Ye, B., Wu, B., Su, Y., Sun, T., & Guo, X. (2022). Recent advances in the application of natural and synthetic polymer-based scaffolds in musculoskeletal regeneration. *Polymers*.

Yin, Y. J., Luo, X. Y., Cui, J. F., Wang, C. Y., Guo, X. M., & Yao, K. D. (2004). A study on biomineralization behavior of N-methylene phosphochitosan scaffolds. *Macromolecular Bioscience, 4*(10), 971–977. Available from https://doi.org/10.1002/mabi.200400063.

Zhou, G., Chang, W., Zhou, X., Chen, Y., Dai, F., Anwar, A., & Yu, X. (2020). nanofibrous nerve conduits with nerve growth factors and bone marrow stromal cells precultured in bioreactors for peripheral nerve regeneration. *ACS Applied Materials & Interfaces, 12*(14), 16168–16177. Available from https://doi.org/10.1021/acsami.0c04191.

CHAPTER 8

Biomimetic coatings for drug delivery

Tejas Girish Agnihotri*, Shyam Sudhakar Gomte*, Vasu Peddinti*, Biswajit Rout* and Aakanchha Jain*
Department of Pharmaceutics, National Institute of Pharmaceutical Education and Research (NIPER)-Ahmedabad, Gandhinagar, Gujarat, India

8.1 Introduction

The word "biomimetics" was coined by Otto Schmitt in the year 1957. He used this terminology under the purview of biophysical science. Biomimesis, biomimicry, biologically inspired design, and biognosis are some of the interchangeable terms for biomimetics; however, biomimetics is the most sought-after terminology used in a wide range of therapeutic applications (Sheikhpour et al., 2017; Vincent, 2009). In the recent past, scientists have unearthed a comprehensive understanding of biological systems at a cellular and molecular level which provided a propelling force to the area of biomimetics. Today's drug delivery system (DDS) research is focused on targeted drug delivery, which can transport medications into the cytoplasm of specific cells sparing any healthy tissues or organs. The rise of nanotechnology enabled the prospect of drug encapsulation into nanocarriers. With the advent of nanotherapeutics, issues with insoluble pharmaceuticals, biodegradable therapeutic agents, and medications with high toxicity for biological systems were significantly alleviated (Vauthier & Labarre, 2008). Under the oncological field, nanotherapeutics showed promising effects in counteracting cancer with enhanced permeation and retention effect (EPR) taking a lead role. The circulation time of nanoparticles (NPs) can be effectively increased by the PEGylation of nanocarriers. Still, the degradation of drugs into lysosomes marred the capability of PEG coating to carry out cellular uptake (Amoozgar & Yeo, 2012; Mishra et al., 2016; Sheikhpour et al., 2017). Scientists have exercised varied solutions in the form of functionalization of PEGylated nanocarrier

*All the authors contributed equally to this work.

Smart Biomimetic Coatings
DOI: https://doi.org/10.1016/B978-0-443-21738-8.00008-4

systems by peptides, proteins, aptamers, vitamins, and other suitable ligands. As a result, biomimetics in targeted DDSs required surface modification with certain amino acids, polysaccharides, and lipids to establish inherent abilities in biomimetic drug carriers. To achieve this, it is necessary to pay close attention to the fundamental core materials, size, and form of drug carriers to imitate natural cells for cellular internalization. Based on the fundamental material, there are two primary categories of biomimetic drug carriers: the first one is existent biological entities such as inactivated viral vectors, and bacterium vectors, and the second is synthetic drug carriers, which are biomimetic-manufactured NPs with features comparable to biological materials. The latter closely resembles in vivo conditions (Sheikhpour et al., 2017).

There have been many literature reports outlining the studies pertaining to biomimetic processes, biomimetic surface engineering techniques, and nanocarrier systems with an aim to elicit sustained release of drugs and prolong the circulation time of nanocarriers in plasma while protecting from immune system activation (Vauthier & Labarre, 2008; Venkatesh et al., 2005; Yoo et al., 2011). In this chapter, the widespread applications of biomimetics in relation to drug delivery through different nanocarriers like dendrimers, polymeric micelles, NPs, liposomes, and hydrogels have been discussed (Fig. 8.1).

Different strategies of biomimetic coating have also been discussed with special emphasis on self-assembled, polysaccharide, and peptide-based

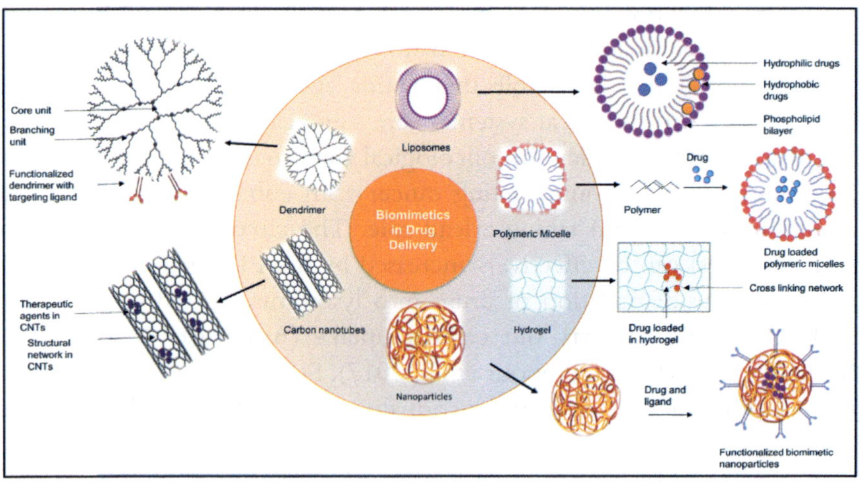

Figure 8.1 Overview of biomimetics in different nanocarriers.

coating in the subsequent sections. Some of the limitations pertaining to biomimetics have also been provided in short, at the end.

8.2 Biomimetics in drug delivery

In recent times, scientists mainly focuses on targeted drug delivery where they can directly transport the therapeutic agents into the cytoplasm of cells and prevents healthy cells or organs from adverse effects. With the advancements in nanotechnology, therapeutic agents can be easily loaded into nanocarriers and targeted delivery can be attained. Additionally, the difficulties faced by therapeutic agents like poor solubility and potential toxicity can be easily overcome by nanocarriers. Furthermore, the surface modification provides the delivery of NPs into the targeted site through the receptor-mediated endocytosis process and effective targeted drug delivery can be achieved (Ding et al., 2023). Thus biomimetics are specifically created for their abilities in advanced drug delivery by functional surface modification by lipids, saccharides, and amino acids. The entry of biomimetics in drug delivery helps to attain targeted drug delivery with reduced side effects (Amoozgar & Yeo, 2012; Choi et al., 2003; Hatakeyama et al., 2013; Mishra et al., 2016). The following section particularly talks about the biomimetics in combination with dendrimers, liposomes, metallic NPs, polymeric micelles, and hydrogel.

8.2.1 Biomimetic dendrimers

Dendrimers are derived from synthetic polymers presented in a tree shape which is a highly branched three-dimensional network of macromolecules that is employed for a particular purpose as drug delivery vehicles in DDSs. It consists of a spherical shape with continuous repeating units initiated from the central core. They are intricate structures containing well-defined size, shape, and molecular weight and several functional moieties are present on their exterior region that are beneficial for targeted drug delivery. In addition, they provide enhanced water solubility, biocompatibility, and bioavailability to therapeutic agents (Cheng et al., 2008; Garg et al., 2011; Tripathy & Das, 2013). Three major issues with dendrimers that are needed to be addressed before their biomedical applications include composition, charge, and a number of generations. Cationic dendrimer possesses more toxic effects than anionic or neutral dendrimers (Cordon et al., 2013). The structural surface modification can be done on dendrimers in their terminal region to fabricate the biomimetics for targeted drug delivery (Sheikhpour et al., 2017). Chawla et al. fabricated RofA (roflumilast analogue)-PAMAM-based dendrimer for enhanced sustained delivery. The RofA-laden dendrimer showed entrapment efficiency and loading at about 72% and 63%, respectively. The in vitro release study showed the sustained release behavior of the prepared formulation. The drug release kinetics showed a non-Fickian diffusion from the prepared dendrimer complex. In addition, RofA-laden dendrimer has enhanced solubility and increased antiinflammatory activity (Chawla et al., 2022). In another study, Lee et al. prepared hyaluronic acid (HA)-coated dendrimer-loaded gold NPs of doxorubicin (HA-AuDEN) for the treatment of ovarian cancer. The prepared formulation showed delayed release at pH 7.4 and exhibited burst release in the acidic environment at pH 5.6 in the presence of glutathione (GSH). Also, the formulation showed increased cellular uptake with IC_{50} of 2.72 μM. The in vivo antitumor activity and biodistribution study was done on the SK-OV-3 xenograft tumor-bearing mouse model and found enhanced tumor growth inhibition and reduced cardiotoxic effects (Lee et al., 2022). Moreover, Hashemi et al. prepared dendrimers based on 1,3,5-benzenetricarbonyl trichloride and citric acid as a core to alter the graphene oxide (GO) surface. Further, green fluorescence was added to the prepared dendrimers to detect the possible interaction between tumor cells and healthy cell lines. The fabricated dendrimers were characterized by several characterization techniques such as scanning electron microscopy (SEM), transmission electron microscopy (TEM), X ray diffraction (XRD), ultraviolet (UV), dynamic light scattering (DLS), atomic force microscopy (AFM), and Raman spectroscopy. It was observed from the experiments that it showed no emission in the UV lamp and conversely showed green fluorescence at 471 nm due to its functionalization. The drug release from the prepared formulation showed pH-dependent release with enhanced drug release in an acidic environment. So, graphene oxide—functionalized dendrimer helps to release the drug in an efficient manner and can be used as a potential candidate for the delivery of various therapeutic agents (Hashemi & Namazi, 2021). Additionally, Yandrapu et al. developed thiolated dendrimers for the controlled drug delivery of acyclovir. Initially, thiolated dendrimers were prepared by conjugation of PAMAM with cysteamine with various molar ratios. The acyclovir-laden dendrimer showed sustained release behavior with enhanced mucoadhesive strength. It can be a potential mucoadhesive carrier for the delivery of different agents (Yandrapu et al., 2013). In another study, Oledzka et al. fabricated

PAMAM dendrimer loaded with camptothecin for the management of cancer. The in vitro drug release suggests the controlled drug release with greater than 80% of drug release in 7 days. It showed higher anticancer activity against non–small-cell lung cancer (A549) cell lines. PAMAM dendrimers can be a potential carrier system for the delivery of anticancer agents (Oledzka et al., 2023). In one of the research studies, in other instance, Jia et al. developed PAMAM dendrimers for the transdermal delivery of non steroidal antiinflammatory drugs (NSAIDs) like diflunisal and ketoprofen. The in vitro skin permeation studies with rat skin suggests that PAMAM dendrimers effectively increased the permeation of both drugs in 24 hours as compared to free drugs. Moreover, bioavailability of ketoprofen and diflunisal was significantly improved in dendrimer complex as compared to free drug suspension. It was found that dendrimer helped to enhance the penetration of drugs through skin barrier and can be beneficial for the development of novel transdermal formulations (Jia et al., 2011).

8.2.2 Biomimetic metallic nanoparticles

Nonspecific drugs have the potential to impact healthy cells in addition to the intended site of disease. Consequently, the creation of appropriate carriers that might improve the effectiveness of therapy at particular locations and decrease resistance to medications by augmenting the concentration of drugs at the designated sites to attain elevated targeted efficiency and minimal overall toxicity is an essential requirement. In this particular scenario, the utilization of targeted drugs has garnered the interest of researchers and has resulted in significant advancements. According to recent research, NPs have significant aptitude as carriers for drugs. This is due to their tiny size and distinctive physical and chemical properties, which render these individuals desirable materials for medical use (Wilczewska et al., 2012). In contemporary times, various types of NPs such as solid lipid NPs, liposomes, polymeric NPs, biomimetic NPs, and metallic NPs have been extensively utilized as DDSs (Jin et al., 2018). Cell membrane-coated NPs possess a plethora of source cell-specific functionalities such as "self" markers, immune system communication, natural targeting, and target tracking to specific regions. These attributes allow for the acquisition of desirable traits such as enhanced biocompatibility, reduced immunogenicity, extended circulation, and targeted tumor localization. As a result, they are utilized with precision for drug delivery

(Niu et al., 2022). At present, the prevailing cell membranes utilized to elicit biomimetic characteristics in a DDS encompass membranes derived from erythrocytes, leukocytes, platelets, stem cells, cancer cells, and hybrid membranes (Guo et al., 2021).

Platelets are short-lived, nucleus-free components of the blood that originate from megakaryocytes. Their life span ranges from 5 to 7 days only. Regulations of hemostasis and thrombosis are the two main functions of platelets in addition to their participation in the immune system, regulation of tumor growth, and extravasation of blood vesicles (Holinstat, 2017). Platelets have a complex surface membrane that contains several active moieties that enable them to interact with a variety of moieties. These moieties provide the platelets the ability to interact with several substrates. Platelets, for instance, express CD47, which is a cell surface glycoprotein that binds to a signal-regulatory protein. As a consequence of this binding, the phagocytosis of platelets by dendritic cells and macrophages is reduced. This enables platelets to remain in circulation for a long period of time (Olsson et al., 2005). Platelets also contain a protein called glycoprotein Ib (GPIb), which is a membrane protein that has the ability to bind directly to harmful microbes. As a consequence of this, platelet aggregation takes place as a component of the host's response to the removal of the bacteria (Cruz et al., 2005). Similar to erythrocytes, platelets are diminutive cells lacking a nucleus, thereby facilitating their retrieval (Zhang, Zhao, et al., 2022). The extensive biointerfacing abilities exhibited by platelets have served as a source of inspiration for the creation of drug carriers that emulate platelets and selectively deliver drug payloads to afflicted areas, thereby augmenting the therapeutic effectiveness of the treatment (Wang et al., 2020). Rao et al. prepared gold nanorods that were camouflaged with platelet membranes. These biomimetic NPs showed excellent photothermal properties due to the presence of gold NPs, whereas the presence of platelet membrane provided these NPs with an effective tumor-targeting ability and prolonged their blood circulation time. This biomimetic system also demonstrated a unique property that improved photothermal therapy in a feedback manner by recruiting more and more membrane-coated gold nanorods at the tumor site (Rao et al., 2018). For the treatment of head-and-neck squamous cell carcinoma, Bu et al. developed a unique metal oxide (Fe_3O_4) NP that was covered with a hybrid membrane composed of cancer stem cells and palate cells. The biomimetic NP was utilized for photothermal therapy in addition to having magnetically active properties. NPs exhibited immune evasion properties as a result of the inclusion of platelet membranes, whereas the inclusion of stem cell membranes caused them to more effectively aggregate in tumor sites (Bu et al., 2019).

Biomimetic NPs have recently gained significant attention among researchers due to their ability to mimic the body's natural circulation, specifically through the use of a "camouflage" technique utilizing red blood cell membranes (RBCMs). Through the implementation of a bionic approach, NPs are able to attain inconspicuous properties within an organism by utilizing RBCMs to isolate the particle from its surroundings. This mechanism effectively circumvents macrophage recognition, thereby prolonging the particle's life span within the bloodstream (Zhang, Zhao, et al., 2022). A group of researchers developed a biomimetic nanoreactor that implemented starvation-activated therapy for the treatment of colon cancer. The preparation of the nanoreactor involved the encapsulation of glucose oxidase and the prodrug tirapazamine within a metal-organic NP that was subsequently coated with an erythrocyte membrane. The reactor demonstrated a high level of efficacy in inducing apoptosis of cancerous cells through targeted delivery of glucose oxidase enzyme and anticancer medication. The inclusion of erythrocyte coating facilitated enhanced evasion of the immune system by the nanocarriers, leading to a prolonged retention period within the organism. The induction of hypoxia due to glucose oxidase facilitated the conversion of tirapazamine into its activated state (Zhang et al., 2018). Qiao et al. conducted a study wherein they prepared a biomimetic nanodrug using a metal-organic framework (MOF) that was camouflaged by an erythrocyte membrane. The metallic nanocarriers were utilized to encapsulate drugs such as doxorubicin and transforming growth factor β-receptor inhibitors. The NPs were observed to accumulate effectively within the cancerous region and exhibit an extended circulation time, owing to the presence of a biomimetic erythrocyte coating that enables them to evade the immune system. The β-receptor inhibitors were found to mitigate the hypoxic state of the cancerous environment, thereby hindering the development of drug resistance induced by hypoxia. The utilization of biomimetic metallic NPs coated with erythrocyte membrane is a potentially effective approach for treating cancers that exhibit chemoresistance (Qiao et al., 2022).

In 2020 a group of researchers developed zeolitic imidazolate framework, a type of MOF, which was cloaked with a cell membrane. This system was utilized for the purpose of enzyme delivery. To assess the pliability of the methodology, various cellular membranes, such as RBCs and macrophages, were employed to envelop the MOF, thereby conferring upon it the biomimetic attribute. Utilization of biomimetic MOFs was employed for the purpose of encapsulating the urease enzyme within its structure. The effectiveness of the biomimetic carriers was subsequently investigated through the utilization of various animal models. The study revealed that formulations coated with RBC membrane were efficacious in significantly reducing serum uric acid levels. Conversely, formulations coated with macrophages exhibited the ability to neutralize inflammatory cytokines and acted in synergy with uricase to decrease insoluble uric acid concentrations in the local inflammatory site. The researchers have deduced from their investigation that the incorporation of a biomimetic coating into the nanoformulation results in enhanced biocompatibility and stability. Additionally, the coating serves to safeguard and maintain enzymatic activity. As such, this approach presents a promising opportunity to enhance the efficacy of enzyme-based treatments for various medical ailments (Zhuang et al., 2020).

In recent years, the escalating incidence of infection provoked by drug-resistant bacteria has made it crucial to come up with a novel, targeted DDS that is tailored to these pathogens. With the aforementioned consideration in mind, Wang et al. came up with a novel biomimetic metallic gold–silver nanocage that was enclosed by bacterial pretreated macrophage. This innovative approach facilitates the targeted transportation of photothermally active metallic NPs to the site of infection. The primary role of macrophages is to identify microbial infections through the expression of specific receptors, such as toll-like receptors, which have a propensity to bind to microbes. The biomimetic system was prepared by initially subjecting macrophages to specific bacteria, which resulted in the overexpression of specific pathogen receptors on macrophage membranes (MMs). Subsequently, the MMs were employed to encapsulate the nanocages. The camouflaged metallic nanocages exhibited a remarkable ability to precisely target bacteria. The metallic nanocage exhibited the capacity to produce elevated temperatures upon exposure to near-infrared radiation, thereby inducing photothermal injury to the microorganisms. The authors of the study also demonstrated that the hollow configuration of the metallic nanocage could be effectively employed for the targeted delivery of an antibacterial agent to the site of infection in a regulated fashion (Wang et al., 2018).

In contrast to conventional techniques for NP coating with cell membranes, a group of researchers fabricated a biomimetic gold NPs (Au-NPs) through the conjugation of an arginine–glycine–aspartate (RGD) peptide, which was derived from an extracellular matrix (ECM) protein. The study described the development of novel NPs with the aim to induce the differentiation of human mesenchymal stem cells (hMSCs) and promote the formation of chondrocytes and cartilage tissues. The inclusion of RGD peptide facilitated the ability of the metallic NPs to imitate the ECM. Additionally, it streamlined their internalization into hMSCs through integrin-mediated endocytosis. The present investigation embodies an exemplary approach for the production of biomimetic NPs aimed at modulating cellular proliferation. The novel biomimetic NPs exhibit significant potential for utilization across a wide range of fields, including, but not limited to, biomedical applications and tissue engineering (Li et al., 2017).

8.2.3 Biomimetic polymeric micelles

Polymeric micelles are defined as self-assembled nanocarriers that form in a liquid matrix composed of amphiphilic macromolecules. These macromolecules are generally composed of di- or tri-block copolymers having both hydrophilic and hydrophobic blocks (Chaudhuri et al., 2022). The chemical composition of block copolymers in micelles allows for the design or changes of physicochemical properties of encapsulated drugs, the pathophysiology of disease, and individual drug release pathways in specific sites. Additionally, the chemical structure of the core might be adjusted to improve drug encapsulation, increase the stability of micelles, and control the amount of drug released from polymeric micelles (Aliabadi & Lavasanifar, 2006; Sheikhpour et al., 2017; Xu et al., 2005). Polymeric micelles have received a lot of interest in the field of therapy and diagnosis for their ability to transport therapeutic and/or diagnostic agents such as low-molecular-weight compounds, DNA, RNA, peptides, or contrast/imaging agents effectively. They have several advantages over other carriers in terms of physicochemical and biological properties, such as nanoscale size for drug delivery, hydrophobic core-hydrophilic shell structure for loading water-insoluble drugs, sustained or controlled release, and targeting to specific sites in vivo (Kedar et al., 2010; Miyata et al., 2011). To avoid unfavorable biological responses to polymeric micelles, a biocompatible hydrophilic shell reducing nonspecific interactions with biological components is required, which is commonly composed of PEG due to its nontoxicity, low immunogenicity, and tightly bound water layer. However, some unfavorable biological reactions to PEGylation have lately been described and PEGylation may also limit nanocarrier binding and uptake into target cells. To avoid problems associated with PEGylation, biomimicking polymeric micelles were preferred due to their great biocompatibility and excellent potential for therapeutic applications (Wu et al., 2014). Hu et al. designed redox-sensitive polymeric micelles with aggregation-induced emission imaging as an excellent anticancer drug carrier system for concurrent chemotherapy and biological imaging. The amphiphilic copolymer (TPE-SS-PLAsp-*b*-PMPC) used in the method could self-assemble into spherical micelles, and these biomimetic micelles showed high biocompatibility and excellent antiprotein adsorption capabilities, indicating a high potential for biomedical applications. The anticancer drug doxorubicin (DOX) could be encapsulated during the self-assembly process, and these drug-loaded micelles demonstrated intelligent drug release and increased antitumor activity due to the rapid disintegration in reaction to high levels of GSH in the environment. Additionally, fluorescence imaging of these AIE micelles enabled the detection of intracellular DOX release. The in vivo anticancer study showed that the drug-loaded micelles showed better anticancer activity and less toxic effects compared to the free drug. These findings made it clear that this intelligent biomimetic micelle system would be an excellent candidate for chemotherapy and bioimaging (Hu et al., 2018). Lymph nodes have been identified as a promising target for cancer immunotherapy, because cellular immunity is essential for cancer vaccines to be effective. The effectiveness of vaccines in eliciting anticancer immune responses is limited by the ineffective delivery of vaccines to lymph nodes and the inadequate lysosomal escape of antigens. To increase antitumor immune response, Yang et al. prepared dendritic cell membrane/histidine-modified stearic acid-grafted chitosan (HCtSA)/ovaalbumin (OVA) micelles, as pH-responsive mimicking vaccines to target lymph nodes and induce cell-mediated immunity. The prepared micelles showed pH-dependent antigen release and accumulation of micelles in the lymph nodes resulted in increased uptake by dendritic cells. Importantly, produced micelles enhanced the release of antitumor-related cytokines and significantly reduced tumor development in addition to inducing strong T-cell immunological responses. Overall, biomimetic micelles showed significant promise for targeted immunotherapy (Yang et al., 2020).

In another instance, Jang et al. developed a mixture of deoxycholic acid (DA3) and low-molecular-weight polyethyleneimine (PEI 1.8 kDa), which has a property that resembles that of cell-penetrating peptides, for the concurrent administration of an anticancer drug and siRNA. The conjugate has the ability to form a micelle-like core–shell structure that allows them to encapsulate and dissolve the water-insoluble drug paclitaxel (PTX). The cationic micelles that have been drug-loaded can then interact with siRNA to produce stable complexes (PTX/DA3/siRNA). The PTX/DA3/siRNA showed a considerable decrease of tumor growth when it was administered to mice with tumors, indicating potential clinical utility (Jang et al., 2012). Liu et al. used biodegradable PBLG as a hydrophobic core and biomimetic PMPC as a hydrophilic shell to prepare polymeric micelles. Anticancer drugs like doxorubicin (DOX) could be encapsulated into the micelle through hydrophobic interactions. Due to the EPR effect, these drug-loaded micelles displayed greater tumor-specific accumulation in breast cancer mouse models than free drugs, which improved therapeutic efficacy, decreased systemic toxicity, and promoted apoptosis in tumor tissues. The in vivo results showed that these biomimetic polymeric micelles would be an effective strategy for the treatment of systemic cancer treatment (Liu et al., 2016).

The hemocompatibility of stimuli-responsive nanocarriers such as polymeric micelles that self-assemble from amphiphilic copolymers containing amino groups has been known to compromise by the positive charge induced by the amino group which can have a considerable impact on the blood components. To address this issue, Lin et al. came up with a biomimetic phosphorylcholine strategy to enhance the hemocompatibility of the positively charged micelles which are stimuli responsive. To produce self-assembling, pH-responsive phosphorylcholine micelles that are bio-imitated, amphiphilic copolymers with varying numbers of tertiary amino groups were used. These micelles had no noticeable impact on RBCs, coagulation, or platelet activation. Additionally, the prepared micelles showed less adsorption of albumin on their surface along with a very less extent of phagocytosis. Results showed that this biomimetic phosphorylcholine is an effective way for enhancing the positively charged nanocarriers' hemocompatibility (Lin et al., 2019). A major cause of renal failure in its final stages is glomerulonephritis. The two important factors that contribute to glomerulonephritis include the increasing number of mesangial cells and the infiltration of macrophages. To resolve this, Zhang et al. formulated novel biomimetic pH-sensitive nanomicelles (MM/HA-DXM) for treating glomerulonephritis. Due to the coating with MM, these nanomicelles could avoid RES phagocytosis and then, as a result of an active homing effect, be drawn to an inflammatory glomerulus. The weakly acidic glomerulonephritis milieu subsequently broke nanomicelles and released HA and dexamethasone (DXM) locally. HA converted M1 macrophages to M2 macrophages which are antiinflammatory in nature. On the other side, DXM prevented an increasing number of mesangial cells. Additionally, in vivo results showed decreased proteinuria levels when treated with the prepared nanomicelles indicating excellent therapeutic efficacy on glomerulonephritis (Zhang, He, et al., 2022). Wu et al. formulated a new biomimetic nanomicelles deoxycholic acid—phosphorylcholine—chitosan conjugate (DCA—PCCs) using Atherton—Todd reaction. In vitro results showed low toxicity to NIH/3T3 mouse embryonic fibroblasts and excellent hemocompatibility. Quercetin was used as a model drug to study drug loading and release studies from the prepared nano-sized micelles. Results showed that nanomicelles could serve as a potential nanocarrier to deliver hydrophobic medications without triggering adverse biological reactions (Wu et al., 2014). Glucosamine and cholic acid, which are of natural origin, were used to prepare amphiphilic block polymers. Zhang et al. prepared three types of diblock copolymers, which consisted of glucosamine and cholic acid and have varying hydrophilic and hydrophobic chain lengths. The prepared block polymers showed the ability of self-assembly to form polymeric micelles consisting of a bile acid core, which is bitter in nature, and a sweet sugar shell. The prepared micelles improved the solubility of hydrophobic drugs rendering them less toxic (Zhang et al., 2017).

8.2.4 Biomimetic liposomes

Liposomes can be defined as spherical, self-assembled phospholipid bilayer structures with a diameter ranging from 100 to 250 nm. Owing to their biocompatibility, biodegradability, and their unique structure, both types of drugs, hydrophilic as well as hydrophobic drugs can be incorporated into liposomes with a greater payload (Agnihotri et al., 2023; Liu, Chen, et al., 2022; Rommasi & Esfandiari, 2021). The bilayer is responsible for protecting drugs from enzymatic degradation and chemical degradation in vivo. Depending on the number of bilayers and size of liposomes, they can be divided into unilamellar vesicles and multilamellar vesicles. Liposomes can also be differentiated based on the lipid content, surface charge, and method of preparation. Targeted specific liposomes can be formulated as biomimetic ones by conjugating ligands or moieties, especially in the oncological field. This could further ease the process of intracellular uptake of drugs in a controlled fashion either actively or passively (Gong et al., 2023). There have been numerous instances where biomimetic liposomes were developed specifically to target cancer and related diseases.

Pitchaimani et al. formulated a modified liposome DDS called NKsome with natural killer (NK) cell–ghost interaction, which can undergo a natural immune response in the treatment of cancer. NK cell, a major component of the innate immunity system, is chiefly responsible for eliciting defense against microbial infections and acts like immunosurveillance mediators. NK cells also take a major role in cytotoxicity either by releasing perforins and granzymes or by death receptor-mediated apoptosis. In this study, doxorubicin was incorporated into NKsome and was found to be efficient targeted delivery with enhanced anticancer activity seen in MCF7 cells induced in vivo model (Pitchaimani et al., 2018). On a similar note, a dual-targeted biomimetic liposomal system was developed with the incorporation of paclitaxel and DNA in HA and folic acid-conjugated liposomes. The formulated system was superior on B16 cells in terms of transfection efficiency, cellular uptake, and protection from degradation by DNAse-I (Liu et al., 2014). Cell-surface glycan dynamics are engaged in a variety of physiologic and pathological activities, including oncogenesis and metastasis. In spite of huge efforts, distinguishing and labeling glycans from distinct cancer cells or cancer subtypes remain a significant difficulty. The scientists were able to formulate pH-responsive azidosugar liposomes disguised with natural cancer-cell membranes for tumor cell-selective glycan engineering using a biomimetic cell membrane-coating technique. Biomimetic liposomes with cancer cell -membrane camouflage were able to inhibit protein corona formation and elude macrophage phagocytosis, allowing metabolic glycans labeling in vivo (Liu, Chen, et al., 2022). Breast cancer metastasis has plagued society to the extent that the 5-year survival rate was found to be only 20%. Nano-DDS could target tumor regions in an attempt to mitigate the spread of cancer through a well-known process called the EPR effect (Agnihotri et al., 2022; Janrao et al., 2022). However, due to the lower size and poor vasculature of the metastatic lesion, nanotherapeutics often fail short to curb the metastasis process. Cao et al. made use of macrophages as a biomimetic coating over liposomal surfaces containing a drug. The coating of the MM facilitated the cellular uptake process of liposomes containing emtansine. In vitro study on 4T1 cells and in vivo study on lung metastasis mice models corroborated the potential of macrophage-coated liposomes in the treatment of breast cancer metastasis to the lungs (Cao et al., 2016). Gao et al. prepared polyelectrolyte microcapsules based on the layer-by-layer (LBL) technique and further, it was coated with biotinylated PEGylated liposomes. This system was proved to be resistant to protein binding thereby eliciting targeted action with an increased tendency of binding to neutravidin and acting like an artificial cellular structure under the biomimetic liposomal category (Gao et al., 2011). In other instance, glycocalyx-mimicking liposomes were formulated with PEG as a spacer which was attached to two hydrophobic tails. The system was intended for prolonging circulation time and eliciting tissue-targeted delivery. The prepared liposomes were similar in structure to the P-selectin glycoprotein ligand present on WBCs with a view of binding liposomes to P-selectin receptors which are present on blood platelets. Overall, in vitro findings suggested the key potential of formulated biomimetic liposomes in treating cardiovascular injuries (Zhu et al., 2007). In rheumatoid arthritis, synovial fibroblasts perform a key role in inducing inflammation for which activation of NF-κB signaling is also responsible. You et al. formulated liposomal delivery system wherein, NF-κB inhibitory peptide (NBD) was encapsulated and further coated with HAP-1 peptide. HAP-1 peptide is known for targeting synovial fibroblasts thereby inhibiting NF-κB signaling while NEMO binding domain (NBD) peptide binds to NEMO domain and disrupts IκB kinase complex formation. Through in vitro and in vivo findings, it was found that the liposomal system was successful in inhibiting NF-κB activation further reducing cytokine release, thus alleviating synovial inflammation and could be a viable alternative for arthritis treatment (You et al., 2018). In another instance, scientists investigated a liposomal delivery system with a novel peptide, ART-1 which can address inflammatory actions seen in rheumatoid arthritis. ART-1 was already found to specifically target synovial endothelial cells in arthritic rats. In this study, scientists compared in vitro and in vivo findings for ART-1 coated and uncoated liposomal systems. Further ART-1 coated liposomes encapsulated with IL-27 were also formulated and tested similarly. The findings demonstrated that ART-1 coated IL-27 encapsulated liposomes were superior in terms of targeting and inhibitory effects (Han et al., 2021). In an interesting study conducted by Wu et al., liposomes were functionalized with a stem cell membrane and curcumin was incorporated inside. The biomimetic vesicles had a controlled release, higher stability, and a longer circulation time. Curcumin loading improved the survival rate of ischemic stroke mice with a single shot (from 30% to over 90%). The worldwide method's adaptability was demonstrated by the alteration of differentially charged liposomes and the creation of erythrocyte membrane-derived vesicles. Overall, the cell membrane-derived biomimetic vesicles enabled targeted distribution and adaptability through a simple technique and easy fabrication (Wu et al., 2020). To counteract the problems of inadequate cell-specific targeting and suboptimal drug levels at the targeted site, Ferguson et al. came up with an innovative concept called dual affinity to RBCs and target cells (DART) wherein liposomes were conjugated to two ligands, one with affinity to RBCs and other to target cells (pulmonary endothelial cells). DART liposomes were initially bound with RBCs and then transferred to endothelial cells in the target organ when the bound RBCs squeeze through capillaries. The findings showed 70% injected dose (ID) of DART liposomes accumulated in the lungs within minutes of intravascular (i.v.) injection in mice, which was more than thrice the% ID ceiling reached by a variety of earlier technologies. This behavior was replicated by humanized DART liposomes in ex vivo perfused human lungs. Furthermore, DART improved delivery selectivity to target endothelial cells over local phagocytes within the target organ by a factor of six. DART's significant increase in organ- and cell-type targeting may thus be useful in localizing medications for a variety of medicinal purposes (Ferguson et al., 2022). Microbes like bacteria and fungi are known to produce exotoxins and endotoxins which can render severe infection by disrupting immunity of persons. To neutralize these toxins, various nanostructured decoys have been developed which can mimick lipid cell membrane. On a similar ground, Henry et al. formulated liposomal system which consisted of sphingomyelin and high amount of cholesterol which could absorb toxins produced by bacteria and alpha-hemolysin. These liposomes were also found to have sequestering role of toxins which were produced by *staphyllococci* and *streptococci*. Liposomes were found to improve septicemia on i.v. administration to mice, while on intransal administration, they also protected mice from pneumonia caused by *S. pneumoniae* serotype 2 (Henry et al., 2015).

In conclusion, the biomimetic alteration of the liposomes, as well as biomimetic techniques of liposomes formulation, improved the therapeutic ability of liposomes in terms of targeting drug delivery. The two prime limitations of liposomes, that is, the limited stability of drug-loaded carriers against enzyme degradation and the premature release of encapsulated drugs before they reach target cells, can be potentially addressed by biomimetic liposomes.

8.2.5 Biomimetic hydrogels

Hydrogels are three-dimensional structures made of water-loving polymers that have the capability of entrapping large quantities of water inside of them. These structures are known as hydrogels. These components may have either natural or synthetic origins, depending on the applications. In addition, hydrogels are able to maintain their shape due to the fact that they have a tendency to absorb a significant amount of water (Lin & Metters, 2006). The hydrogel matrix can be altered to exhibit distinct characteristics that enable swift and reversible reactions to diverse physiochemical stimuli, rendering it suitable for the continuous and controlled dispensation of medication for an extended duration. The aforementioned characteristic renders them advantageous for the transportation of biomolecules (Lin & Metters, 2006). Contemporary studies have been primarily centered on the development of biomimetic hydrogels with the objective of augmenting the biological efficacy of artificial hydrogels in the capacity of scaffolds for tissue manipulation. These hydrogels are designed to imitate the ECM. The goal is to improve unique cell responses and facilitate the healing of tissues. Mimicry can manifest itself through either physical or chemical methods. The concept of physical imitation involves the replication of the structural and mechanical characteristics of the ECM. This matrix plays a crucial role in facilitating cell morphology. The concept of chemical mimicry involves the integration of bioactive compounds into hydrogel matrices, a process that plays a pivotal role in facilitating the binding of protein and subsequent signal transduction pathways (Zhu et al., 2013). In recent years, advancements have been made in the development and production of biomimetic hydrogels for use as scaffolds in different types of tissue engineering, especially bone and cartilage tissue engineering.

Bone and cartilage damage may arise due to various factors, including, but not limited to, trauma, rheumatism, and damages related to sports activities (Ren et al., 2015). According to reports, a substantial number of patients who undergo knee arthroscopy have some cartilage-related defects. Additionally, around 15% of individuals who are over 60 show symptoms of this kind of damage. The regenerative capacity of damaged cartilage is restricted due to its deficient vascularization (Vilela et al., 2015).

Similarly, the healing of bone is often hindered by the limitations of frequently employed methods, like autografting and allografting, regardless of the extensive vascularization of the tissue (Tomlinson & Silva, 2013). Hence, the development of a technique that can effectively and durably restore impaired bone and cartilage cells is of notable clinical importance for individuals suffering from bone or cartilage defects.

Exosomes are nothing but single-membrane extracellular vesicles with a 30–150 nm size and are implicated in various diseases. Recent studies have indicated that paracrine discharge of exosomes derived from bone marrow mesenchymal stem cells (BMSC) possesses significant chondroprotective characteristics. Cheng et al. employed this observation in their research and synthesized a biomimetic hydrogel through the utilization of methacrylic acid and gelatine as precursor materials. The researchers utilized exosomes derived from BMSC and incorporated them into the biocompatible hydrogel. The hydrogel demonstrated exceptional capacity for carrying the exosomes, which can be attributed to its three-dimensional porous characteristics. The results of the in vitro examination demonstrated that the hydrogel exhibited biocompatibility and sustained exosome release, which consequently enhanced its effectiveness. The study demonstrated that the hydrogel matrix's DART's sustained release of exosomes resulted in an augmentation of chondrocyte proliferation and the synthesis of the cartilage ECM. Also, the hydrogel exhibited encouraging results in rat models with respect to cartilage regeneration. This study expands the therapeutic options available for the clinical management of patients suffering from cartilage injuries. A group of researchers prepared a biomimetic hydrogel for cartilage tissue repair. The product was developed by using the ECM of MSCs which had already undergone predifferentiation into chondrocytes. This injectable hydrogel was found to be biocompatible. Moreover, it was demonstrated that the hydrogel possessed the capability to stimulate chondrogenesis in MSCs and had the ability to generate tissue resembling hyaline cartilage after in vivo implantation. The study demonstrated the efficacy of hydrogel in the restoration and rejuvenation of cartilage. In yet another study, Jin and colleagues used HA, dextran, and tyramine as initial components to create a chondrocyte-incorporated biomimetic hydrogel. Studies on the biomimetic hydrogel for cartilage tissue engineering showed that it stimulated chondrocyte proliferation as well as glycosaminoglycan and collagen synthesis. As injectable scaffolds for cartilage tissue they, therefore, showed considerable promise. Paul and coworkers created a biodegradable and biocompatible hydrogel using nanosilicates. This hydrogel was found to promote the proliferation of human MSCs into the osteogenic lineage, without any help from additional osteo-inductive agents. The hydrogel was synthesized by integrating nanosilicates into a photo-crosslinked hydrogel composed of gelatine and methacrylate anhydride. The incorporation of nanosilicates resulted in a notable improvement in the osteogenic differentiation of human MSCs that were encapsulated. Moreover, this nanoengineered hydrogel exhibited elevated biocompatibility, ascertained through in vivo experimentation utilizing an immunocompetent rat model. The hydrogels also exhibited minimal localized immune responses, thereby demonstrating their potential for utilization in tissue engineering endeavors. In a study done by Shi et al., a bone mimetic hydrogel was prepared by using gelatine and methacrylic anhydride as starting materials. Along with nanosilicate and nanohydroxyapatite, the BMSC and nanohydroxyapatite were incorporated into the hydrogel. It was discovered that this injectable hydrogel was biocompatible, and its biomimicking capacity was owing to the presence of nanohydroxyapatite. Additionally, the presence of nanosilicate helped in giving optimal injectability and promoting osteogenesis, which amplified the osteogenic activity of MSC. It was discovered through in vivo research that stem cell-loaded hydrogel has remarkable bone healing capabilities. The use of this biomimetic hydrogel as a graft material for the repair of bone deformities is now under investigation.

Biomimetic hydrogel has also found applications in treating wound healing. The method of wound repair is a prevalent physiological phenomenon that involves a series of molecular occurrences subsequent to the emergence of a tissue injury, aimed at protecting the wound from the external environment. Hydrogels possess basic characteristics that facilitate the healing of injured tissue by providing a moist environment. This characteristic has been extensively studied in the context of wound management to promote autolytic debridement. Over the last few decades, a plethora of hydrogels has been created and adapted to correspond with the temporal progression of specific phases of wound healing (Fan et al., 2021). Zhang et al. were successful in their attempt to develop a novel biomimetic hydrogel for wound dressing purposes by making use of lignin and poly (ionic liquids). The self-healing capacity of the hydrogel can be attributed to the covalent link that exists between the lignin, which acts as an antioxidant, and the poly (ionic liquids), which has an action similar to that of an antibiotic. The researcher found that the hydrogel is mechanically stable which makes it ideal for use as a dressing agent. Besides that, it possesses several desirable features, including those that aid wound healing (Zhang et al., 2020). In a similar study, Liu et al. developed a biomimetic self-healing hydrogel by using carboxy chitosan, a nontoxic, biodegradable material, and polyethyl glycol (PEG) as a cross-linker. The novel hydrogel had a strain-stiffening property and could withstand excessive strain yet preserve its structural integrity. The study also showcased that the self-healing property of hydrogel was due to the presence of dynamic cross-linkage between chitosan and PEG which enabled the hydrogel to rebuild and regain its mechanical integrity after being damaged. The in vivo test showed that this biomimetic hydrogel had excellent wound-healing properties as well (Liu, Lin, et al., 2022). Table 8.1 represents the overview of biomimetic nanocarriers and their respective research findings.

8.3 Strategies for biomimetic coating in drug delivery

8.3.1 Polysaccharide-based coating

The increasing prevalence of bone defect cases presses an urgent need for the development of cost-effective bone tissue engineering technologies. Bone growth factors like bone morphogenetic protein-2 (BMP-2) are essential in bone tissue engineering. The dosage and route of administration of BMP-2 and other osteogenic factors further dictate the course of action in vivo. A modest dosage of BMP-2 delivered slowly and consistently enhances bone defect repair while the burst release of a large dosage of BMP-2 has negative local and systemic effects. The biomimetic calcium phosphate (BioCaP) coating process ensures that BMP-2 is released slowly, gradually, and locally, mimicking its natural release from the bone matrix under physiological circumstances. As a result, BioCaP coatings have long been thought to be a suitable medicinal carrier for growth factors (Lin et al., 2020). In bone tissue engineering, polymer-based scaffolds are widely employed materials for their physicochemical, functional, and structural properties. However, these materials lack osteoconductivity and inflammatory response may be seen in synthetic polymers which can hamper their utilization in the tissue engineering field. To counter this problem, Palaveniene and coworkers formulated a 3D naturally polymer-based scaffold using regenerated cellulose. Osteoconductive characteristic was achieved by immobilizing cuttlebone microparticles and subsequent coating by simulated body fluid in a concentrated form. Chemically, cuttlebone is

Table 8.1 Overview of biomimetic nanocarriers and respective research findings.

Sr. no.	Biomimetic nanocarrier	Therapeutic agent	Cell line study	Outcomes	References
1	PAMAM dendrimers-phosphorylcholine (PC)	Adriamycin (ADR)	–	Low cytotoxicity of PAMAM dendrimers & sustained delivery of ADR	Jia et al. (2011)
2	Macrophage membrane liposomes	Doxorubicin (DOX)	U87 GBM cell line	Treatment of GBM	Mendanha et al. (2023)
3	Biomimetic PLGA nanoparticles	All-trans retinoic acid (ATRA)	Murine macrophage cell line RAW264.7	Antifibrosis therapy	Xia et al. (2023)
4	Biomimetic nanoparticles	Indocyanine green (ICG) and NLG919 (an effective IDO-1 enzyme inhibitor)	–	Increased immunogenicity of the tumor through photothermal and increased the infiltration of cytotoxic T lymphocytes in the tumor, thus increasing the immunotherapy response.	Li et al. (2023)
5	Biomimetic pH-sensitive nanomicelles	Hyaluronic acid (HA)-dexamethasone (DXM)	Cell line HBZY-1 and RAW 264.7 macrophages	Treatment of glomerulonephritis	Zhang, He, et al. (2022)
6	Biomimetic micelles	Simvastatin	–	Atherosclerosis treatment	Shen et al. (2021)
7	Biomimetic micelles	Ovalbumin (OVA)	–	Enhanced immunotherapy	Yang et al. (2020)
8	Biomimetic hydrogel	Chondroitin sulfate and gelatin	–	Enhancing tissue regeneration	Nguyen et al. (2023)
9	Biomimetic hydrogel	Graphene oxide	–	Increased mechanical stability and lubrication in joint replacement	Hou et al. (2023)

composed of beta-chitin and macro, micro, and trace elements, which were required for mineralization. This coating facilitated cell attaching ability to scaffold by redepositing carbonate apatite crystallites on a scaffold. Further, in vitro study on osteoblast-like MG63 cells confirmed its potential use as a biomimetic coating for bone tissue engineering applications (Palaveniene et al., 2020). On a similar note, Zhou et al. developed a silk fibroin—chitosan—hydroxyapatite (SF—CS—nHA) bone scaffold which was biomimetic in nature and further modified it with a coating of polydopamine incorporating exosomes derived from BMSC (Fig. 8.2).

SF, obtained from silk was chosen to mimic type-I collagen in the bone while chitosan, which is similar to glycosaminoglycan in humans has been used for cell proliferation and adhesion. HA (nanometer scale) resembles carbonated nanocrystals in the human bone mineral structure. In this study, the physicochemical properties of this composite were investigated by SEM, contact angle test, and energy spectrum analysis (Fig. 8.3).

In vitro as well as in vivo study (rabbit radial defect model) was performed for the same. The findings confirmed that coated composite was superior to its control in terms of bone repair efficiency and new bone formation capability (in vivo findings) alongside osteogenic differentiation and proliferation of BMSC (in vitro findings). Thus it was concluded that the amalgamation of exosomes with polydopamine-coated biomimetic bone scaffold could be a better alternative for bone regeneration (Zhou, Deng, et al., 2023).

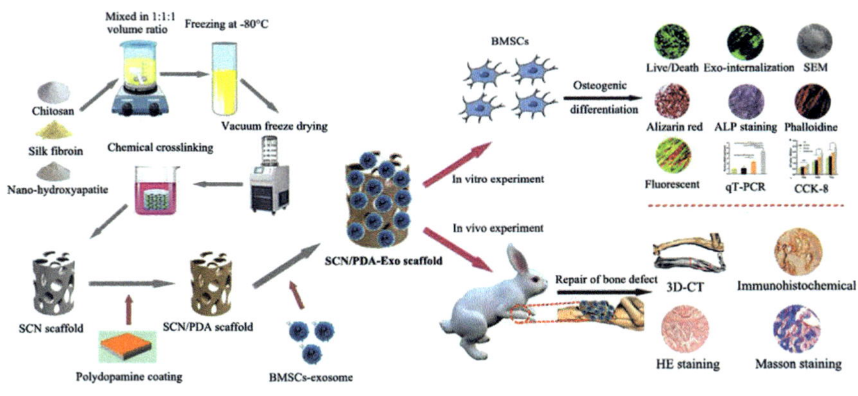

Figure 8.2 Schematic illustration of the study. *From Zhou, Y., Deng, G., She, H., Bai, F., Xiang, B., Zhou, J., & Zhang, S. (2023). Polydopamine-coated biomimetic bone scaffolds loaded with exosomes promote osteogenic differentiation of BMSC and bone regeneration.* Regenerative Therapy, *23, 25—36. https://doi.org/10.1016/j.reth.2023.03.005.*

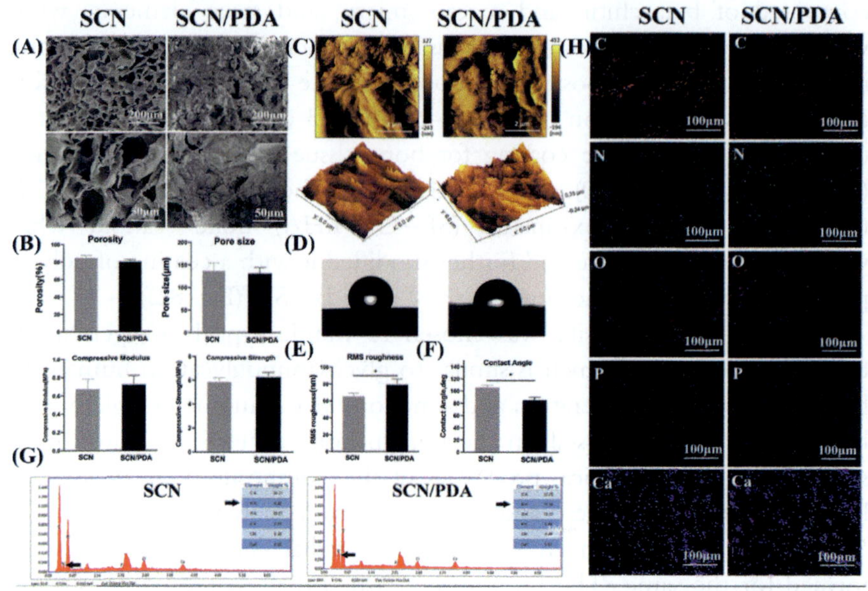

Figure 8.3 Scaffold characterization. (A) SEM image of the scaffold. (B) Relevant characterization parameters of the scaffold. (C and E) Surface roughness of the scaffold analyzed by AFM. (D and F) The scaffold surface hydrophilicity was measured by a contact angle tester. (G and H) EDS analysis of the scaffold. *AFM*, Atomic force microscopy; *EDS*, energy dispersive spectrometry; *SEM*, scanning electron microscopy. *From Zhou, Y., Deng, G., She, H., Bai, F., Xiang, B., Zhou, J., & Zhang, S. (2023). Polydopamine-coated biomimetic bone scaffolds loaded with exosomes promote osteogenic differentiation of BMSC and bone regeneration.* Regenerative Therapy, 23, *25–36. https://doi.org/10.1016/j.reth.2023.03.005.*

Polysaccharide-coated biomimetics has also found applications in skin tissue engineering. Along the same line, ECM mimetic scaffolds have attained significant attention, which can exemplify an interplay of cell-matrix communication, tissue modeling, and cellular equilibrium state. Singh and coworkers formulated in vitro skin scaffold wherein the system composed of biomimetic ECM was coated with carrageenan on electrospun nanofibers. Carrageenan, a natural algal polysaccharide, resembled with that of glucosaminoglycan, which is a component of human skin ECM while electrospun nanofibers serve the purpose of mimicking 3D topographic structure of ECM. Overall, the coated biomimetic system mediated a 3D microenvironment for the human skin ECM, facilitating the necessary growth, adhesion, proliferation, and infiltration of fibroblasts. Summarily, the research findings provided a viable and better approach for skin ECM scaffold having immense therapeutic implications in the skin tissue-engineering field (Singh et al., 2021).

The research into implant materials has been directed at developing biocompatible and antimicrobial materials which possess disinfection properties without activating immune response to microbes. Attempts have been made to prevent microbes' adhesion thereby breaking down the biofilm. One potential method for combating implant-associated biofilm infections is surface treatment with polyelectrolytes. Polyelectrolytes are charged polymers with ionizable groups connected to polymer chains that have a significant adsorption propensity on solid surfaces. Chitosan, due to its biodegradability, biocompatibility, and safer profile in humans has been widely used as an antimicrobial agent. Due to its polycationic nature, the positively charged NH_3 group disrupts microbial cellular membranes by interacting with negatively charged components in microbial cells. Chitosan and 77KS, a lysine-derived surfactant, generated polyelectrolyte complexes inverting their charge from positive to negative by increasing 77KS concentrations and resulting in amoxicillin-embedded aggregates. This complex dispersion was used to coat polydimethylsiloxane (PDMS) films, with an additional layer of anionic and hydrophilic HA to improve protein repulsion and antimicrobial activity. It was subjected to different analytical techniques like X-ray photoelectron spectroscopy, zeta potential measurement, and water contact angle measurement and confirmed the presence of two layers on PDMS film. The system showed better antifouling properties which were confirmed by adsorption experiments. The successful exploration of a formed system in terms of microbiological and biocompatibility testing, on silicon disks paved the way for developing stents, catheters, prostheses, etc. (Ajdnik et al., 2021). To address the problem of implant failure in orthopedic surgery, Liu et al. employed LBL self-assembled nanosheet coating over a hybrid implant which can specifically target WNT16, which is associated with glucocorticoid-induced osteopenia. To inhibit WNT16 signaling, laponite was used along with quaternized chitosan and HA as a coating solution. This facilitated hydrophilicity and provided optimum roughness. Through findings, it was also revealed that developed implant improved cell viability and osteogenic differentiation of BMSC with promising antibacterial effects on methicillin-resistant *Staphylococcus aureus* and *Escherichia coli in vitro* and in vivo (Liu et al., 2023). To treat inflammatory diseases, MSCs are one of the better alternatives due to their tissue-repairing properties and immunosuppressing nature, except for their potential to cause platelet aggregation during allogenic transplantation of MSCs hampering the clinical utility. To overcome the aforementioned problem, Rangasami et al. employed LBL coating approach with gelatin and heparin polymers having positive and negative charges, which could effectively complex with the glycocalyx of MSCs. This would further diminish thrombotic activation by suppressing complement induction. They also found that the biomimetic coating of MSCs was able to retain the immunosuppressing characteristics and differentiation properties of MSCs on exposure to inflammatory episodes (Rangasami et al., 2023).

8.3.2 Peptide-based coatings

Zein is a good protein-based pharmaceutical excipient that has undergone extensive study as a DDS carrier. The effective delivery of zein and in vivo applications are, however, constrained by its poor targeting ability. To improve homotypic target ability, Huang et al. prepared the B16 cancer cell membrane coated-zein biomimetic DDS by employing the coextrusion method. By using SDS-PAGE protein electrophoresis and AFM, it was demonstrated that the B16 cell membrane had been successfully coated. As a model drug, paclitaxel (PTX) was chosen. Cell cytotoxicity and migration experiments were used to examine the drug delivery efficiency of DDS. Qualitative and quantitative experiments were also used to assess the cellular uptake capacity and these studies showed that the prepared DDS has homologous targeting ability (Huang et al., 2023). Bai et al. prepared a biomimetic peptide which is having both muscle adhesion and osteogenic properties for regulating interfacial osteoclasts and osteoblasts under inflammation. The prepared peptide system was coated on titanium implants. In lipopolysaccharide (LPS)-induced systemic inflammatory conditions, the peptide-coated implants reduced inflammation and osteoclastogenesis thereby enhancing interfacial osteogenesis and osseointegration after implantation (Bai et al., 2020).

Zhou et al. developed antimicrobial peptides (AMPs) having osteogenic fragments and these complexed on the surface of silver NPs (AgNPs) through hydrogen bonding and SF was coated to carry AgNPs@AMPs to get infection triggered antibacterial and osteointegration. The SF-based coating encouraged the expression of osteogenic genes and collagen production while facilitating the adhesion, diffusion, and proliferation of BMSCs on the surface (Fig. 8.4).

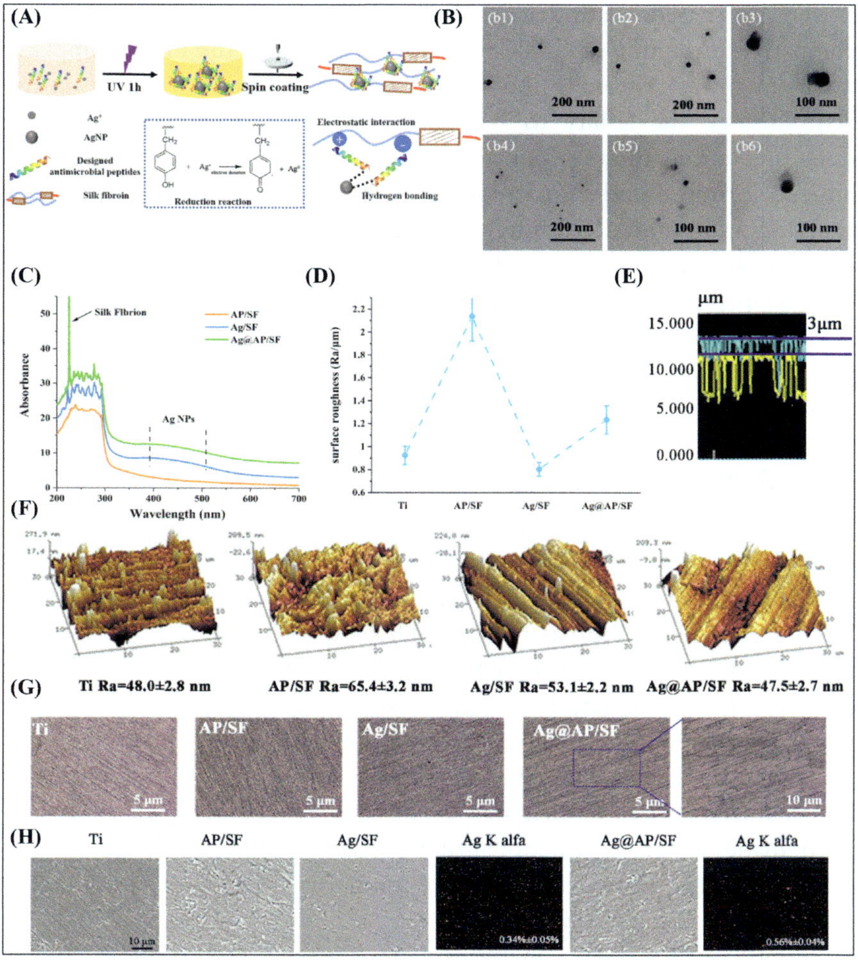

Figure 8.4 (A) The schematic diagram illustrated the formation of silver nanoparticles and the construction of a SF-based coating with antibacterial and bone-promoting functions; (b1–b3) AgNPs reduced by SF, (b4–b6) AgNPs reduced by SF/AMPs; (C) UV–vis spectra; (D) surface toughness (E) layer thickness of Ag/Ap specimen; (F) AFM observation of the surface morphology; (G) surface morphology; (H) SEM observation and EDS analysis of the coated specimens. *AFM*, Atomic force microscopy; *EDS*, energy dispersive spectrometry; *SEM*, scanning electron microscopy. *From Zhou, Y., Deng, G., She, H., Bai, F., Xiang, B., Zhou, J., & Zhang, S. (2023). Polydopamine-coated biomimetic bone scaffolds loaded with exosomes promote osteogenic differentiation of BMSC and bone regeneration.* Regenerative Therapy, 23, *25–36. https://doi.org/10.1016/j.reth.2023.03.005.*

The SF-based coating improved osseointegration at weeks 4 and 8 compared to the untreated Ti implants, according to the in vivo implantation outcomes. Overall, the AgNPs@AMPs-loaded SF-based coating demonstrated the ability to synergistically inhibit bacteria and enhance osseointegration, offering enormous promise for use in the treatment of bone deformities and associated infections (Zhou, Bai, et al., 2023). By adopting a biomimetic technique to intrafibrillar-mineralized collagen, Ye et al. created hybrid scaffolds that were then coated with an antibacterial designer peptide (GL13K) which is having both cationic and amphipathic characteristics. The fabricated scaffolds were capable of killing gram-negative and gram-positive bacteria and were cytocompatible with mesenchymal stromal cells produced by human bone marrow (Ye et al., 2021).

8.3.3 Self-assembled coatings

Tissue engineering faces a significant challenge in creating extracellular multiple-layered scaffolds which mimic the intricate, lattice-like architecture of tissues. These multilayer scaffolds can mimic natural tissues (Lutolf & Hubbell, 2005). Biomaterial scaffolds used for tissue regeneration templates should be able to stimulate the proper cellular responses, direct the creation of new operational tissues, and provide assistance to organ networks to achieve the results (Green & Elisseeff, 2016). However, there are several significant difficulties in tissue engineering. Controlling the surface characteristics of biomaterials is one such issue. Significant efforts have been made so far to functionalize the surfaces of biomaterials in tissue engineering to control their surface properties. Surface self-assembly is one of these strategies (Fig. 8.5).

Some well-known methods of surface modification include Langmuir–Blodgett deposition, self-assembled monolayer assembly, LBL

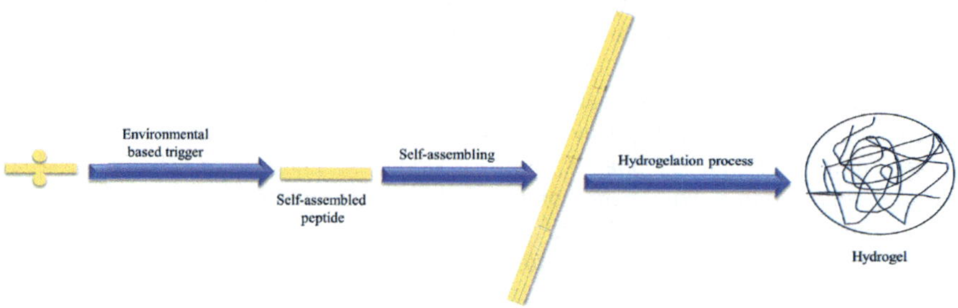

Figure 8.5 Schematic representation of the process involved in the self-assembled coating in hydrogel drug delivery.

self-assembly, etc. (Langmuir & Schaefer, 1937; Nuzzo & Allara, 1983). LBL assembly technique is a flexible and straightforward method for multilayer self-assembly. It enables the fabrication of controlled multiple-layer coatings using a wide range of materials, making it suitable for diverse biomedical applications (Borges & Mano, 2014; Richardson et al., 2015). The application of LBL is utilized for diverse purposes that require distinct methods of processing. There exist multiple techniques for LBL deposition, including dipping, spraying, fluid assembly, spin coating, and electromagnetically driven layering. The selection of LBL processing methodology is vital as it governs the surface characteristics of the shaped materials and also is an important factor in attaining optimal production and efficient utilization of modified materials. Various techniques of assembly typically result in unique patterns and traits of the assembled materials (Zhang et al., 2020). Numerous investigations have been conducted on the development of biomimetic coating by the self-assembly process. Shi et al. conducted a study in which they fabricated a dual membrane microcapsule that was inspired by mitochondria. The microcapsules were produced using a double template strategy, employing LBL self-assembly and mineralization techniques. The inner organic layer of the microcapsule was created using LBL self-assembly of protamine and oxidized alginate, with a template of calcium carbonate. The second template layer, the silica layer, was then formed on the protamine coat through biomimetic silicification. Ultimately, the outer layer was generated by the biomimetic mineralization of titanium precursor. The templates were subsequently eliminated to obtain a biomimetic capsule (Shi et al., 2011). In a comparable investigation, a cohort of scholars fabricated hybrid biomimetic microcapsules composed of protamine and titania through the utilization of LBL self-assembly and biomineralization methodology. Calcium carbonate ($CaCO_3$) microparticles were employed as a template to construct the initial positive layer of protamine. Subsequently, the affirmative stratum was employed as a prototype for the application of a subsequent negative layer of titania upon it. The procedure was replicated several times to obtain microcapsules with the correct thickness. The hollow microcapsules were formulated through the elimination of $CaCO_3$ microparticles utilizing EDTA at the conclusion of the process (Jiang et al., 2009). The authors, Silva et al. utilized a combination technique of template leaching and LBL process to fabricate three-dimensional nanostructured products for cartilage repair. The constructs were based on chondroitin sulfate and positively charged chitosan multilayers.

The obtained 3D scaffolds showed a high porosity and a high-water uptake capacity. It could maintain the chondrogenic phenotype and chondrogenic differentiation of multipotent bone marrow mesenchymal stem cells, revealing the potential for clinical application in the field of cartilage tissue engineering (Silva et al., 2013). Sasaki and colleagues have recently demonstrated the successful construction of hepatic tissue, showcasing the practical application of the LbL coating method. The study employed a methodology that facilitated the preparation of a composite layer comprising gelatine and fibronectin. This composite layer exhibited the potential to enhance the production of cytochrome P450 and human albumin in an in vitro setting (Sasaki et al., 2017).

8.4 Conclusion and future perspectives

With the flourishing number of studies on biomimetic drug carriers, it is clear that drug efficiency in targeted drug delivery has been greatly improved. Indeed, there has been a considerable increase in the capacity of drug loading in drug carriers, cellular internalization of drug carriers, and sustained drug release inside target cells. This chapter contemplates upon biomimetic delivery through polymeric micelles, dendrimers, and liposomes wherein the surface was functionalized to protect drugs and elicit targeted delivery without much harm to other tissues/organs. The biomimetic hydrogel has particularly attracted much attention for its resemblance with ECM and its growing clinical applications in bone engineering techniques and the oncological field. At the same time, biomimetics possess certain limitations in drug delivery that are needed to be addressed for improved delivery of therapeutic agents. The compatibility between the blood constituents with biomimetics must be taken into consideration to avoid any adverse effects. The residence time of biomimetics inside the cell for a longer period may create toxicity issues that must be resolved prior to their clinical applications (Sheikhpour et al., 2017). Biological systems are very complex and the mechanism between the biological environment and biomimetics should be extensively investigated. Stability is also one of the prime concerns in the case of biomimetics. They should be stable for a longer period and biomimetic-based formulations should be stable for effective therapeutic delivery. The prepared biomimetic formulation should be biocompatible and should not produce any kind of side effects. Biomimetic-derived nanocarriers also face challenges in their large-scale production where reproducibility is one of the major issues and proper sterile conditions are required for production purposes. For biomimetic drug delivery, well-standardized protocols and characterization techniques are needed to be established and long-term storage issues need to be resolved (Soprano et al., 2022). In conclusion, we expect that by investigating the aforementioned challenges, we can accelerate the clinical transformation of biomimetic-coated nanocarriers, which will benefit human health and be economically valuable.

Acknowledgment

All the authors are thankful to the director of the National Institute of Pharmaceutical Education and Research, Ahmedabad for providing literature search facilities.

References

Agnihotri, T. G., Alexander, A., Agrawal, M., Dubey, S. K., & Jain, A. (2023). In vitro-in vivo correlation in nanocarriers: From protein corona to therapeutic implications. *Journal of Controlled Release*, *354*, 794–809. Available from https://doi.org/10.1016/j.jconrel.2023.01.063, http://www.elsevier.com/locate/jconrel.

Agnihotri, T. G., Gomte, S. S., & Jain, A. (2022). Emerging theranostics to combat cancer: A perspective on metal-based nanomaterials. *Drug Development and Industrial Pharmacy*, *48*(11), 585–601. Available from https://doi.org/10.1080/03639045.2022.2153862, http://www.tandfonline.com/loi/iddi20#.Vmuk8Lfovcs.

Ajdnik, U., Luxbacher, T., Vesel, A., Štern, A., Žegura, B., Trček, J., & Zemljič, L. F. (2021). Polysaccharide-based bilayer coatings for biofilm-inhibiting surfaces of medical devices. *Materials*, *14*(16). Available from https://doi.org/10.3390/ma14164720, https://www.mdpi.com/1996-1944/14/16/4720/pdf.

Aliabadi, H. M., & Lavasanifar, A. (2006). Polymeric micelles for drug delivery. *Expert Opinion on Drug Delivery*, *3*(1), 139–162. Available from https://doi.org/10.1517/17425247.3.1.139.

Amoozgar, Zohreh, & Yeo, Yoon (2012). Recent advances in stealth coating of nanoparticle drug delivery systems. *WIREs Nanomedicine and Nanobiotechnology*, *4*(2), 219–233. Available from https://doi.org/10.1002/wnan.1157.

Bai, Jiaxiang, Wang, Huaiyu, Chen, Hao, Ge, Gaoran, Wang, Miao, Gao, Ang, Tong, Liping, Xu, Yaozeng, Yang, Huiling, Pan, Guoqing, Chu, Paul K., & Geng, Dechun (2020). Biomimetic osteogenic peptide with mussel adhesion and osteoimmunomodulatory functions to ameliorate interfacial osseointegration under chronic inflammation. *Biomaterials*, *255*120197. Available from https://doi.org/10.1016/j.biomaterials.2020.120197.

Borges, J., & Mano, J. F. (2014). Molecular interactions driving the layer-by-layer assembly of multilayers. *Chemical Reviews*, *114*(18), 8883–8942.

Bu, Lin-Lin, Rao, Lang, Yu, Guang-Tao, Chen, Lei, Deng, Wei-Wei, Liu, Jian-Feng, Wu, Hao, Meng, Qian-Fang, Guo, S. -S., Zhao, X. -Z., Zhang, W. -F., Chen, G., Gu, Z., Liu, W., & Sun, Z. -J. (2019). Cancer Stem Cell-Platelet Hybrid Membrane-Coated Magnetic Nanoparticles for Enhanced Photothermal Therapy of Head and Neck Squamous Cell Carcinoma. *Advanced Functional Materials*, *29*(10). Available from https://doi.org/10.1002/adfm.201807733.

Cao, H., Dan, Z., He, X., Zhang, Z., Yu, H., Yin, Q., & Li, Y. (2016). Liposomes coated with isolated macrophage membrane can target lung metastasis of breast cancer. *ACS Nano*, *10*(8), 7738–7748. Available from https://doi.org/10.1021/acsnano.6b03148, http://pubs.acs.org/journal/ancac3.

Chaudhuri, A., Ramesh, K., Kumar, D. N., Dehari, D., Singh, S., Kumar, D., & Agrawal, A. K. (2022). Polymeric micelles: A novel drug delivery system for the treatment of breast cancer. *Journal of Drug Delivery Science and Technology*, 77. Available from https://doi.org/10.1016/j.jddst.2022.103886, http://www.editionsdesante.fr/category.php?id_category = 48.

Chawla, Malvika, Kaushik, R. D., Malik, Mayank Kumar, Pundir, Vishakha, Singh, Jaspal, & Rehmaan, Hafeezur (2022). Development and optimization of RofA-PAMAM dendrimer complex materials for sustained drug delivery. *Materials Today Communications*, *33*104881. Available from https://doi.org/10.1016/j.mtcomm.2022.104881.

Cheng, Y., Wang, J., Rao, T., He, X., & Xu, T. (2008). Pharmaceutical applications of dendrimers: Promising nanocarriers for drug delivery. *Frontiers in Bioscience*, *13*(4), 1447–1471. Available from https://doi.org/10.2741/2774, https://www.fbscience.com/archives.

Choi, S. W., Kim, W. S., & Kim, J. H. (2003). Surface modification of functional nanoparticles for controlled drug delivery. *Journal of Dispersion Science and Technology*, *24* (3–4), 475–487. Available from https://doi.org/10.1081/DIS-120021803.

Cordon, C. S., Piva, M. B. R., Melo, C. M., Pinhal, M. A. S., & Suarez, E. R. (2013). Nanoparticles as platforms of molecular delivery in diagnosis and therapy. *OA Cancer*, *1*(2). Available from https://doi.org/10.13172/2053-3918-1-2-986.

Cruz, M. A., Chen, J., Whitelock, J. L., Morales, L. D., & López, J. A. (2005). The platelet glycoprotein Ib-von Willebrand factor interaction activates the collagen receptor $\alpha 2\beta 1$ to bind collagen: Activation-dependent conformational change of the $\alpha 2$-I domain. *Blood*, *105*(5), 1986–1991. Available from https://doi.org/10.1182/blood-2004-04-1365, https://www.journals.elsevier.com/blood.

Ding, Zhendong, Chen, Weiming, Jiang, Fengyu, Mo, Mengmiao, Bi, Yongguang, & Kong, Fansheng (2023). Synthesis, characterization and in vitro digestion of folate conjugated chitosan-loaded proanthocyanidins nanoparticles. *Food Research International*, *163*112141. Available from https://doi.org/10.1016/j.foodres.2022.112141.

Fan, F., Saha, S., & Hanjaya-Putra, D. (2021). Biomimetic hydrogels to promote wound healing. *Frontiers in Bioengineering and Biotechnology*, *9*. Available from https://doi.org/10.3389/fbioe.2021.718377, http://journal.frontiersin.org/journal/bioengineering-and-biotechnology#archive.

Ferguson, L. T., Hood, E. D., Shuvaeva, T., Shuvaev, V. V., Basil, M. C., Wang, Z., Nong, J., Ma, X., Wu, J., Myerson, J. W., Marcos-Contreras, O. A., Katzen, J., Carl, J. M., Morrisey, E. E., Cantu, E., Villa, C. H., Mitragotri, S., Muzykantov, V. R., & Brenner, J. S. (2022). Dual affinity to RBCs and target cells (DART) enhances both organ- and cell type-targeting of intravascular nanocarriers. *ACS Nano*, *16*(3), 4666–4683. Available from https://doi.org/10.1021/acsnano.1c11374, http://pubs.acs.org/journal/ancac3.

Gao, J., Reibetanz, U., Venkatraman, S., & Neu, B. (2011). Biofunctionalization of polyelectrolyte microcapsules with biotinylated polyethylene glycol-grafted liposomes. *Macromolecular Bioscience*, *11*(8), 1079–1087. Available from https://doi.org/10.1002/mabi.201100040.

Garg, T., Singh, O., Arora, S., & Murthy, R. S. R. (2011). Dendrimer—A novel scaffold for drug delivery. *International Journal of Pharmaceutical Sciences Review and Research*, 7(2),

211–220. Available from http://globalresearchonline.net/journalcontents/volume7issue2/Article-039.pdf.

Gong, X. F., Li, Y. J., Wang, D., Cao, H., Yang, Z., Wang, H., & Wang, L. (2023). Process-biomimetic macromolecular materials for in vivo applications. *Progress in Materials Science*, *131*. Available from https://doi.org/10.1016/j.pmatsci.2022.101015, https://www.journals.elsevier.com/progress-in-materials-science.

Green, J. J., & Elisseeff, J. H. (2016). Mimicking biological functionality with polymers for biomedical applications. *Nature*, *540*(7633), 386–394. Available from https://doi.org/10.1038/nature21005, http://www.nature.com/nature/index.html.

Guo, M., Xia, C., Wu, Y., Zhou, N., Chen, Z., & Li, W. (2021). Research progress on cell membrane-coated biomimetic delivery systems. *Frontiers in Bioengineering and Biotechnology*, *9*, 772522.

Han, Y., Pang, X., & Pi, G. (2021). Biomimetic and bioinspired intervention strategies for the treatment of rheumatoid arthritis. *Advanced Functional Materials*, *31*(38). Available from https://doi.org/10.1002/adfm.202104640, http://onlinelibrary.wiley.com/journal/10.1002/(ISSN)1616-3028.

Hashemi, Hamed, & Namazi, Hassan (2021). Understanding the pH dependent fluorescence and doxorubicin release from graphene oxide functionalized citric acid dendrimer as a highly efficient drug delivery system. *Materials Today Communications*, *28*102593. Available from https://doi.org/10.1016/j.mtcomm.2021.102593.

Hatakeyama, H., Akita, H., & Harashima, H. (2013). The polyethyleneglycol dilemma: Advantage and disadvantage of PEGylation of liposomes for systemic genes and nucleic acids delivery to tumors. *Biological and Pharmaceutical Bulletin*, *36*(6), 892–899. Available from https://doi.org/10.1248/bpb.b13-00059Japan, https://www.jstage.jst.go.jp/article/bpb/36/6/36_b13-00059/_pdf.

Henry, B. D., Neill, D. R., Becker, K. A., Gore, S., Bricio-Moreno, L., Ziobro, R., Edwards, M. J., Mühlemann, K., Steinmann, J., Kleuser, B., Japtok, L., Luginbühl, M., Wolfmeier, H., Scherag, A., Gulbins, E., Kadioglu, A., Draeger, A., & Babiychuk, E. B. (2015). Engineered liposomes sequester bacterial exotoxins and protect from severe invasive infections in mice. *Nature Biotechnology*, *33*(1), 81–88. Available from https://doi.org/10.1038/nbt.3037, http://www.nature.com/nbt/index.html.

Holinstat, M. (2017). Normal platelet function. *Cancer and Metastasis Reviews*, *36*(2), 195–198. Available from https://doi.org/10.1007/s10555-017-9677-x, http://www.wkap.nl/journalhome.htm/0167-7659.

Hou, Y., Jin, M., Liu, Y., Jiang, N., Zhang, L., & Zhu, S. (2023). Biomimetic construction of a lubricious hydrogel with robust mechanics via polymer chains interpenetration and entanglement for TMJ disc replacement. *Chemical Engineering Journal*, *460*, 141731.

Huang, Wenquan, Li, Zhiqiang, Liu, Weiqi, Liu, Shiyuan, Zhou, Rujin, & Jiang, Yanbin (2023). Preparation of B16 cancer cell membrane coated α-zein biomimetic drug delivery system for the enhancement of homotypic target ability. *Industrial Crops and Products*, *194*116301. Available from https://doi.org/10.1016/j.indcrop.2023.116301.

Hu, J., Zhuang, W., Ma, B., Su, X., Yu, T., Li, G., Hu, Y., & Wang, Y. (2018). Redox-responsive biomimetic polymeric micelle for simultaneous anticancer drug delivery and aggregation-induced emission active imaging. *Bioconjugate Chemistry*, *29*(6), 1897–1910. Available from https://doi.org/10.1021/acs.bioconjchem.8b00119, http://pubs.acs.org/journal/bcches.

Jang, Y. L., Yun, U. J., Lee, M. S., Kim, M. G., Son, S., Lee, K., Chae, S. Y., Lim, D. W., Kim, H. T., Kim, S. H., & Jeong, J. H. (2012). Cell-penetrating peptide mimicking polymer-based combined delivery of paclitaxel and siRNA for enhanced tumor growth suppression. *International Journal of Pharmaceutics, 434*(1–2), 488–493. Available from https://doi.org/10.1016/j.ijpharm.2012.04.083.

Janrao, C., Khopade, S., Bavaskar, A., Gomte, S. S., Agnihotri, T. G., & Jain, A. (2022). Recent advances of polymer based nanosystems in cancer management. *Journal of Biomaterials Science, Polymer Edition*. Available from https://doi.org/10.1080/09205063.2022.2161780, http://www.tandfonline.com/loi/tbsp20.

Jiang, Y., Yang, D., Zhang, L., Sun, Q., Sun, X., Li, J., & Jiang, Z. (2009). Preparation of protamine-titania microcapsules through synergy between layer-by-layer assembly and biomimetic mineralization. *Advanced Functional Materials, 19*(1), 150–156. Available from https://doi.org/10.1002/adfm.200800974China, http://www3.interscience.wiley.com/cgi-bin/fulltext/121542316/PDFSTART.

Jia, L., Xu, J. P., Wang, H., & Ji, J. (2011). Polyamidoamine dendrimers surface-engineered with biomimetic phosphorylcholine as potential drug delivery carriers. *Colloids and Surfaces B: Biointerfaces, 84*(1), 49–54. Available from https://doi.org/10.1016/j.colsurfb.2010.12.012.

Jin, K., Luo, Z., Zhang, B., & Pang, Z. (2018). Biomimetic nanoparticles for inflammation targeting. *Acta Pharmaceutica Sinica B, 8*(1), 23–33. Available from https://doi.org/10.1016/j.apsb.2017.12.002, http://www.elsevier.com/wps/find/journaldescription.cws_home/725753/description#description.

Kedar, U., Phutane, P., Shidhaye, S., & Kadam, V. (2010). Advances in polymeric micelles for drug delivery and tumor targeting. *Nanomedicine: Nanotechnology, Biology, and Medicine, 6*(6), 714–729. Available from https://doi.org/10.1016/j.nano.2010.05.005.

Langmuir, I., & Schaefer, V. J. (1937). Monolayers and multilayers of chlorophyll. *Journal of the American Chemical Society, 59*(10), 2075–2076. Available from https://doi.org/10.1021/ja01289a506.

Lee, C.-S., Kim, T. W., Kang, Y., Ju, Y., Ryu, J., Kong, H., Jang, Y.-S., Oh, D. E., Jang, S. J., Cho, H., Jeon, S., Kim, J., & Kim, T. H. (2022). Targeted drug delivery nanocarriers based on hyaluronic acid-decorated dendrimer encapsulating gold nanoparticles for ovarian cancer therapy. *Materials Today Chemistry, 26*101083. Available from https://doi.org/10.1016/j.mtchem.2022.101083.

Li, W., Ma, T., He, T., Li, Y., & Yin, S. (2023). Cancer cell membrane–encapsulated biomimetic nanoparticles for tumor immuno-photothermal therapy. *Chemical Engineering Journal, 463*, 142495.

Lin, X., Chen, J., Liao, Y., Pathak, J. L., Li, H., & Liu, Y. (2020). Biomimetic calcium phosphate coating as a drug delivery vehicle for bone tissue engineering: A mini-review. *Coatings, 10*(11), 1–19. Available from https://doi.org/10.3390/coatings10111118, https://www.mdpi.com/2079-6412/10/11/1118/pdf.

Lin, C. C., & Metters, A. T. (2006). Hydrogels in controlled release formulations: Network design and mathematical modeling. *Advanced Drug Delivery Reviews, 58*(12–13), 1379–1408. Available from https://doi.org/10.1016/j.addr.2006.09.004.

Lin, Hu, Wang, Quan, Zhong, Rui, Li, Zhen, Zhao, Weifeng, Chen, Yuanwei, Tian, Meng, & Luo, Xianglin (2019). Biomimetic phosphorylcholine strategy to improve the hemocompatibility of pH-responsive micelles containing tertiary amino groups. *Colloids and Surfaces B: Biointerfaces, 184*110545. Available from https://doi.org/10.1016/j.colsurfb.2019.110545.

Liu, P., Chen, G., & Zhang, J. (2022). A review of liposomes as a drug delivery system: Current status of approved products, regulatory environments, and future perspectives. *Molecules (Basel, Switzerland), 27*(4). Available from https://doi.org/10.3390/molecules27041372, https://www.mdpi.com/1420-3049/27/4/1372/pdf.

Liu, G. X., Fang, G. Q., & Xu, W. (2014). Dual targeting biomimetic liposomes for paclitaxel/DNA combination cancer treatment. *International Journal of Molecular Sciences, 15*

(9), 15287–15303. Available from https://doi.org/10.3390/ijms150915287, http://www.mdpi.com/1422-0067/15/9/15287/pdf.

Liu, Y., Lin, S. H., Chuang, W. T., Dai, N. T., & Hsu, S. H. (2022). Biomimetic strain-stiffening in chitosan self-healing hydrogels. *ACS Applied Materials and Interfaces, 14* (14), 16032–16046. Available from https://doi.org/10.1021/acsami.2c01720, http://pubs.acs.org/journal/aamick.

Liu, Z., Tang, Q., Liu, R. T., Yu, M. Z., Peng, H., Zhang, C. Q., Zhu, Z. Z., & Wei, X. J. (2023). Laponite intercalated biomimetic multilayer coating prevents glucocorticoids induced orthopedic implant failure. *Bioactive Materials, 22*, 60–73. Available from https://doi.org/10.1016/j.bioactmat.2022.09.013, http://www.keaipublishing.com/en/journals/bioactive-materials/.

Liu, G., Zhuang, W., Chen, X., Yin, A., Nie, Y., & Wang, Y. (2016). Drug carrier system self-assembled from biomimetic polyphosphorycholine and biodegradable polypeptide based diblock copolymers. *Polymer, 100*, 45–55. Available from https://doi.org/10.1016/j.polymer.2016.08.012, http://www.journals.elsevier.com/polymer/.

Li, Jingchao, Li, Xiaomeng, Zhang, Jing, Kawazoe, Naoki, & Chen, Guoping (2017). Induction of chondrogenic differentiation of human mesenchymal stem cells by biomimetic gold nanoparticles with tunable RGD density. *Advanced Healthcare Materials, 6* (14)1700317. Available from https://doi.org/10.1002/adhm.201700317.

Lutolf, M. P., & Hubbell, J. A. (2005). Synthetic biomaterials as instructive extracellular microenvironments for morphogenesis in tissue engineering. *Nature Biotechnology, 23* (1), 47–55. Available from https://doi.org/10.1038/nbt1055.

Mendanha, D., de Castro, J. V., Casanova, M. R., Gimondi, S., Ferreira, H., & Neves, N. M. (2023). Macrophage cell membrane infused biomimetic liposomes for glioblastoma targeted therapy. *Nanomedicine: Nanotechnology, Biology and Medicine, 49*, 102663.

Mishra, P., Nayak, B., & Dey, R. K. (2016). PEGylation in anti-cancer therapy: An overview. *Asian Journal of Pharmaceutical Sciences, 11*(3), 337–348. Available from https://doi.org/10.1016/j.ajps.2015.08.011, http://www.journals.elsevier.com/asian-journal-of-pharmaceutical-sciences/recent-articles/.

Miyata, K., Christie, R. J., & Kataoka, K. (2011). Polymeric micelles for nano-scale drug delivery. *Reactive and Functional Polymers, 71*(3), 227–234. Available from https://doi.org/10.1016/j.reactfunctpolym.2010.10.009.

Nguyen, T. T., Nguyen, P., Pham, T. L.-B., Le, H. K., Nguyen, M.-T., Nhi, T. T. Y., Feng, S., Chen, J., & Tran, N. Q. (2023). Dual composition Chondroitin Sulfate and gelatin biomimetic hydrogel based on tyramine crosslinking for tissue regenerative medicine. *European Polymer Journal, 189*, 111975.

Niu, Q., Liu, Y., Zheng, Y., Tang, Z., Qian, Y., Qi, R., Shen, J., & Zhao, P. (2022). Co-delivery of nigericin and decitabine using hexahistidine-metal nanocarriers for pyroptosis-induced immunotherapeutics. *Acta Pharmaceutica Sinica B, 12*(12), 4458–4471. Available from https://doi.org/10.1016/j.apsb.2022.11.002, http://www.elsevier.com/wps/find/journaldescription.cws_home/725753/description#description.

Nuzzo, R. G., & Allara, D. L. (1983). Adsorption of bifunctional organic disulfides on gold surfaces. *Journal of the American Chemical Society, 105*(13), 4481–4483. Available from https://doi.org/10.1021/ja00351a063.

Oledzka, Ewa, Paśnik, Klaudia, Domańska, Izabela, Zielińska-Pisklak, Monika, Piotrowska, Urszula, Sobczak, Marcin, Szeleszczuk, èukasz, & Laskowska, Anna (2023). Poly(amidoamine) dendrimer/camptothecin complex: from synthesis to in vitro cancer cell line studies. *Molecules (Basel, Switzerland), 28*(6), 2696. Available from https://doi.org/10.3390/molecules28062696.

Olsson, M., Bruhns, P., Frazier, W. A., Ravetch, J. V., & Oldenborg, P. A. (2005). Platelet homeostasis is regulated by platelet expression of CD47 under normal conditions and in passive immune thrombocytopenia. *Blood*, *105*(9), 3577–3582. Available from https://doi.org/10.1182/blood-2004-08-2980, https://www.journals.elsevier.com/blood.

Palaveniene, A., Songailiene, K., Baniukaitiene, O., Tamburaci, S., Kimna, C., Tihminlioğlu, F., & Liesiene, J. (2020). The effect of biomimetic coating and cuttlebone microparticle reinforcement on the osteoconductive properties of cellulose-based scaffolds. *International Journal of Biological Macromolecules*, *152*, 1194–1204. Available from https://doi.org/10.1016/j.ijbiomac.2019.10.213, http://www.elsevier.com/locate/ijbiomac.

Pitchaimani, A., Nguyen, T. D. T., & Aryal, S. (2018). Natural killer cell membrane infused biomimetic liposomes for targeted tumor therapy. *Biomaterials*, *160*, 124–137. Available from https://doi.org/10.1016/j.biomaterials.2018.01.018, http://www.journals.elsevier.com/biomaterials/.

Qiao, C., Wang, X., Liu, G., Yang, Z., Jia, Q., Wang, L., Zhang, R., Xia, Y., Wang, Z., & Yang, Y. (2022). Erythrocyte membrane camouflaged metal–organic framework nanodrugs for remodeled tumor microenvironment and enhanced tumor chemotherapy. *Advanced Functional Materials*, *32*(6). Available from https://doi.org/10.1002/adfm.202107791, http://onlinelibrary.wiley.com/journal/10.1002/(ISSN)1616-3028.

Rangasami, V. K., Asawa, K., Teramura, Y., Le Blanc, K., Nilsson, B., Hilborn, J., Varghese, O. P., & Oommen, O. P. (2023). Biomimetic polyelectrolyte coating of stem cells suppresses thrombotic activation and enhances its survival and function. *Biomaterials Advances*, *147*. Available from https://doi.org/10.1016/j.bioadv.2023.213331, https://www.sciencedirect.com/journal/biomaterials-advances/about/aims-and-scope.

Rao, Lang, Bu, Lin-Lin, Ma, Liang, Wang, Wenbiao, Liu, Huiqin, Wan, Da, Liu, Jian-Feng, Li, Andrew, Guo, Shi-Shang, Zhang, Lu, Zhang, Wen-Feng, Zhao, Xing-Zhong, Sun, Zhi-Jun, & Liu, Wei (2018). Platelet-facilitated photothermal therapy of head and neck squamous cell carcinoma. *Angewandte Chemie.*, *130*(4), 998–1003. Available from https://doi.org/10.1002/ange.201709457.

Ren, K., He, C., Xiao, C., Li, G., & Chen, X. (2015). Injectable glycopolypeptide hydrogels as biomimetic scaffolds forcartilage tissue engineering. *Biomaterials*, *51*, 238–249. Available from https://doi.org/10.1016/j.biomaterials.2015.02.026, http://www.journals.elsevier.com/biomaterials/.

Richardson, J. J., Björnmalm, M., & Caruso, F. (2015). Technology-driven layer-by-layer assembly of nanofilms. *Science*, *348*(6233), 2491.

Rommasi, F., & Esfandiari, N. (2021). Liposomal nanomedicine: Applications for drug delivery in cancer therapy. *Nanoscale Research Letters*, *16*(1). Available from https://doi.org/10.1186/s11671-021-03553-8, http://www.springer.com/materials/nanotechnology/journal/11671.

Sasaki, K., Akagi, T., Asaoka, T., Eguchi, H., Fukuda, Y., Iwagami, Y., Yamada, D., Noda, T., Wada, H., Gotoh, K., Kawamoto, K., Doki, Y., Mori, M., & Akashi, M. (2017). Construction of three-dimensional vascularized functional human liver tissue using a layer-by-layer cell coating technique. *Biomaterials*, *133*, 263–274. Available from https://doi.org/10.1016/j.biomaterials.2017.02.034, http://www.journals.elsevier.com/biomaterials/.

Sheikhpour, M., Barani, L., & Kasaeian, A. (2017). Biomimetics in drug delivery systems: A critical review. *Journal of Controlled Release*, *253*, 97–109. Available from https://doi.org/10.1016/j.jconrel.2017.03.026, http://www.elsevier.com/locate/jconrel.

Shen, M., Li, H., Yao, S., Wu, X., Liu, S., Yang, Q., Zhang, Y., Du, J., Qi, S., & Li, Y. (2021). Shear stress and ROS-responsive biomimetic micelles for atherosclerosis via ROS consumption. *Materials Science and Engineering: C*, *126*, 112164.

Shi, J., Zhang, L., & Jiang, Z. (2011). Facile construction of multicompartment multienzyme system through layer-by-layer self-assembly and biomimetic mineralization. *ACS Applied Materials and Interfaces*, *3*(3), 881–889. Available from https://doi.org/10.1021/am101241u.

Silva, J. M., Georgi, N., Costa, R., Sher, P., Reis, R. L., van Blitterswijk, C. A., Karperien, M., & Mano, J. F. (2013). Nanostructured 3D constructs based on chitosan and chondroitin sulphate multilayers for cartilage tissue engineering. *PLoS One*, *8*(2). Available from https://doi.org/10.1371/journal.pone.0055451Portugal, http://www.plosone.org/article/fetchObjectAttachment.action?uri = info%3Adoi%2F10.1371%2Fjournal.pone.0055451&representation = PDF.

Singh, Prerana, Maparu, Auhin Kumar, Shah, Savita, Rai, Beena, & Sivakumar, Sri (2021). Biomimetic algal polysaccharide coated 3D nanofibrous scaffolds promote skin extracellular matrix formation. *Materials Science and Engineering: C*, *119*111580. Available from https://doi.org/10.1016/j.msec.2020.111580.

Soprano, E., Polo, E., Pelaz, B., & del Pino, P. (2022). Biomimetic cell-derived nanocarriers in cancer research. *Journal of Nanobiotechnology*, *20*(1). Available from https://doi.org/10.1186/s12951-022-01748-4, https://jnanobiotechnology.biomedcentral.com.

Tomlinson, R. E., & Silva, M. J. (2013). Skeletal blood flow in bone repair and maintenance. *Bone Research*, *1*, 311–322. Available from https://doi.org/10.4248/BR201304002, http://www.nature.com/boneres/.

Tripathy, S., & Das, M. K. (2013). Dendrimers and their applications as novel drug delivery carriers. *Journal of Applied Pharmaceutical Science*, *3*(9), 142–149. Available from https://doi.org/10.7324/JAPS.2013.3924India, http://www.japsonline.com/admin/php/uploads/1064_pdf.pdf.

Vauthier, C., & Labarre, D. (2008). Modular biomimetic drug delivery systems. *Journal of Drug Delivery Science and Technology*, *18*(1), 59–68. Available from https://doi.org/10.1016/S1773-2247(08)50008-6, http://www.editionsdesante.fr/category.php?id_category = 48.

Venkatesh, S., Byrne, M. E., Peppas, N. A., & Hilt, J. Z. (2005). Applications of biomimetic systems in drug delivery. *Expert Opinion on Drug Delivery*, *2*(6), 1085–1096. Available from https://doi.org/10.1517/17425247.2.6.1085.

Vilela, C. A., Correia, C., Oliveira, J. M., Sousa, R. A., Espregueira-Mendes, J., & Reis, R. L. (2015). Cartilage repair using hydrogels: A critical review of in vivo experimental designs. *ACS Biomaterials Science and Engineering*, *1*(9), 726–739. Available from https://doi.org/10.1021/acsbiomaterials.5b00245, http://pubs.acs.org/journal/abseba.

Vincent, J. F. V. (2009). Biomimetics – A review. *Proceedings of the Institution of Mechanical Engineers, Part H: Journal of Engineering in Medicine*, *223*(8), 919–939. Available from https://doi.org/10.1243/09544119JEIM561.

Wang, Shuyan, Duan, Yaou, Zhang, Qiangzhe, Komarla, Anvita, Gong, Hua, Gao, Weiwei, & Zhang, Liangfang (2020). Drug targeting via platelet membrane–coated nanoparticles. *Small Structures*, *1*(1)2000018. Available from https://doi.org/10.1002/sstr.202000018.

Wang, Can, Wang, Yulan, Zhang, Lingling, Miron, Richard J., Liang, Jianfei, Shi, Miusi, Mo, Wenting, Zheng, Shihang, Zhao, Yanbing, & Zhang, Yufeng (2018). Pretreated macrophage-membrane-coated gold nanocages for precise drug delivery for treatment of bacterial infections. *Advanced Materials*, *30*(46)1804023. Available from https://doi.org/10.1002/adma.201804023.

Wilczewska, A. Z., Niemirowicz, K., Markiewicz, K. H., & Car, H. (2012). Nanoparticles as drug delivery systems. *Pharmacological Reports*, *64*(5), 1020–1037. Available from https://doi.org/10.1016/S1734-1140(12)70901-5, http://www.if-pan.krakow.pl/pjp/pdf/2012/5_1020.pdf.

Wu, M., Guo, K., Dong, H., Zeng, R., Tu, M., & Zhao, J. (2014). In vitro drug release and biological evaluation of biomimetic polymeric micelles self-assembled from amphiphilic deoxycholic acid-phosphorylcholine-chitosan conjugate. *Materials Science and Engineering C, 45*, 162–169. Available from https://doi.org/10.1016/j.msec.2014.09.008.

Wu, H., Jiang, X., Li, Y., Zhou, Y., Zhang, T., Zhi, P., & Gao, J. (2020). Engineering stem cell derived biomimetic vesicles for versatility and effective targeted delivery. *Advanced Functional Materials, 30*(49). Available from https://doi.org/10.1002/adfm.202006169, http://onlinelibrary.wiley.com/journal/10.1002/(ISSN)1616-3028.

Xia, S., Liu, Z., Cai, J., Ren, H., Li, Q., Zhang, H., Yue, J., Zhou, Q., Zhou, T., & Wang, L. (2023). Liver fibrosis therapy based on biomimetic nanoparticles which deplete activated hepatic stellate cells. *Journal of Controlled Release, 355*, 54–67.

Xu, J. P., Ji, J., Chen, W. D., & Shen, J. C. (2005). Novel biomimetic polymersomes as polymer therapeutics for drug delivery. *Journal of Controlled Release, 107*(3), 502–512. Available from https://doi.org/10.1016/j.jconrel.2005.06.013.

Yandrapu, S. K., Kanujia, P., Chalasani, K. B., Mangamoori, L., Kolapalli, R. V., & Chauhan, A. (2013). Development and optimization of thiolated dendrimer as a viable mucoadhesive excipient for the controlled drug delivery: An acyclovir model formulation. *Nanomedicine: Nanotechnology, Biology, and Medicine, 9*(4), 514–522. Available from https://doi.org/10.1016/j.nano.2012.10.005.

Yang, X., Yu, T., Zeng, Y., Lian, K., Zhou, X., Ke, J., Li, Y., Yuan, H., & Hu, F. (2020). PH-responsive biomimetic polymeric micelles as lymph node-targeting vaccines for enhanced antitumor immune responses. *Biomacromolecules, 21*(7), 2818–2828. Available from https://doi.org/10.1021/acs.biomac.0c00518, http://pubs.acs.org/journal/bomaf6.

Ye, Z., Zhu, X., Mutreja, I., Boda, S. K., Fischer, N. G., Zhang, A., Lui, C., Qi, Y., & Aparicio, C. (2021). Biomimetic mineralized hybrid scaffolds with antimicrobial peptides. *Bioactive Materials, 6*(8), 2250–2260. Available from https://doi.org/10.1016/j.bioactmat.2020.12.029, http://www.keaipublishing.com/en/journals/bioactive-materials/.

Yoo, J. W., Irvine, D. J., Discher, D. E., & Mitragotri, S. (2011). Bio-inspired, bioengineered and biomimetic drug delivery carriers. *Nature Reviews. Drug Discovery, 10*(7), 521–535. Available from https://doi.org/10.1038/nrd3499.

You, Changcheng, Zu, Jianing, Liu, Xiaoqi, Kong, Pengyu, Song, Chengchao, Wei, Rongzhi, Zhou, Changlong, Wang, Yufu, & Yan, Jinglong (2018). Synovial fibroblast-targeting liposomes encapsulating an NF -κB-blocking peptide ameliorates zymosan-induced synovial inflammation. *Journal of Cellular and Molecular Medicine, 22*(4), 2449–2457. Available from https://doi.org/10.1111/jcmm.13549.

Zhang, M., Du, Y., Wang, S., & Chen, B. (2020). A review of biomimetic nanoparticle drug delivery systems based on cell membranes. *Drug Design, Development and Therapy, 14*, 5495–5503. Available from https://doi.org/10.2147/DDDT.S282368, https://www.dovepress.com/getfile.php?fileID = 64709.

Zhang, Huijuan, He, Qingqing, Wang, Jingjing, Wang, Yaping, Xuan, Xiangyang, Sui, Mingli, Zhang, Zhenzhong, & Hou, Lin (2022). Biomimetic micelles to accurately regulate the inflammatory microenvironment for glomerulonephritis treatment. *Pharmacological Research, 181*106263. Available from https://doi.org/10.1016/j.phrs.2022.106263.

Zhang, K., Jia, Y. G., Tsai, I. H., Strandman, S., Ren, L., Hong, L., Zhang, G., Guan, Y., Zhang, Y., & Zhu, X. X. (2017). "Bitter-sweet" polymeric micelles formed by block copolymers from glucosamine and cholic acid. *Biomacromolecules, 18*(3), 778–786. Available from https://doi.org/10.1021/acs.biomac.6b01640, http://pubs.acs.org/journal/bomaf6.

Zhang, L., Wang, Z., Zhang, Y., Cao, F., Dong, K., Ren, J., & Qu, X. (2018). Erythrocyte membrane cloaked metal-organic framework nanoparticle as biomimetic nanoreactor for starvation-activated colon cancer therapy. *ACS Nano*, *12*(10), 10201–10211. Available from https://doi.org/10.1021/acsnano.8b05200, http://pubs.acs.org/journal/ancac3.

Zhang, Wenyuan, Zhao, Man, Gao, Yali, Cheng, Xu, Liu, Xiaoying, Tang, Shukun, Peng, Yanbo, Wang, Na, Hu, Dandan, Peng, Haisheng, Zhang, Jinqiu, & Wang, Qun (2022). Biomimetic erythrocytes engineered drug delivery for cancer therapy. *Chemical Engineering Journal*, *433*133498. Available from https://doi.org/10.1016/j.cej.2021.133498.

Zhou, W., Bai, T., Wang, L., Cheng, Y., Xia, D., Yu, S., & Zheng, Y. (2023). Biomimetic AgNPs@antimicrobial peptide/silk fibroin coating for infection-trigger antibacterial capability and enhanced osseointegration. *Bioactive Materials*, *20*, 64–80. Available from https://doi.org/10.1016/j.bioactmat.2022.05.015, http://www.keai-publishing.com/en/journals/bioactive-materials/.

Zhou, Y., Deng, G., She, H., Bai, F., Xiang, B., Zhou, J., & Zhang, S. (2023). Polydopamine-coated biomimetic bone scaffolds loaded with exosomes promote osteogenic differentiation of BMSC and bone regeneration. *Regenerative Therapy*, *23*, 25–36. Available from https://doi.org/10.1016/j.reth.2023.03.005, http://www.journals.elsevier.com/regenerative-therapy/.

Zhuang, J., Duan, Y., Zhang, Q., Gao, W., Li, S., Fang, R. H., & Zhang, L. (2020). Multimodal enzyme delivery and therapy enabled by cell membrane-coated metal-organic framework nanoparticles. *Nano Letters*, *20*(5), 4051–4058. Available from https://doi.org/10.1021/acs.nanolett.0c01654, http://pubs.acs.org/journal/nalefd.

Zhu, J., Hu, J., & Marchant, R. E. (2013). *Biomimetic hydrogels as scaffolds for tissue-engineering applications Biomimetic Biomaterials: Structure and Applications* (pp. 238–275). United States: Elsevier Ltd. Available from http://www.sciencedirect.com/science/book/9780857094162, 10.1533/9780857098887.2.238.

Zhu, J., Xue, J., Guo, Z., Zhang, L., & Marchant, R. E. (2007). Biomimetic glycoliposomes as nanocarriers for targeting P-selectin on activated platelets. *Bioconjugate Chemistry*, *18*(5), 1366–1369. Available from https://doi.org/10.1021/bc700212b, http://pubs.acs.org/journal/bcches.

Zhang, L., Wang, Z., Zhang, Y., Cao, F., Dong, K., Ren, J., & Qu, X. (2018). Erythrocyte membrane cloaked metal-organic framework nanoparticle as biomimetic nanoreactor for starvation-activated colon cancer therapy. ACS Nano, 12(10), 10201–10211. Available from [illegible]

[illegible]

CHAPTER 9

Biomimetic coatings anticorrosion applications

N. Mehranshad[1], Sh. Roshan[1], B. Ramezanzadeh[2] and H. Eivaz Mohammadloo[3]

[1]Department of Polymer Engineering and Color Technology, Amirkabir University of Technology, Tehran, Iran
[2]Department of Surface Coating and Corrosion, Institute for Color Science and Technology, Tehran, Iran
[3]Color, Resin and Surface Coatings Department, Iran Polymer and Petrochemical Institute, Tehran, Iran

9.1 Introduction

In 1957 Otto Schmitt coined the word "biomimetic" for the first time. As he gave his explanation, he pointed out that biomimetics is neither a subject matter nor a point of view, but rather a relation to biophysics science. It is the application of biological theory and technology to technological problems (Vincent, 2009). Moreover, biomimetics, bionics, biognosis, and bionics are synonyms for biomimetics. Among these words, the word "biomimetics" appears to be the most prominent and useful (Sheikhpour et al., 2017).

An inspiration for biomimetic coatings comes from nature. Natural materials, like lotus leaves, are mimicked with these coatings. Medicinal, energy production, and environmental applications of biomimetic coatings are all possible.

Humanity draws inspiration from nature when developing technology. The micro-nanostructures of many biological surfaces exhibit skills and attributes beyond those of conventional engineerings, such as lotus leaves, butterfly wings, rose petals, and shark skin. Bioinspired materials are produced by mimicking biological materials by exploiting these skills and properties. As a result of their inspiration from nature, these materials are referred to as biomimetic materials by scientists. Researchers have introduced biomimetic materials with a wide range of advanced properties over the last few decades.

Lotus coatings are examples of biomimetic coatings. Because of their microstructure, lotus leaves are capable of repelling dirt and water. Building coatings that resist dirt buildup and self-clean have been produced with this effect. The result is not only the improvement of these structures' appearance but also a reduction in maintenance costs and the impact on the environment (Collins & Safiuddin, 2022).

Smart Biomimetic Coatings
DOI: https://doi.org/10.1016/B978-0-443-21738-8.00009-6

Superhydrophobic surfaces have been produced using biomimicry. To solve problems or provide services, biomimicry uses artificial means to reproduce naturally occurring phenomena from the environment.

9.2 Surface wettability behavior

9.2.1 Theoretical models

9.2.1.1 Smooth surface

It was at the very beginning that ideal solids, both flat and chemically homogeneous, were subjected to some basic laws. In their study of Young and Laplace's surface tension, it was noted that the surface energy reflects the cohesion of the condensed phase beneath (liquid or solid).

As the name implies, γ_{IJ} refers to the quantity that exists between phases *I* and *J* (which are represented by solids, liquids, and vapors, respectively). Force per unit of length, or energy per unit of area, defines surface tension as force per unit of length. To minimize the corresponding (positive) surface energy, this force is applied along the *IJ* surface. A drop's equilibrium contact angle θ_{eq} with a surface and its three surface tensions are determined by Young's equation:

$$\gamma_{SV} = \gamma_{SL} + \gamma_{LV}\cos\theta_{eq} \tag{9.1}$$

On a smooth solid surface, θ_{eq} is Young's contact angle or the equilibrium contact angle. This angle is commonly found between 0 and 90 degrees (i.e., on hydrophilic surfaces). Surface tensions between liquid and solid (with two condensed phases) are relatively smaller than those between solid and air (with one), due to the smaller difference between phases in the first case. This implies that θ_{eq} has an acute angle, as shown by a positive cosine in Eq. (9.1).

In addition, roughness, chemical heterogeneity, surface reconstruction, swelling, and dissolution are not taken into account for an ideal solid surface. It is thought that surface roughness is one of the parameters that determine the surface contact angle. Molecular flatness is rare in solids. A molecularly flat solid is typically formed by solidifying a liquid film, either free-standing or supported on another liquid. If such conditions exist, roughness can be compared with thermal roughness at liquid interfaces, which is generally a few angstroms. Glass can be taken as an example. Glass generally solidifies from its molten state after being deposited onto the molten tin.

However, on a micrometric scale, a solid's bulk is generally rough compared with its surface. Roughness can be caused by striations or microgrooves which are created during fabrication (e.g., when lamination is performed). It is also possible for coatings to cause roughness, especially when they dewet and produce microdroplets as a result (Yu et al., 2015).

9.2.1.2 Rough surface

The coefficient θ_{eq} is the major determinant of wettability on rough surfaces, including hydrophobicity and hydrophilicity. Typically, surface roughness is correlated with apparent contact angle using two distinct models: the Wenzel model (Wenzel, 1936) and the Cassie–Baxter model (Wenzel, 1949).

9.2.1.3 Contact angle hysteresis

The Gibbs principle suggests that flaws in solids can pin contact lines. Because of the nonwetting and wetting defects in front and rear contact, droplets remain at rest on a slope. As a result of this dissymmetry in contact angles, the front has a high curvature while the back has a smaller curvature, which causes a Laplace pressure difference. As a result, gravity can be overcome by this force for a small drop (Kumar & Gupta, 2015).

Chemical heterogeneities and roughness can help pin the drop in place. Contact angles can vary even on chemically homogeneous surfaces due to the edges of defects. Small and large contact angles are also possible for solids possessing both kinds of defects. It is possible to block a liquid drop with a groove and to reverse the effect with a tip. Consequently, liquid deposition processes determine contact angles. When a gently deposited drop comes in contact with nonwetting flaws, it spreads and then stops, thereby preventing further probes of the surface. During its evaporated state, the drop will appear to adhere to wetting defects a short time later. The contact line will remain fixed if sufficient liquid is added to the drop, but the contact angle will increase if the sufficient liquid is removed.

The same is true if this liquid is removed from the drop. Thus the contact angle hysteresis (CAH) can be quantified by two steps: (1) drop volumes are gradually increased, and contact lines remain stuck until a critical volume is abruptly exceeded, after which they design and move to the next set of pinning flaws. An advancing contact angle, or θ_a, is observed in such circumstances. (2) A receding contact angle θ_r can be observed, however, by sucking liquid from the drop and flattening it until it retracts to the next series of wetting events that stop and pin the line. Typically, the CAH for Young equilibrium falls within those two ranges.

$$\Delta\theta = \theta_a - \theta_r \tag{9.2}$$

It is possible to consider CAH as beneficial or detrimental depending on the conditions. In light of this, it is essential to gain a deeper understanding of it; however, it remains a mystery how the microscopic and macroscale images are linked (measurement of hysteresis and its average value for many flaws). In general, $\Delta\theta = \theta_a - \theta_r$ on a rough solid varies greatly between almost zero and the order of θ_a itself in terms of CAH (Yu et al., 2015).

9.2.2 Wetting regimes

9.2.2.1 The Wenzel model

According to Wenzel, if liquid contact occurs on a rough surface, roughness should enhance either film formation or contact angle if the liquid follows the profile of the rough surface. In a wet-contact mode, water droplets are pinned to the surface, causing high CAH. In the case of high CAH, the sliding angle becomes deficient since the water droplets cannot slide on the surface. Wenzel's equation gives the contact angle on this sort of surface.

$$\cos\theta^{w} = r\cos\theta_{eq} \tag{9.3}$$

The Wenzel contact angle is given by θ^{w}, and the equilibrium contact angle is given by θ_{eq} on a smooth surface of the same material. According to Eq. (9.3), r signifies the roughness factor. this factor is measured by the ratio between apparent and true surface area. A roughness contribution is contained in r and a surface chemistry contribution is contained in θ_{eq} (Liu et al., 2010a). Using Eq. (9.3), we can see that a surface that is hydrophobic (θ_{eq} >90 degrees) becomes more hydrophobic as the degree of roughness increases, whereas a surface that is hydrophilic (θ_{eq} <90 degrees) becomes more hydrophilic as the roughness increases.

It is undoubtedly true that adding surface roughness will enhance the intrinsic wetting properties of materials with smooth surfaces. There may be situations, however, where the value of the right side in Eq. (9.3) is greater than 1 for surfaces with high roughness or porous structures. As a consequence, the Cassie–Baxter model would predominate on such occasions where the Wenzel model would be inadequate (Yu et al., 2015).

9.2.2.2 The Cassie–Baxter model

Chemochemical heterogeneities of the surface play an important role in the Cassie–Baxter case. Surfaces with multiple states can be thought of as nonwetting if air-related parts of them are not coated. Due to the low adhesive force, a water drop can easily roll off in such a situation. In this case, the sliding angle is a good indicator of the CAH. Under plentiful observations, lotus leaves exhibit both superhydrophobicity and a further self-cleaning effect, which are clear examples of the Cassie–Baxter model. Using Cassie–Baxter, we can define apparent contact angle, $\boldsymbol{\theta^{CB}}$, as:

$$\cos\theta^{CB} = f\left(\cos\theta_{eq} + 1\right) - 1 \tag{9.4}$$

The fraction of surface contact between liquid and solid is given by f, where f is numerically smaller than 1. A threshold contact angle can be used to define the composite contact condition, using $\cos\theta_t = (f - 1)(r - f)$. A composite contact condition is established when $\theta_{eq} > \theta_t$. To form a wetting contact, extra energy is needed, which is referred to as the Wenzel model. It is also possible to convert a metastable Cassie–Baxter nonwetting state into a stable Wenzel wetting state on surfaces of moderate hydrophobicity (90 degrees $< \theta_{eq} < \theta_t$). Further, according to an alternative criterion for Cassie–Baxter states, there are two conditions that lead to Cassie–Baxter states: (1) droplet weight that is not supported by the fluid contact line exceeds body forces and (2) there is enough height in microstructures to prevent liquid from touching them (Extrand, 2004).

Liquid contact angles will be affected by additional surface roughness. Because of this, there is a growth in angles greater than 90 degrees on a flat surface, while angles below 90 degrees may move either way. As a result, water drops tend to adhere to surfaces that match the Wenzel model of total wetting more than flat surfaces of the same material (Quéré et al., 2003). In contrast, those on a "slippery" surface conforming to the Cassie–Baxter model will roll off easier than those on a level surface. It is likely that a surface with a high inherent CAH will create a "sticky" surface while conforming with the Cassie–Baxter model at the same time (Shirtcliffe et al., 2004).

It is also possible for the Cassie–Baxter/Wenzel state to have a large hysteresis since there is as much interfacial area on a flat surface as there is on a solid (Law, 2022). Therefore CAH cannot be an effective criterion for surface wetting in such circumstances. With just a slight incline, water drops easily roll off Cassie–Baxter bridging surfaces. Water drops can become trapped in valleys when they fall from a height. It is not just the intrinsic hydrophobicity of a surface that determines the change from a Cassie—Baxter state to a wetted Wenzel state, but also the distance between and shape of the roughness features (Yu et al., 2015).

9.2.3 Wetting transition

A variety of factors can contribute to the superhydrophobicity of surfaces, and the ones that have high contact angles are no doubt due to this. However, when a high contact angle is formed, the wetting state is not clearly presented in most cases. It is still unclear whether the liquid droplet rests on the solid surface or the air depending on the Wenzel and Cassie—Baxter states; however, they might be suitable for superhydrophobic surfaces. Furthermore, CAH can be lower in the CB state than in the Wenzel state, which may lead to greater stability in the CB state (Bernhard, 1965; Wenzel, 1949). It appears that the two states differ. In the presence of a large CAH, a transition might occur, and this reduces the stability or metastability of wetting (Mizukoshi et al., 2007; Wenzel, 1936, 1949). With a "superhydrophobic" surface, advancing contact angles might exceed 150 degrees and receding contact angles might be below 150 degrees. For hydrophobic surfaces, it may be the case that the advancing contact angle exceeds 90 degrees and the receding contact angle is less than 90 degrees. The advancing and receding contact angles can change the wetting state of these states, so they are not 100% superhydrophobic or hydrophobic. The structure and chemical properties of the surface are incongruent and inhomogeneous, resulting in this effect. The hysteresis of contact angles and pinning of liquid droplets can be caused by structural and chemical properties as well as adhesive forces. Our discussion of wetting states continues based on contact angles (Yan et al., 2011).

9.3 Biomimetic surface properties

9.3.1 Wettability

The contact angle is a measure of wetting or the angle between a solid surface and a liquid surface. Liquids that wet surfaces have a contact angle of $0 < \theta < 90$, while liquids that do not wet surfaces (referred to as nonwetting liquids or hydrophobic surfaces) have a contact angle of $90 < \theta < 180$. In order for a surface to be considered superhydrophobic, θ must be close to 180 (Nosonovsky & Bhushan, 2005).

The property of being highly water-repellent is also referred to as "superhydrophobicity." There is no clear definition of superhydrophobicity in the literature, nor is it consistently used. It refers to surfaces that have static contact angles greater than 140 degrees. It is also mentioned that low CAH, low water roll-off angles, and low water-holding capacities as implications of extremely water-repellent materials (Mohamed et al., 2015). Producing surfaces with a contact angle enlarged more than 120 degrees is only possible by any texture or by way of hydrophobic surface chemistry on smooth surfaces (Cerman et al., 2009; Solga et al., 2007).

It is also necessary to have a rough surface to achieve superhydrophobicity. An enlarged water—air interface results in reduced capillary forces between the droplet and surface when a surface is micro- or nanometer-structured (Herminghaus, 2000). This results in almost spherical droplets that usually roll off easily. De Gennes et al. referred to these surfaces as "low energy surfaces" (De Gennes et al., 2004).

Quere et al. have defined droplet behavior on low-energy surfaces (Quéré et al., 2003). Hansen and Autumn found that the particle's contact area with the underlying solid is significantly reduced, leading to a very low adhesion force (Hansen & Autumn, 2005). The particle adheres to the droplet instead of the surface when a droplet appears, yielding to the prevalent capillary forces. This results in the particle being carried away. In combination with surface roughness, hydrophobicity has been shown to create surfaces with contact angles exceeding 170 degrees (close to the theoretical maximum of 180 degrees). A droplet may move easily over a surface despite having a very high contact angle, according to Chen et al. A surface with a contact angle of 169 degrees was presented by them, on which even when the surface was held upside down, droplets stuck (Chen et al., 1999; Solga et al., 2007).

To attain superhydrophobic properties, a surface should meet the following requirements when analyzed based on various roughness distributions. The first requirement is that asperities must have a high aspect ratio in order for the surface area to be large. A second recommendation is to avoid sharp edges, so as not to pin the triple line. The third asperity should be tightly packed in to prevent destabilization of the composite interface by reducing the distance between them. The fourth factor is that asperities should be small in comparison to the typical size of droplets. Finally, to achieve an initial $\theta > 90$, a hydrophobic film must be applied over a hydrophilic surface. Surfaces that are superhydrophobic can be created using these recommendations (Nosonovsky & Bhushan, 2005).

9.3.2 Roughness

A rough surface can have a greater contact angle with nonwetting liquids than a flat surface, as has been observed with leaves of plants in which water does not stay on their surface, for instance, lotus leaves. In addition to the fact that rough surfaces have sharp edges, roughness affects the contact angle due to the increase in the solid–liquid interface area. An interface composed of solid, liquid, and air may be unstable or stable depending on how high the roughness of the surface is.

In addition to roughness, the manner of surface preparation, as well as the cleanliness of the surface contribute to the contact angle (Adamson, 1990; Nosonovsky & Bhushan, 2005; Schwartz et al., 1992). An increase in surface roughness can lead to a surface becoming more hydrophobic or hydrophilic. A droplet spreading on a rough surface was modeled by Wenzel based on the net energy decrease. In hydrophobic surfaces, the roughness increases the contact angle, while in hydrophilic surfaces, it decreases it. Rough surfaces have larger solid–liquid interface areas, leading to more net energy. Using a composite solid–liquid–air interface, Cassie and Baxter have suggested that cavities may form on rough surfaces, affecting the contact angle and forming a composite solid–liquid–air interface (Nosonovsky & Bhushan, 2005).

Using the Wenzel model, roughness changes the contact angle according to experimental evidence. Polypropylene's contact angle (104 degrees for a smooth surface) increases with increasing roughness, according to Erbil et al.

The contact angle is influenced by roughness in two different ways: by the increase of the area of solid–liquid interfaces and by the effect of sharp edges. Surfaces with a rough texture have a greater contact angle than those with a flat texture, and superhydrophobic surfaces may approach 180 degrees. A plant with high roughness and high contact angles, like lotus leaves, is known to have this effect, which can be used to produce water-repellent surfaces. When sharp edges are present, they pin the triple line. This results in contact angles that progress and recede at different rates (CAH), which hinders fluid flow. For most applications, where fluid flow is essential, this is not desirable. There is an increased contact angle when surfaces are very rough, which is caused by a composite system of solid, liquid, and air (Nosonovsky & Bhushan, 2005).

9.3.3 Topography

An important factor for tissue engineering (TE) success is the interface between cells and substrates. In addition to influencing endothelial cell proliferation and metabolism, the topography of the substrate also influences endothelial cell morphology, migration, and the secretion of cytokines and chemokines (Monteiro et al., 2022).

A new TE approach considers the surface topography of biomaterial-based grafts as a crucial property. The composition of protein layers can be impacted dramatically by topographical features, such as grooves, ridges, pits, and pillars. A number of surface properties, including surface compliance, have been demonstrated to have a significant impact on specific interactions between cells and surfaces. The shape, size, spacing, and curvature of topographical features should be considered when designing strategies to minimize foreign body reactions. Thus the cell behavior and ultimately the response of the tissue can be controlled by controlling the signals relayed to the nucleus.

During the attachment, proliferation, and differentiation of cells on biomaterials, surface topography impacts them at the micrometer and sub-micrometer levels (Altankov et al., 1996; Baleani et al., 2000; Baneyx et al., 2002; Vogel & Sheetz, 2006). Increasing the porosity and roughness of biomaterial surfaces promotes bone ingrowth, proliferation, and attachment (Harvey et al., 2013).

9.4 Biomimetic materials

One or both of the two polymers (proteins and polysaccharides) exist as the main component of biological materials. Many biological materials have less density compared with hand-made ones. In fact, biological materials can show the same mechanical properties if their density is close enough to the hand-made materials. In most biological structures, the better orientation of their bonds and tightly controlled structure can compensate for their lower density. Silk is an example of biological material which is stronger, tougher in tension, and stiffer compared to steel (Ashby et al., 2004).

9.4.1 Single polymer materials

Several materials are based on cellulose and would be considered biomimetic although they are in the category of fibers. One of the earliest fibers utilized by humans was silk. The first biomimetic fiber was nylon which was discovered accidentally (Vincent, 2009).

Dan Urry et al. use chemical synthetic methods to produce elastin analogs. Based on their data, these materials can transfer energy in different ways which raises it chance to have controllable mechanical characteristics to be utilized in different molecular machines. They also provided polymers that can adsorb vibrational energy released through submarine machinery (Huang et al., 2000).

Tissue scaffolds that are used in skin growth are made from elastin analogs. In addition, researchers are trying to find out new ways to develop and produce enough synthetic biological materials for clinical development (Currey & Taylor, 1974).

9.4.2 Water-based systems

Water is one of the main contents of biological materials and it is an essential organization of biological systems (Pollack, 2003). However, the technology and new generation of coating have progressed to eliminate water and superhydrophobic coatings came into use. Researchers have focused on solving the problem of hydrophobic systems for many years till they generated water-based systems. Nowadays it is possible to synthesize silk in a water environment (Hamodrakas et al., 2002; Vincent & Wegst, 2004; Yamanaka et al., 2013).

9.4.3 Ceramic composites

The cheapest way for enhancing biological tissues is calcium carbonate, hydroxyapatite, dolomite silica, etc. in crystalline or semicrystalline form. Nacre as the simplest biological ceramic is made of thin sheets of aragonite and polymer between the sheets (Currey & Taylor, 1974; Jackson et al., 1277). The polymer can increase the resistance of the system to fracture under high shear conditions (Jackson et al., 1988, 1989). Based on the literature, the only biomimetic nacre is formed from laminae 200 μm of silicon carbide and graphite filled the free space of the plates (Jackson et al., 1989). The absence of polymer makes it act as thermal fatigue resistant system (Cook & Gordon, 1964).

The toughness and hardness of the nacreous structures cannot touch the ceramic materials. *Euplectella* sponge is another biomimetic ceramic with a complex and tough structure. The existing space between its layers is filled by soft protein (Walter et al., 2007). It is complexity and layered structure cause an increase in durability.

9.4.4 Fibrous composites

There are many biological fibrous such as cellulose, chitin, collagen, and keratin. But the only one that can be called biomimetic is the one developed by Gordon and Jeronimides (Gordon & Jeronimidis, 1980). The wood analog invented by them did not embrace high energy absorption. In this kind of wood, the thickness of the wall usually contains 80% of the total wall thickness and it is usually oriented in one direction such as cellulose wounding at an angle of about 15. This wounding structure enhances the toughness.

In early models, several glass fibers were stuck together by resin and showed 50 times tougher compared with man-made materials. The fibrous materials were designed for protection against explosives and bullets. If they were so light to be used in cellular materials, they would be suitable for textile industries. The use of fibrous materials as protective shields may increase the cost of them but its benefit is in their lower weight compared to the traditional shield. In addition, the main reason for their usage is to accept penetration and adsorb the energy despite the traditional ones designed to resist penetration (Bernhard, 1965).

9.5 Processing technologies

9.5.1 Layer-by-layer deposition

Deposition of layer-by-layer (LBL) films relies on changing the charge of the substrate. This permits multilayered films to be constructed (Chen & McCarthy, 1999). The process is usually carried out by assembling layers through spontaneous adsorption, while substrate sizes can vary. In contrast to imprinting methods, a plasma treatment chamber or chemical vapour deposition (CVD) chamber is not required for replicating the master. It is therefore relatively straightforward and potentially economical to use this type of method. Often, nanoparticles are added to deposition to achieve a superhydrophobic surface (Soeno et al., 2004). Surface patterns can, however, become more difficult to control in this way. Functional surfaces were produced in a series of research projects conducted by Cohen and Rubner using the LBL method (Bravo et al., 2007; Cebeci et al., 2006; Lee et al., 2006; Wu et al., 2007).

Their typical process of creating transparent superhydrophobic films containing SiO_2 nanoparticles of varying sizes was LBL processing (Bravo et al., 2007). Several aqueous solutions were used to immerse the substrates repeatedly to effectively form three layers of the film: the adhesion layer, the body layer, and the top layer (Fig. 9.1). First, the substrate was dipped into a cationic solution, followed by a solution of anionic ions with the proper assistant operation. For the adhesion layers, poly(allylamine hydrochloride) (PAH) and

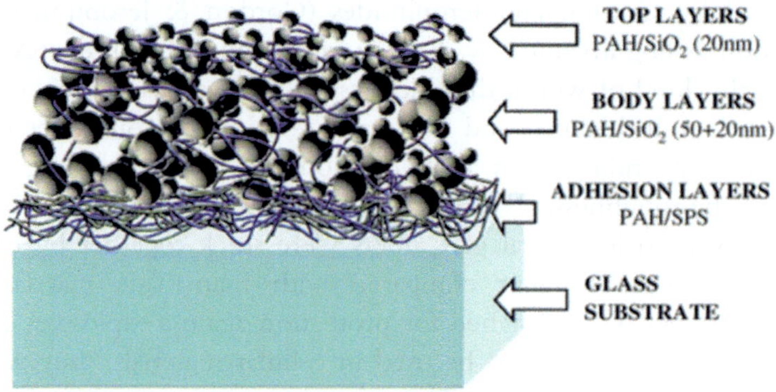

Figure 9.1 Three main assemblies of the multilayer film shown in a simplified schematic. *Reprinted with permission from Yan, Y. Y., Gao, N., & Barthlott, W. (2011). Mimicking natural superhydrophobic surfaces and grasping the wetting process: A review on recent progress in preparing superhydrophobic surfaces.* Advances in Colloid and Interface Science, *169(2), 80–105.*

poly(sodium 4-styrenesulfonate) were used to create cationic and anionic solutions, which could enhance the polymer–nanoparticle bonding. The cationic solution was created with PAH, while the anionic solution was made with two types of silica nanoparticles (50 and 20 nm). PAH was used for the cationic solution on top and distilled water solution containing silica particles of 20 nm for the anionic solution. A multilayered thin film optimized for optical transmission maintained optical transmission levels exceeding 90% and achieved contact angles of 160 degrees with a CAH of as little as 10 degrees. The LBL techniques used by Zhai's group were also used to fabricate a switchable superhydrophilic/hydrophobic surface (Chunder et al., 2009). Using precise control over film thickness and roughness, PAH and silica nanoparticle multilayered films were applied to the surface. A low surface energy material—(1 H,1 H,2 H,2H-perfluorooctyl)silane(perfluorosilane)—was applied to the surface as well as poly(N-isopropylacryamide) (PNIPAAm), a thermos-responsive polymer that exhibits low critical solution temperature in aqueous solutions. In microfluidic channels, the combination of surface roughness and chemical composition could potentially create superhydrophobic/superhydrophilic valves. The lotus leaf was mimicked by Jindasuwan et al. to produce superhydrophobic surfaces. Through LBL deposition of polyelectrolytes onto glass substrates, they deposited superhydrophobic films. A semifluorinated silane was then applied to reduce the surface energy after SiO_2 nanoparticles were deposited to modify the surface roughness (Yan et al., 2011).

9.5.2 Colloidal assembling and aggregation

To make superhydrophobic surfaces, colloidal particles can be assembled or aggregated during chemical deposition, sol–gel processing, and lithography (Amigoni et al., 2009; Bravo et al., 2007; Lvov et al., 1997; Manca et al., 2009; Sato et al., 2009). A colloidal assembly is formed when monodispersed particles are chemically bonded or are held together by van der Waals forces. It is possible to obtain multilayered roughness (Sun et al., 2007) by controlling the size of the assembling particles and having different scales. Substrates are usually immersed in the particle solution or spin-coated with the solution (Hsieh et al., 2008). Several studies have demonstrated that monodispersed silica particles can be spin-coated over a wide area, such as Min et al. (Min et al., 2008). Fig. 9.2A illustrates a typical transmission electron microscope image of the nanoparticles as they were made. Images of the spheres were analyzed using image analysis software (Scion Image) and calculated as 72 ± 6 nm. In Fig. 9.2B, you can see a top-view SEM image of the multilayered crystal structure that was spun-coated for 10 minutes at 10,000 rpm. An example of a nonclose-packed spin-coated colloidal crystal is shown in Fig. 9.2C. By filling in the triangular crevices created by the second layer's spheres, the spheres of the top-layer completed the structure.

There was a single layer of spheres individually distributed on this occasion. During spin-coating, the time and speed could be adjusted to control the thickness of the colloidal crystals.

Multilayered colloidal crystals based on self-assembly techniques were the key to achieving the superhydrophobic states mentioned earlier.

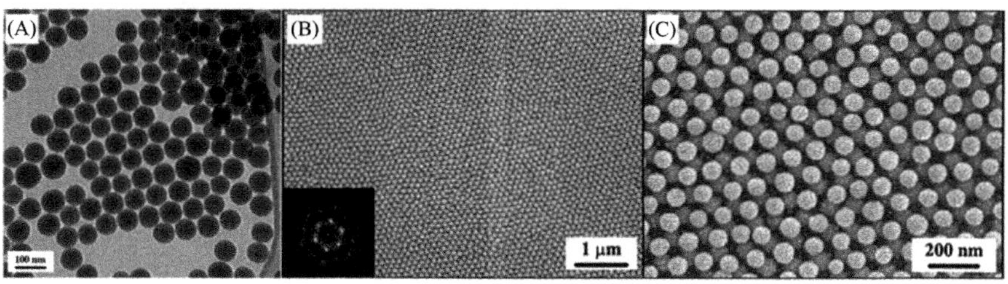

Figure 9.2 (A) Silica nanoparticles synthesized. (B) Image of a spin-coated multilayer colloidal crystal taken with a scanning electron microscope. (C) The sample in (B) was taken at a higher magnification. *Reprinted with permission from Yan, Y. Y., Gao, N., & Barthlott, W. (2011). Mimicking natural superhydrophobic surfaces and grasping the wetting process: A review on recent progress in preparing superhydrophobic surfaces.* Advances in Colloid and Interface Science, 169*(2), 80–105.*

The patterns on superhydrophobic surfaces are formed by the self-assembly of colloidal particles under the influence of internal forces. Choosing a solid substrate that has a specific and favorable interface for self-assembled monolayers (SAMs) requires the forming of a stable monolayer film. Therefore despite taking the substrate away from the solution from which the SAMs formed, the formed film must remain attached firmly to the substrate. Repeatedly conducting SAMs can create multilayered structures (Lai et al., 2010; Lim et al., 2009; Lin & Tang, 2015).

An assembly process of 1D polyaniline nanofibers in the presence of perfluorosebacic acid was described by Zhu et al. for preparing a superhydrophobic dandelion-like microstructure. PANI 1D nanofibers are self-assembled via hydrogen bonding, stacking, and hydrophobic interactions to form 3D microstructures, the result of hydrogen bonding, stacking, and hydrophobic interactions. A fullerene derivative containing three long aliphatic chains was hierarchically self-assembled using supramolecular chemistry by Shen et al. (Lin & Tang, 2015). As shown in Fig. 9.3, compared

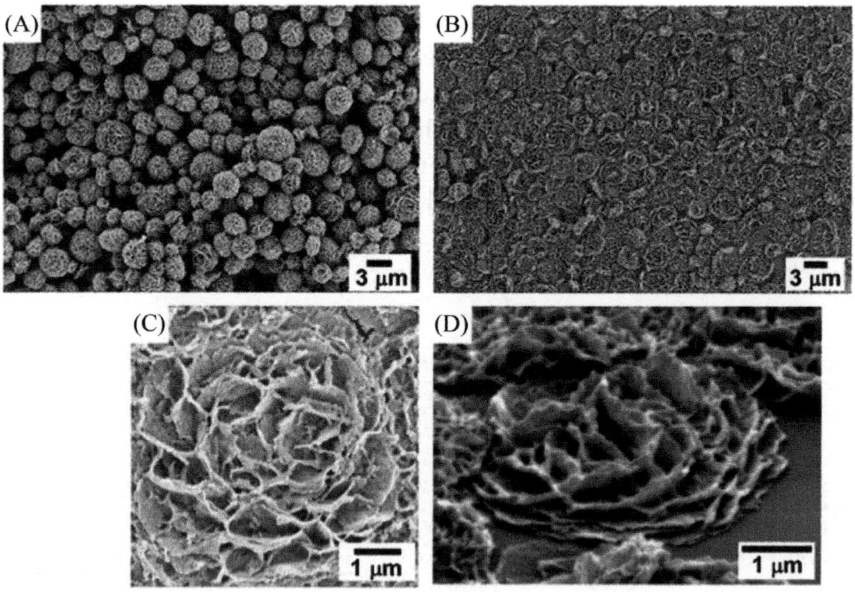

Figure 9.3 An image of the globular assembly of fullerene derivatives painted with SEM (A), Au nanoflakes transcribed from globular objects (B), a top view (C), and a 34.7-degree angle (D). *Reprinted with permission from Yan, Y. Y., Gao, N., & Barthlott, W. (2011). Mimicking natural superhydrophobic surfaces and grasping the wetting process: A review on recent progress in preparing superhydrophobic surfaces.* Advances in Colloid and Interface Science, 169*(2), 80–105.*

to SAMs of thiols, assembled fullerene derivatives provided rough surfaces, whereas SAMs of thiols provided superhydrophilic or superhydrophobic surfaces (Yan et al., 2011).

Furthermore, SAMs can be chemically modified to be superhydrophobic by introducing superhydrophobic properties into micro- or nanostructures. For nanostructures, ZnO nanorods were formed using a solution method and conventional silicon wet-etching (to fabricate microstructures). In addition, surfaces without SAMs and those with SAMs could have contact angles that differ by up to 167 degrees. Tridecafluoro-1,1,2,2-tetrahydrooctyltrichlorosilane (FOTS) was used as a SAM to treat transparent and superhydrophobic glass surfaces (Lee et al., 2008). As a result of combining colloidal lithography and plasma etching, tower-shaped nanostructures were produced that display superhydrophobic properties when treated with fluoroalkylsilane (FAS) SAMs. Using waterborne solutions, Motornov et al. produced superhydrophobic surfaces using nanoparticle aggregates deposited (cast) from nanoparticles (Motornov et al., 2008).

Fig. 9.4A–C illustrates what the particle aggregates looked like in hierarchical colloids with three levels. There was a wide range of lengths in the grafted copolymer layer composed of P4VP and poly(styrene-block-4-vinylpyridine) P(S-b-4VP) chains (Fig. 9.4D). Hydrophilic particles were initially formed, but as the coating warmed above polystyrene (PS) glass transition temperature, they became hydrophobic, even becoming superhydrophobic (Yan et al., 2011).

An intricate coating of silica nanoparticles was used by Xue et al. to create superhydrophobic surfaces on cotton textiles (Xue et al., 2009). Polymerization of tetraethylorthosilicate was followed by amino-functionalization and epoxy-functionalization to produce nanoparticles. It was then dipped in an ethanol solution of amino-functionalized silica nanoparticles and finally in an ethanol solution of epoxy-functionalized silica nanoparticles with proper nipping, after being epoxy-functionalized by a mixture of epichlorohydrin and alkaline solution beforehand. After the covalent bonding of the silica particles to cotton fibers, there were epoxy groups on the fibers' surface to be used for surface grafting. Final finishing could be carried out by layering stearic acid, 1 H, 1 H, 2 H, 2H-perfluorodecyltrichlorosilane (PFTDS), or both on the rough surface of cotton textiles. A schematic representation of the methodology can be found in Fig. 9.5.

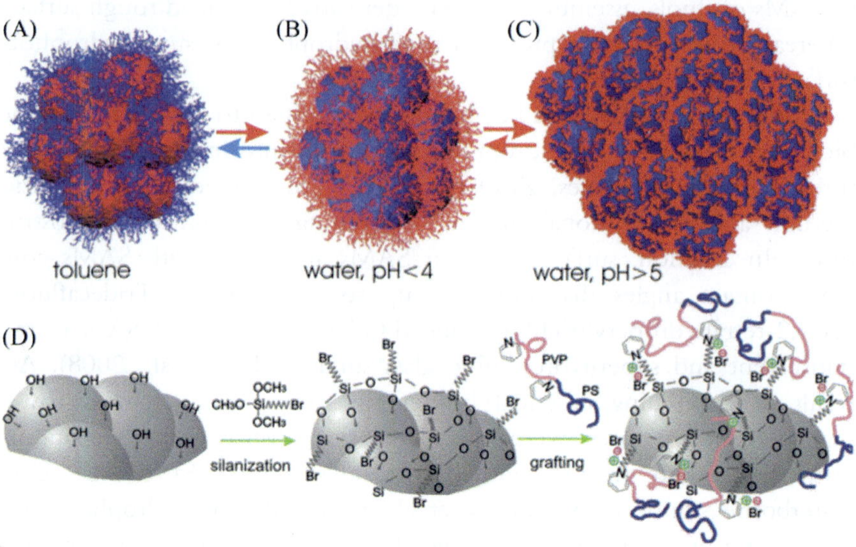

Figure 9.4 Synthesized hybrid nanoparticles exhibit different morphologies. (A) Toluene, a good solvent for PS and a poor solvent for P4VP was used to coat primary aggregates coated by collapsed P4VP chains (red) and stretched PS chains (blue); (B) primary aggregates coated with collapsed PS and stretched P4VP in water at pHb4, a good solvent for P4VP, but a poor solvent for PS; (C) secondary aggregate in water at pHN5; (D) grafting block copolymer brushes on primary silica particle aggregates. *Reprinted with permission from Yan, Y. Y., Gao, N., & Barthlott, W. (2011). Mimicking natural superhydrophobic surfaces and grasping the wetting process: A review on recent progress in preparing superhydrophobic surfaces.* Advances in Colloid and Interface Science, 169*(2), 80–105.*

Based on those examples, it can be seen that colloidal assembly and aggregation is a very effective ways of modifying surface energy and extending the roughness of the surface structure to create extremely wettable surfaces. As a result of these chemical reactions, the colloidal aggregates can generally remain connected to the substrate for a considerable period of time, contributing to the durability of the formed structure. Production equipment and operation procedures do not necessarily need to be complex.

Hence, colloidal assembling and aggregation offer a significant advantage over traditional imprinting methods and even some CVD processes. Besides providing sufficient surface coverage, it also produces a precise order of structure. It is essential, however, to graft desired properties into colloidal solutions and to maintain stable and uniform operations to widely apply the process (Yan et al., 2011).

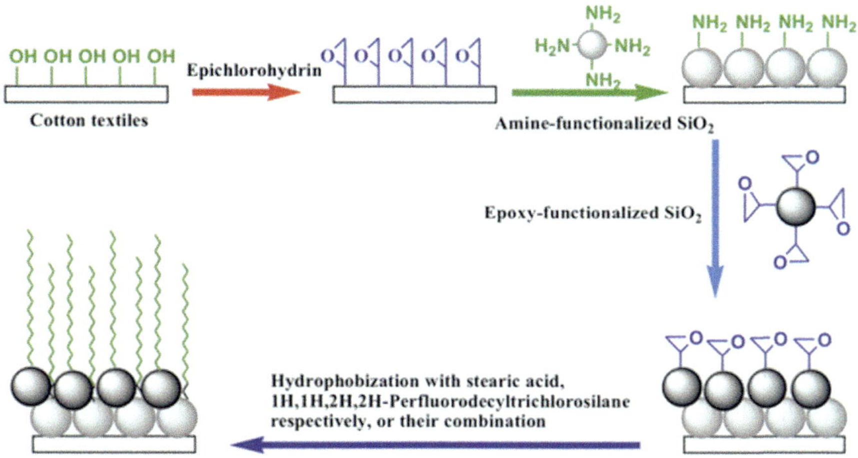

Figure 9.5 The procedure for preparing superhydrophobic surfaces on cotton. *Reprinted with permission from Yan, Y. Y., Gao, N., & Barthlott, W. (2011). Mimicking natural superhydrophobic surfaces and grasping the wetting process: A review on recent progress in preparing superhydrophobic surfaces.* Advances in Colloid and Interface Science, 169*(2), 80–105.*

9.5.3 Sol–gel process

Based on Wenzel or Cassie–Baxter's theories, sol–gel methods have been used to mimic the surface structure of lotus leaves since the very early stages of creating superhydrophobic surfaces (Bico et al., 1999; Mahltig & Böttcher, 2003; Sheen et al., 2009; Shirtcliffe et al., 2003). In this process, chemicals are used as precursors to form a gel-like network and are then deposited onto the selected substrate. A superhydrophobic surface can be created by adding materials that have low surface energy, as well as micro- and nanoparticles. Transparent and superhydrophobic films on glass surfaces can be created using this type of method because it is compatible with glass (Hikita et al., 2005; Shang et al., 2005; Tadanaga et al., 2000, 2003). It is always necessary to control processes like spin-coating to ensure a generally regular surface pattern on the network.

An example reported recently involved the formation of silica films with optical transparency and superhydrophobicity by using a eutectic liquid in a sol–gel process (Xue et al., 2009). A common sol–gel solvent (such as ethanol) had an extremely high vapor pressure compared to the eutectic liquid (urea and choline chloride). During the process of filmmaking under ambient conditions, the eutectic liquid remained in the film, allowing better control over film thickness and surface roughness. After the eutectic liquid was extracted from the eutectic solution, porous silica thin films were formed with asperities. The base catalyst consisted of tetraethoxysilane, ethanol, HCl, and H_2O. By treating the polymers with FAS, superhydrophobicity was achieved, resulting in a contact angle of 170 degrees and a hysteresis of 2–3 degrees. Using ethanol to dilute the sol solution and spin-coat, it on substrates further improves the transparency of superhydrophobic films. This SEM image (Fig. 9.6) shows spin-coated surfaces that have been diluted with ethanol by 1:1, 3:1, 5:1, and 7:1 and coated with a sol dilution by 1:1, 3:1, 5:1. As spin-coated films were diluted, their surface roughness and thickness decreased continuously while their superhydrophobicity remained. Consequently, the films were more transparent (Yan et al., 2011).

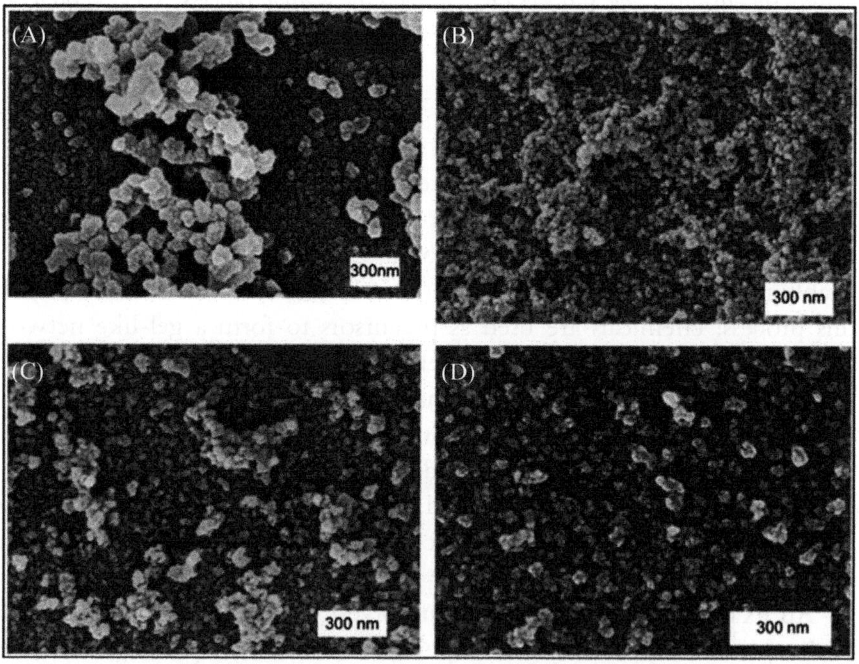

Figure 9.6 Image of a dilute-sol-coated glass slide taken by SEM. There is a 1:1 ratio of ethanol to sol in (A), a 3:1 ratio in (B), a 5:1 ratio in (C), and a 7:1 ratio in (D). *Reprinted with permission from Yan, Y. Y., Gao, N., & Barthlott, W. (2011). Mimicking natural superhydrophobic surfaces and grasping the wetting process: A review on recent progress in preparing superhydrophobic surfaces.* Advances in Colloid and Interface Science, 169*(2), 80–105.*

9.5.4 Electrospinning and electrospraying

Microstructures and nanostructures can be fabricated using electrospinning and electrospraying, two similar but different techniques. In terms of creating superhydrophobic surfaces, however, both methods are very susceptible to mistakes. Several techniques have been developed to produce continuous polymer fibers at the micro- and nanoscale, including electrospinning (Wang et al., 2008). A rough surface can be created more effectively by prompting its roughness (Tuteja et al., 2007). Properly preparing the polymer's molecular weight and solution concentration is necessary for forming uniform fibers (Ma et al., 2005). Electrospraying can also be used on other materials besides fibers, however. Electrospraying deposits polymer films in the form of spheres, fibers, or other shapes (Mizukoshi et al., 2007). However, the electrospinning process produces fibers, while the electrospraying process produces beads. Using electrospinning, Ding et al. produced superhydrophobic ZnO nanostructures. To obtain ZnO fibrous films, electrospun PVA/zinc acetate solution was electrospun into composite poly(vinyl alcohol)/ZnO nanofibrous films.

A FAS coating was applied to the rough surface to induce superhydrophobicity. In Fig. 9.7A and B, you can see images captured by field emission scanning electron microscopy. There were approximately 100 nanometers in diameter of the fibers that formed the structure's base. An average diameter of 69 nm grain-like ZnO particles originated on the fiber surface, and these particles consisted of the secondary structure. The water contact angle was 0 degree before FAS coating, indicating the superhydrophilicity of fibrous ZnO films. FZnO films coated with FAS showed apparent superhydrophobicity after FAS coating with a contact angle of up to 165 degrees and a sliding angle of approximately 5 degrees. FZnO fibers with grain-like ZnO particles on the fiber surface were observed in FE-SEM images in Fig. 9.7C and D (Yan et al., 2011).

A recent study by Hen et al. about coaxial electrospinning produced nano/microfibers that were core-sheath structured but had different properties from those that were individually colored and sheathed. Combining Teflon AF (2,2-bis-trifluoromethyl4,5-difluoro-1,3-dioxole with tetrafluoroethylene) with an electrospinnable core material enabled it to be electrospun successfully. Fig. 9.8A shows a coaxial nozzle as an annular tube surrounded by a central tube. Using a coaxial nozzle, separate polymer solutions were fed into the coaxial nozzle for both the core and the sheath. Fig. 9.8B shows an emergent compound pendant droplet. At a

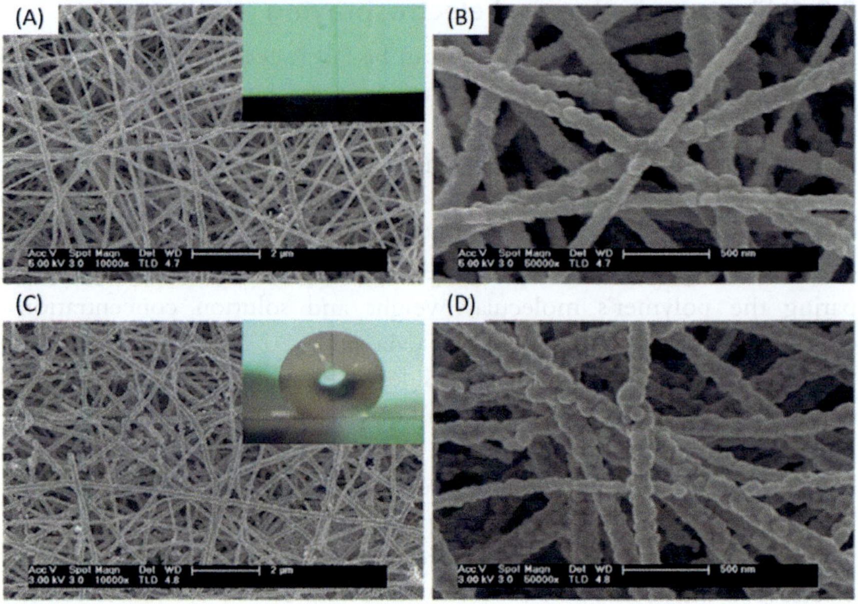

Figure 9.7 Films of fibrous ZnO (A) and FZnO (B) made by FE-SEM. An inset shows the profile of a water droplet on the films. The corresponding magnifications for (A) and (B) are (B) and (D), respectively. *Reprinted with permission from Yan, Y. Y., Gao, N., & Barthlott, W. (2011). Mimicking natural superhydrophobic surfaces and grasping the wetting process: A review on recent progress in preparing superhydrophobic surfaces.* Advances in Colloid and Interface Science, *169(2), 80–105.*

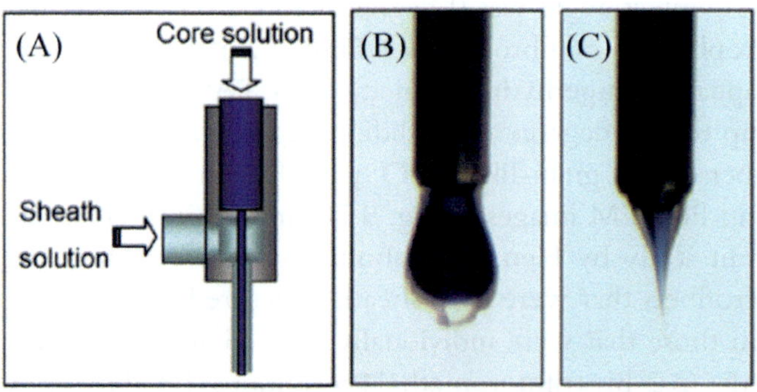

Figure 9.8 Electrospinning with axial motion. (A) Diagram of the coaxial nozzle; (B) core-sheath droplet without bias; (C) Taylor cone and coaxial jet formation at 12.5 kV. *Reprinted with permission from Yan, Y. Y., Gao, N., & Barthlott, W. (2011). Mimicking natural superhydrophobic surfaces and grasping the wetting process: A review on recent progress in preparing superhydrophobic surfaces.* Advances in Colloid and Interface Science, *169(2), 80–105.*

sufficient voltage, a distorted droplet with a core and sheath material ejected a charged liquid jet called a Taylor cone (Fig. 9.8C). The coaxial electrospinning method was used to fabricate ultrahydrophobic and oleophobic membranes while preserving their mechanical strength. The authors also reported a large-scale superhydrophobic mat surface made by electrospinning with four jets. Adding polyamide 6 (PA6) fibers to PS fibers enhanced the electrospun surface's mechanical properties. Electrospinning the fibers was achieved using four syringes. As part of the electrospinning process, jet ratios of PS/PA6 were tuned to regulate the mechanical properties of PS mats.

An electrospraying method was considered to be used for forming PTFE fibers. As can be seen in Fig. 9.9, the electrospray PTFE coating has a peculiar micro- and nanoscale structure, which provides the rough surface required for superhydrophobic surfaces (Yan et al., 2011).

9.5.5 Phase separation

By changing surrounding conditions such as temperature and pressure, patterned surface structures can be created by colloidal aggregation methods that use phase separation to separate solid particles from metastable mixtures. It is possible to form macroscopic, microscopic, and even nanoscopic surface structures and roughnesses as a result of phase separation. Sol–gel is often associated with this method for creating controllable surface patterns due to its working mechanism (Nakajima et al., 2000;

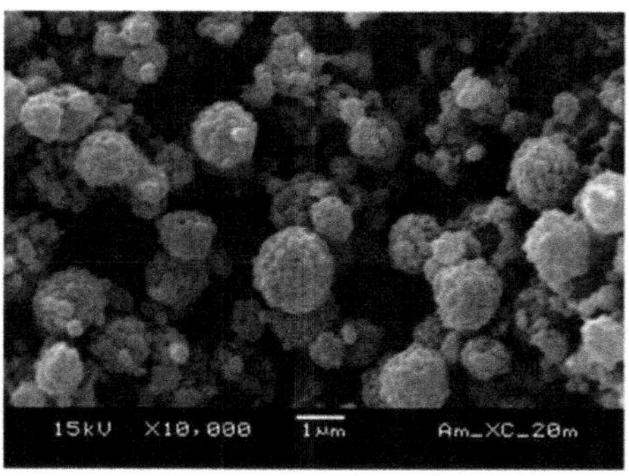

Figure 9.9 Electrospray superhydrophobic PTFE surface imaged using SEM. *Reprinted with permission from Yan, Y. Y., Gao, N., & Barthlott, W. (2011). Mimicking natural superhydrophobic surfaces and grasping the wetting process: A review on recent progress in preparing superhydrophobic surfaces.* Advances in Colloid and Interface Science, 169*(2), 80–105.*

Shirtcliffe et al., 2003). Sol–gel methods do not rely exclusively on phase separation; other techniques, such as plasma treatment (Song et al., 2009), electrospinning, and self-aggregation (Xie et al., 2004), can also support this process. All these methods involve phase separation processes related to colloidal polymerization in some way (Yan et al., 2011).

9.6 Characteristics of biomimetic coatings

9.6.1 Mechanical strength

Composition, structure, and processing conditions all play a role in determining the mechanical properties of biomimetic coatings.

1. **Hardness:** Biomimetic coatings can simulate the hardness of natural materials like shells or teeth. In addition to ensuring wear resistance, this property also protects against abrasion. Despite being eroded by seawater and sediment for a long time, tidal shells still appear intact and are very resistant to damage. Soft-hard phases with special structures are observed on the nonsmooth surface of the shells (Zhao et al., 2022).
2. **Elasticity:** It is also possible to design biomimetic coatings to have high elasticity similar to natural tissues like tendons and ligaments. Flexibility and shock absorption depend on this property.
3. **Adhesion:** For long-term durability and performance, biomimetic coatings must have strong adhesion to the substrate material. A variety of surface modification techniques have been developed in the field of biomaterials and TE to emulate the properties of native extracellular matrices (ECMs). Cell–surface receptors, such as integrins, interact with ECM proteins, regulating cell behavior, resulting in tissue-specific cell spreading, migration, tissue assembly, and differentiation, as well as cell-to-cell communication.

   The development of biomimetic materials is currently based on three major strategies: (1) incorporation and release of bioactive molecules; (2) surface modification of biomaterials with bioadhesive ECM macromolecules or specific binding motifs; and (3) nanoscale patterning (Rahmany & Van Dyke, 2013).
4. **Toughness:** Biomimetic coatings can simulate natural materials with high toughness values similar to bone or wood. Although highly hydrated, plant cell walls demonstrate mechanical stiffness, strength, and toughness (Svagan et al., 2007). As well, the evolution of the biological world over millions of years has developed a rigorous organic/inorganic laminated structure of nacre that can withstand

mechanical shocks and chemical attacks. Several studies have demonstrated that nacre-biomimetic materials are capable of achieving high strength and toughness simultaneously. When the brick-and-mortar layers of nacre are integrated into the matrix, the fracture toughness of the material can exceed that of $CaCO_3$ by three orders of magnitude. Since the organic matrix dissipates strain and the aragonite provides strength, it has a high level of resistance to crack initiation and growth (Zhang et al., 2018). Accordingly, this property contributes to the resistance to fracture and cracking.

5. **Fatigue resistance:** In applications where the coating will experience repeated stress cycles over time, biomimetic coatings can be designed to resist fatigue failure under cyclic loading conditions. According to studies, the thermal fatigue of biomimetic coatings can be improved by coupling materials. A laser surface melting and laser coating technology was used by Zhao et al. to prepare two kinds of biomimetic coupling materials. As a result of the study, biomimetic coupling samples were more resistant to frictional wear and thermal fatigue than those not treated, and laser coating treated samples had superior resistance to thermal fatigue and wear compared with laser melting samples (Zhao et al., 2008).

Overall, biomimetic coatings must have some conducive mechanical properties to be useful in a range of applications. Compared to traditional synthetic materials, these coatings can improve performance and durability by mimicking the structure and properties of natural materials.

9.6.2 Degradation

Biomimetic coatings are used in a variety of applications, including medical implants, drug delivery systems, and environmental remediation. However, like all materials, biomimetic coatings can degrade over time due to various factors such as exposure to environmental conditions, mechanical stress, and chemical reactions.

A biomimetic coating will degrade when exposed to temperatures, humidity, and UV radiation. Coatings can break down due to these factors, and their protective properties can be lost. As a result of exposure to body fluids and enzymes, biomimetic coatings used on medical implants may degrade over time.

Metal implants and biomaterials can be coated with biomimetic coatings, for instance. It is not possible to induce bone growth with the materials used to fill bony defects. Therefore the biomimetic method was used to biologically functionalize such materials, which resulted in a biomimetic coating onto various biomaterials.

In a three-dimensional environment, bone substitutes support osteogenic and angiogenic cell migration and proliferation. It is imperative that the substitute is gradually degraded and replaced by natural bone once a bone and vascular system are established (Sokolsky-Papkov et al., 2007). To fulfill its function, a bone substitute must undergo a certain degradation rate: if it is degraded too rapidly, osteogenic activities will be disrupted and connective tissue healing will dominate; on the other hand, if it decays too slowly, the natural bone will be unable to replace it. The degradation rate of bone substitutes has been modulated in many studies (Liu et al., 2010b; Mistry et al., 2010; Sokolsky-Papkov et al., 2007).

Biomimetic coatings can also degrade under mechanical stress. An implant with a joint replacement coating can suffer from this when exposed to repeated cycles of strain. It can also lead to the coating peeling away from its underlying material over time due to this stress.

For instance, biomimetic implants used inside the body could be subjected to mechanical forces along the femur before the cortical bone has healed completely. As a result of these mechanical stresses, cylinders inserted in the cortical bone may show signs of micromotion, which may explain the degradation of their outer surfaces (Barrere et al., 2003).

The degradation of biomimetic coatings can also be caused by chemical reactions. As an example, coatings may be damaged or lost their protective properties if they are exposed to acidic or alkaline environments. The coating may also degrade more rapidly if it is exposed to certain chemicals or drugs (Yazdani et al., 2018).

The research community is currently investigating new materials and manufacturing techniques to mitigate these issues and improve the durability of biomimetic coatings. To create more durable, complex structures, advanced manufacturing techniques like 3D printing are being used to develop new polymers that are more resistant to environmental conditions and mechanical stress.

9.7 Substrate for fabrication of biomimetic coatings

9.7.1 Biomimetic coatings on polymer substrates

It has become increasingly important to develop calcium phosphate layers on polymer substrates because of their enhanced biocompatibility. A variety of coating techniques are employed, including biomimetic, spray coating, laser deposition, coupling, and low-temperature precipitation. It is most common to use biomimetic coatings among them. For surface modification, however, pretreatment of the substrate is quite a necessity before coating. On the basis of the common polymer substrates, Table 9.1 summarizes biomimetic coatings and their compositions (Koju et al., 2017).

9.7.2 Biomimetic coatings on metallic substrates

A metallic substrate has several intrinsic properties that make it useful for fabricating orthopedic implants and dental implants, such as high fracture toughness, good strength-to-weight ratio, good ductility, and biocompatibility. In terms of implant fabrication, titanium and related alloys are the most common materials. Nevertheless, bone-like apatites can enhance the bioactivity of such materials in vitro and in vivo. Surfaces such as Ti are coated with plasma spray, sol—gel, and other coating techniques to enhance osseointegration. Nevertheless, such coating techniques have disadvantages, including nonuniform thicknesses, poor adhesion to substrates, and high temperatures involved in processing. Ti-based implants face such issues due to biomimetic coating techniques (Barrere et al., 1999, 2002b). There is a growing body of evidence showing that magnesium (Mg) and its related alloys can be suitable implants (Staiger et al., 2006). These materials are important in this field because they combine low Young's modulus, high strength/weight ratio, biodegradability, as well as biocompatibility. They have, however, limited practical applications due to their fast degradation. The degradation rate of magnesium alloy substrates can be tailored through various protective coatings such as calcium phosphate and polymeric films, which would help the alloys to maintain mechanical integrity before the fractured bones have completely healed (Gray-Munro et al., 2009; Keim et al., 2011; Li et al., 2004; Witte et al., 2005; Yang et al., 2008; Zhang et al., 2009). Several biomimetic coatings have been created on popular metallic substrates, as shown in Table 9.2 (Koju et al., 2017).

9.8 Multifunctional biomimetic coatings

The design and fabrication of multifunctional biomimetic coatings have attracted great attention in recent years. This section outlines the potential of integration of relevant biomimetic characteristics and some functions such as self-cleaning, self-healing, anticorrosion, and antireflection

Table 9.1 Important examples of biomimetic coatings on a polymeric substrate.

Number	Authors	Significant outcomes
Biodegradable polymer substrates: A. Poly(0-caprolacetone) (PCL)		
1	Zhang et al. (2005)	• Bone marrow stromal cells infiltrate up to 48 and 114 mm into electrospun PCL and PCL/gelatin scaffold respectively
2	Oyane et al. (2005)	• A dense, uniform, thin, and irremovable layer of interconnected porous apatite structure formed over 2D and 3D structures.
3	Suárez-González et al. (2012)	• Rapid dissolution kinetics in Ca and P mineral deficient environment with higher HCO3 content. • Re-precipitation in Ca and P ions rich environment.
Poly(lactic acid) (PLA)/poly(lactic-*co*-glycolide) (PLGA)		
4	Yang et al. (2001)	• Effective cell proliferation and differentiation at low concentrations on PLA and PLGA films (adsorbed with FN, -RGD-, PLL)
5	Kim et al. (2008)	• PLGA/HA composites exhibited satisfactory osteoconductivity in in vivo transplantation. • In fibrin gel, BMP-2 is released for up to 8 weeks.
Nonbiodegradable polymer substrate: polyetheretherketone (PEEK)		
6	Yu et al. (2005)	• Crystal quantity was proportional to the HA volume fraction, in HA/PEEK composite. • Crystal size increased with prolonged immersion time and HA volume fraction
7	Chi et al. (2013)	• The AIP technique resulted in columnar and crystalline anatase or rutile phase for R-TiO_2/PEEK specimens. • Superior HA formation and osteocompatibility were noted after biomimetic immersion.
8	Zheng et al. (2014)	• Plasma polymerization maintained a Ca/P ratio of 1.58 with no discontinuities. • Defects and cracks appeared after 4-week immersion in 1.5 SBF.

Source: Reprinted with permission from Koju, N., et al. (2017). Biomimetic coating technology for orthopedic implants. *Current opinion in Chemical Engineering*, *15*, 49–55.

Table 9.2 Important examples of biomimetic coatings on metallic substrates.

Number	Authors	Salient features
Nonbiodegradable metallic substrates: titanium and related alloys		
1	Habibovic et al. (2002)	• Immersion in 5x SBF resulted in thin but uniform CaP. • Immersion in SBF with decreased crystal growth inhibitors resulted in fast precipitation of CaP
2	Song et al. (2004)	• When 1.5 SBF was used, apatite induction and formation time was shorter than 1.0 SBF and the film surface oxidation voltage was reduced to 350 V
3	Barrere et al. (2002a)	• The influence of Mg^{2+} and $HCO3^{-}$ ions in 5x SBF to form CaP coating on Ti6Al4V was studied.
4	Barrere et al. (2002a)	• Rapid CaP induction in 1.5 SBF within 18 hours regardless of the amount of predeposited HA.
5	Ma et al. (2003)	• A uniform layer of apatite with a nanocrystalline microporous structure formed. • Apatite thickness saturation in 1.5 SBF after 10 days
Biodegradable metallic substrates: magnesium and related alloys		
6	Witte et al. (2005)	• Bone cell activation in high Mg ion concentration. • However, no bone formation was found in the surrounding soft tissue. • Gas pockets were observed after 1 week of implantation but no adverse effects were recorded
7	Li et al. (2004)	• 99.99% pure magnesium, alkali, and heat treated, exhibited no mass loss when immersed in SBF (high and low concentration of Cl^{-} ions) for 180 days. • While marrow cell growth was not affected, apatite coating hindered the corrosion of Mg substrates
8	Gray-Munro et al. (2009)	• Surface modification minimizes the production of toxic by-products. • Corrosion rate of surface treated Mg alloys in descending order: Clean > Acid Etched > Calcium Phosphate Coated > PLA Coated > Poly(DTH carbonate) Coated
9	Keim et al. (2011)	• A spontaneous biomimetic layer, containing Ca, P, and C, was formed in a cell culture medium. • This reduced Mg release by 60% coupled with enhanced cell adhesion.

Source: Reprinted with permission from Koju, N., et al. (2017). Biomimetic coating technology for orthopedic implants. *Current opinion in Chemical Engineering, 15*, 49–55.

9.8.1 Shape memory and wettability

A lot of surfaces in nature show nonwetting behavior. The most common examples of these types of surfaces are lotus leaves, rose petals, and butterfly wings (Liu et al., 2018).

For many years, the surface with single wettability called traditional superhydrophobic surfaces used as nonwettable coatings. During the time, with development in industry, traditional superhydrophobic surfaces could not overcome the industry's requirements. So, the design of a surface with switchable wettability was noticed by researchers (Liu et al., 2018; Zhang et al., 2019).

Since controlling the surface roughness and structures is more complex than the surface chemistry, in the design of coating with reversible wetting behavior, changing the chemical composition is more usual. For this reason, shape-memory materials can play an important role because of their special advantages (Zhang et al., 2019). However, there is more controllable wetting behavior if both surface chemistry and structure can be changed (Tian & Guo, 2019; Wang et al., 2017a). In the case of shape memory, surface change in microstructure can happen in different ways: pressing and changing the height of roughness, electromagnetic waves absorbent, and stretching and release process (García-Huete et al., 2015).

Shape memory polymers can also be used to achieve a special wetting behavior like water spreading (Jeon et al., 2013). As an example, shape memory polymer Janus pillars can be obtained by evaporation of metal layers on epoxy-based shape memory polymer pillars (Chen et al., 2015). Above the glass transition temperature, the pillars lean back in the upright state, while their movement is limited by the coated metal layer. The combined effect between the presence of the metal layer and shape memory behavior led to tilting angle formation on the surface. This special wetting behavior is a result of both the surface chemistry of Janus and microstructure of pillars.

Superhydrophobic shape memory polymers with controllable surface wettability can be a good candidate for use in intelligent fields.

In traditional superhydrophobic coatings only, the static contact angle can be controlled reversibly. While in superhydrophobic shape memory surfaces, the tilting property can be intelligently controlled. The repeatability of the reversible wetting behavior of shape memory polymers was investigated by Cheng et al. (Lv et al., 2016).

Chen et al. (Chen & Yang, 2014) proved that the shape memory polymers can switch between isotropic/anisotropic behavior. They reported that when the pillars are in the erect direction, the surface shows isotropic behavior, and when they lean back to collapsed form, anisotropic behavior has appeared. By increasing the temperature, the pillars tend to recover their upright state and isotropic behavior would have appeared again.

Shape memory polymers can be designed as super slippery and superoleophobic surfaces. But, up to now, there are rare studies on these types of surfaces. As an example, Wang et al. (2017b) designed a mushroom-like structure with a thiolene/acrylate-based thermos-responsive shape memory polymer. The prepared coating could switch between mushroom/collapsed structures by pressing/recovery process.

Summarizing, current studies results show that simultaneous control of both chemical composition and surface microstructure led to proper control of wetting behavior from superhydrophilicity to superhydrophobicity. Most current research is based on thermos-responsive shape memory polymers; however, investigations of other materials with different sensitivities like being responsive to water, light, and pH, are interesting. A wide range of materials with different sensitivities will help to overcome more challenges in different industries.

9.8.2 Self-healing and toughness

Self-healing is an ability that existed in nature and lead us to achieve great practical application. Scientists developed self-healing polymers with two different healing mechanisms: intrinsic and extrinsic self-healing processes (Rule et al., 2007; Tanvir et al., 2017; Vijayan P & Al-Maadeed, 2016). In the intrinsic mechanism, healing is feasible due to reversible covalent bonds, supramolecular chemistry, or thermos-reversible physical interaction. In this kind of material, establishing a balance between mechanical properties and self-healing performance is important.

In this regard, thermoplastic polyurethane (TPU) was developed with high tensile strength, along with self-healing ability for fabrication on wearable electronics. The reported value of tensile strength for the mentioned TPU was 6.8 MPa. The suggested mechanism for recovery of this film was reversible covalent bonds. Fig. 9.10 shows the transparency and healing performance of the film before 2 h (Kim et al., 2018). In extrinsic self-healing, recovery is possible by the incorporation of nano/microcapsules containing a healing agent into the polymer matrix. The release process of encapsulated healing agents is usually based on demand. They can be sensitive to mechanical damage (Fayyad et al., 2015; Vijayan P et al., 2016).

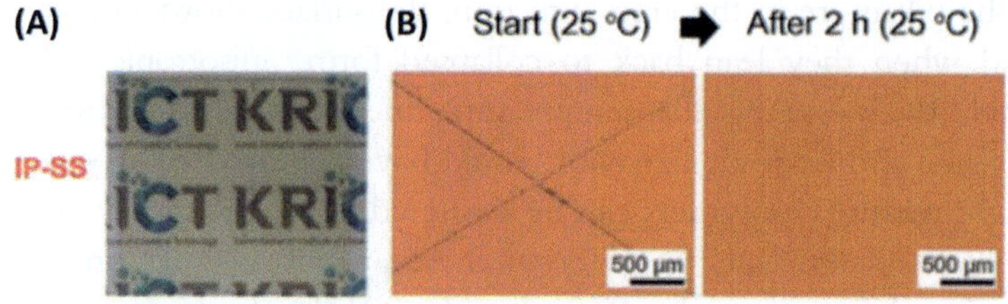

Figure 9.10 (A) digital image of TPU film, (B) optical microscopy images of scratched TPU film before and after healing for 2 h at 25°C. *Reprinted with permission from Kim, S. M., et al. (2018). Superior toughness and fast self-healing at room temperature engineered by transparent elastomers.* Advanced Materials, 30*(1), 1705145.*

Healing agent containers are usually based on polymeric nano/microcapsules inorganic nanoporous aterials, nanotubes, etc (Fayyad et al., 2015).

However, there is a believe that polymeric capsules weaken the mechanical performance of the final system, but there is research that found a strategy to improve the mechanical performance of the final product by using graphene-based Cu_2O filler (Blaiszik et al., 2008; Rana et al., 2016).

9.8.3 Self-cleaning with self-healing surfaces

It is known that there are two prerequisites for preparing superhydrophobic surfaces: low surface energy and hierarchical nano/microstructure but designing durable superhydrophobic coating with photocatalytic self-cleaning properties is challenging. Since TiO_2 can degrade fluoroalkylsilane materials under light irradiation (Wooh et al., 2017). So, using self-healing ability can help them to overcome this issue.

There is a report from Chen and McCarthy (2017) that provided self-healing superhydrophobic coating based on TiO_2 UV-sensitive microcapsules. Having superhydrophobicity with a sliding angle of fewer than 10 degrees combined with capsules to deliver a healing agent can be a good candidate for self-healing/self-cleaning application (Bauer et al., 2010; Vijayan & Puglia, 2019).

In addition, the self-healing process can happen to recover the topographic structures by using living microorganisms (Ionov & Synytska, 2012; Xue & Ma, 2013; Yin et al., 2015).

Manna's group used a method to achieve self-healing ability in porous superhydrophobic coatings. They used crushing loads in superhydrophobic coating to compact it and flatten the rough structure.

Another mechanism for the self-healing process is to recover or repair the chemical components of the surface. MacCallum et al. (2013) used oil to replace air pockets in the rough structure of traditional superhydrophobic surfaces. They treated cotton and polyester fabric with oil to gain a slippery porous surface, showing omni-repellent properties against polar and nonpolar liquids. Xue's group (Vijayan & Puglia, 2019) fabricated self-healing superhydrophobic coating by spraying SiO_2 core–shell nanoparticles/PS as coating and polydimethylsiloxane as hydrophobic interconnection. They reported this coating was able to recover itself in 12 h at ambient temperature or by heat curing after being damaged through plasma treatment.

9.8.4 Self-cleaning and antireflection

Gathering transparency and self-cleaning ability is one of the challenges that still remain despite many efforts. So, there are some unclarified aspects of designing transparent superamphiphobic coating. The main and foremost challenge is that most fabricated coating has lower transmittance compared to the substrate. This property can limit their application especially their usage in solar cell-protecting panels, infrared detector-protecting panels, and self-cleaning green houses. So gathering antireflection properties and superhydrophobicity would be the key point. There are only a few reports that claimed their prepared coating had higher transmittance compared to the substrate (Geng & He, 2014; Geng et al., 2013).

The roughness of superhydrophobic coating can decrease transparency due to light scattering. Silica nanoparticles are one of the key materials that are used in the transparent superhydrophobic coating because of their refractive index. The other reason is the ease of surface modification of these particles via silane functionalization (Deng et al., 2011).

Yang et al. (2012) prepared a porous surface based on diallyldimethylammonium chloride (PDDA)—sodium perfluorooctanoate (PFO)/SiO_2 which lets water pass through it but keeps oil on the top of the surface. The porous antioil coating showed proper transparency compared with the substrate.

Bravo et al. (2007) fabricated transparent films with 20–50 nm silica particles. They prepare these films by deposition of poly (sodium 4-styrene sulfonate) (PSS) and poly (allylamine hydrochloride) via layer-by-layer process. They reported that visible transparency was obtained by controlling the size of aggregation and layering parameters. Another strategy to achieve an antireflective surface is provided by TiO_2 nanoparticles because of their high refractive index, brightness, and stability.

Polymeric materials are another candidate for achieving antireflective superhydrophobic coatings due to their flexibility and controllable toughness. For example, polymethylmethacrylate (PMMA) with a refractive index of 1.49 is a suitable polymer for optical application.

Xu's group (Xu et al., 2012) generated a dip-coating approach to prepare visible/near IR ARCs with PMMA and hallow SiO_2 modified with hexamethyldisilazane (hydrophobic part). They could control and optimize the wetting and optical properties by adjusting the PMMA concentration.

9.8.5 Self-cleaning with low fluid drag

Low fluid drag coatings matter especially in aircraft and marine industries (Fu et al., 2017). In nature, shark skin is an example of a low fluid drag surface but in addition to the low fluid drag property, the shark skin is able to prevent the growth of biofouling on it (Bixler & Bhushan, 2013).

Rice leaves and butterfly wings combine the drag reduction and self-cleaning ability which was named the rice and butterfly wing effect (Bixler & Bhushan, 2012). This effect dramatically reduced drag and enhanced self-cleaning ability.

9.8.6 Self-cleaning and anticorrosion surfaces

A major challenge in self-cleaning coating applications is that they usually suffer from corrosion phenomena. Recently scientists have developed anticorrosive self-cleaning coatings. Based on the published results, nanocasting is the most effective technique to fabricate this kind of coatings (Chang et al., 2013).

Chang et al. (2014) used nanocasting to fabricate hydrophobic epoxy/graphene coating on the steel substrate. They used the template of PDMS imprinted with *Xanthosoma sagittifolium* leaf to create microstructure on the epoxy coating. Besides the water repellency, the graphene nanosheets act as barrier layers and lengthen the passways of water and aggressive ions.

Similarly, Nine's group (Nine et al., 2015) prepared multifunctional anticorrosive/self-cleaning coating with superior mechanical robustness. The prepared coatings contained PDMS, graphene oxide (GO), TiO_2, and diatomaceous earth (DE) particles. Based on their results, PDMS, GO, DE, and TiO_2 contributed to self-cleaning, toughness, barrier, and self-cleaning/superhydrophobicity properties respectively. The presence of nanoparticles could effectively enhance the anticorrosion performance of the final coating.

In addition to nano casting, there are different methods to achieve hierarchical structure. Lv et al. (2018) modified the potassium titanate whisker (PTW) surface with SiO_2 via a sol–gel process. Dopamine was used as an interconnector of SiO_2/PTW to improve the superhydrophobicity of the coating. Amino silicone oil was selected due to the methyl group, repelling water droplets. The rise in water contact angle value positively effects the anticorrosion and self-cleaning ability of the prepared coating.

9.9 Applications of biomimetic materials

9.9.1 Orthopedic implants

In the last two decades, researchers have been researching the coating of various orthopedic implant surfaces using the "biomimetic technique." In order for an implant surface to osseointegrate (form a direct bond with the adjacent bone) without being surrounded by fibrous tissue, the technique is especially useful for forming bone-like calcium-deficient carbonated hydroxyapatite (CDHA) coatings. Simulated body fluid (SBF) is an essential part of the procedure. A seminal review paper published by Kokubo is credited with the popularity of the technique, according to the authors (Kokubo, 1998). In addition, Kokubo came up with the term SBF. With the caveat that such compositions do not contain any organic species, such as proteins or amino acids, it is apparent that artificially produced medium should behave like bodily fluids. SBF and biomimicry may be regarded as synonymous terms. Due to its benign nature, the method has many advantages. High-temperature processes like plasma spray can damage underlying substrates, in contrast to lower temperature processes such as vacuum coating. The use of high temperatures for coating metals does not pose a significant problem, but high temperatures are not suitable for coating low melting point polymers, such as scaffolds for bone regeneration (Koju et al., 2017).

Biomimetic implants are designed to mimic the structure and function of natural tissues and organs. In orthopedics, biomimetic implants are used to replace damaged or diseased bone, cartilage, and other tissues. These implants offer several advantages over traditional implants, including improved biocompatibility, reduced risk of rejection, and better integration with surrounding tissues.

Biomimetic implants are common in orthopedics, such as bioinspired bone scaffolds. The scaffold mimics the structure and composition of natural bone by combining natural and synthetic materials. New bone growth is allowed to occur on the scaffold, allowing the body to repair or regenerate lost or damaged bone. The design of traditional synthetic porous scaffolds ignores the native structure and properties of cells and natural tissues, and they are made of metals, polymers, ceramics, or even composite biomaterials. Due to poor corrosion and wear, mechanical mismatch, unamiable surface environment, and other undesirable properties, these synthetic scaffolds often do not integrate well with the surrounding cells and host tissue. Orthopedic surgery aims to reconstruct the musculoskeletal system (Wu et al., 2014).

Biomimetic cartilage implants are another example. Its function and structure mimic that of natural cartilage—the cushioning and gliding properties that enable the smooth movement of joints. Synthetic materials used to manufacture the implant closely resemble natural cartilage properties.

As an interdisciplinary approach in TE, it aims to design tissues with optimal clinical performance. In TE a variety of factors play a crucial role. These factors include cells, biomaterials, cell culture conditions, and signaling molecules like growth factors. Biomimetic scaffolds are being developed to elicit appropriate cellular responses (Del Bakhshayesh et al., 2019).

Spinal surgery can also benefit from biomimetic implants. Research is underway to develop biomimetic spinal disks that can replace damaged or degenerated disks. Vertebrae are supported and cushioned with these disks, which mimic the structure and function of natural spinal disks.

The use of biomimetic implants has the potential to improve orthopedic conditions in which tissue needs to be replaced or regenerated. Biomimetic implants are expected to become more advanced as research in this field continues.

9.9.2 Preclinical applications

The use of biomimetic coatings in preclinical applications is promising. In vitro, drug testing and other preclinical studies can be conducted more realistically with these coatings because they mimic the natural environment of cells and tissues. Scientists can create realistic 3D cell cultures by using biomimetic coatings, which enable them to study the effects of drugs on cells in a more realistic setting. Moreover, tissue-engineered models can be created with these coatings that better replicate human tissue structure and function. Microfluidic devices can be created using biomimetic coatings enabling researchers to understand cell behavior under controlled conditions.

The primary purpose of biomimetic bioreactors in TE research is to imitate native, physiological conditions and promote tissue regeneration in vitro (Stojkovska et al., 2020).

9.9.3 Carrier for drug

An effective treatment for incurable diseases such as cancer is to apply biomimetics to prove the substantial issues in medicine and pharmaceutics. Recent studies have focused on understanding biological processes and systems in detail. By understanding macromolecular structures and their high-tech processes at cellular and subcellular levels (such as proteins' structure and functions), scientists can model and imitate these natural processes for biomedical applications. As part of biomimetic thinking, it is important to understand cell growth and division, metabolic regulation, cellular interactions, and hormone signaling pathways (Axente et al., 2020).

Currently, research on drug delivery systems is focused on targeted delivery systems, which enable drugs to be transferred into cells without harming healthy organs or tissues. Biomimetic hydrogels, biomimetic micelles, biomimetic liposomes, biomimetic dendrimers, biomimetic polymeric carriers, and biomimetic nanostructures are some of the most common types of therapeutic drug carriers in advanced drug delivery systems (Sheikhpour et al., 2017).

To restore damaged tissues, it is becoming possible to regenerate them using cell-based TE therapies. Bioresorbable delivery materials are combined with autologous cells in these strategies. It is important to note that a delivery scaffold serves several functions: establishing mechanical stability, distributing cells evenly in three dimensions, improving tissue differentiation, handling carefully during delivery and fixation, and providing a range of properties that are suitable for delivery and fixation. Microencapsulation is an immunoprotective process that allows cells to be delivered by injectable matrixes, soft scaffolds, membranes, or solid load-bearing scaffolds. Smart delivery concepts will extend the clinical potential of next-generation therapies by leveraging stem cell regenerative capabilities, morphogenetic growth factors, and biomimetic materials (Sittinger et al., 2004).

9.10 Conclusion and future work

In-depth and comprehensive knowledge about the surface characteristics and structure in biocoatings and their biological mechanism can effectively lead scientists to mimic them to meet modern world requirements. Nowadays, scientists succeed in gathering different functions in a single material. The ability to develop complicated structures on different surfaces has enhanced such as hierarchical structure. Different technologies have appeared in the last few years, and some of them enabled to development of biomimetic coating from the laboratory into the industry. The preparation and development of random roughness or sculptured surfaces and controllable wetting behavior have resulted in multifunctional surfaces. So, the combination of different characteristics such as superhydrophobicity/icephobicity, anticorrosion, antireflection, and self-cleaning ability is possible due to the growing knowledge in this area. However, obtaining optimum conditions for topography and surface chemistry has its own difficulties. While developing biomimetic materials, the crucial demands for lightweight structure in biomedical, military, and transportation have greatly influenced researchers to pay more attention to biomimetic composites. However, there are still many difficulties. The major one is scaling up the mimetic systems from lab conditions to industrial large scale. The second one is designing the multifunctional system with low-cost materials and one-step fabrication methods.

Subsequently, based on experimental data and analysis, the roughness is a more effective factor of wettability behavior compared to surface chemistry. On the other hand, the roughened surfaces may limit their application of them in the outdoor environment due to lack of durability to mechanical damage. Therefore the improvement of durability, robustness, and physical and chemical characteristics is important for future studies. In addition, using environment-friendly materials at low cost is another crucial factor. It is obvious, the bright future of biomimetic polymers will be beheld with the efforts of scientists and researchers.

References

Adamson, A. (1990). Contact angle. *Physical Chemistry of Surfaces*, 385–388.

Altankov, G., Grinnell, F., & Groth, T. (1996). Studies on the biocompatibility of materials: Fibroblast reorganization of substratum-bound fibronectin on surfaces varying in wettability. *Journal of Biomedical Materials Research: An Official Journal of The Society for Biomaterials and The Japanese Society for Biomaterials, 30*(3), 385–391.

Amigoni, S., Taffin de Givenchy, E., Dufay, M., & Guittard, F. (2009). Covalent layer-by-layer assembled superhydrophobic organic − inorganic hybrid films. *Langmuir: The ACS Journal of Surfaces and Colloids*, *25*(18), 11073−11077.

Ashby, M., Bréchet, Y. J. M., Cebon, D., & Salvo, L. (2004). Selection strategies for materials and processes. *Materials & Design*, *25*(1), 51−67.

Axente, E., Elena Sima, L., & Sima, F. (2020). Biomimetic coatings obtained by combinatorial laser technologies. *Coatings*, *10*(5), 463.

Baleani, M., Viceconti, M., & Toni, A. (2000). The effect of sandblasting treatment on endurance properties of titanium alloy hip prostheses. *Artificial Organs*, *24*(4), 296−299.

Baneyx, G., Baugh, L., & Vogel, V. (2002). Fibronectin extension and unfolding within cell matrix fibrils controlled by cytoskeletal tension. *Proceedings of the National Academy of Sciences*, *99*(8), 5139−5143.

Barrere, F., Layrolle, P., van Blitterswijk, C. A., & de Groot, K. (1999). Biomimetic calcium phosphate coatings on Ti6Al4V: A crystal growth study of octacalcium phosphate and inhibition by Mg2 + and HCO3 − . *Bone*, *25*(2), 107S−111S.

Barrere, F., van Blitterswijk, CA., De Groot, K., Layrolle, P. (2002a). Influence of ionic strength and carbonate on the Ca-P coating formation from SBF × 5 solution. Biomaterials, 23(9), 1921−1930.

Barrere, F., Van Der Valk, C. M., & Meijer, G. (2003). Osteointegration of biomimetic apatite coating applied onto dense and porous metal implants in femurs of goats. *Journal of Biomedical Materials Research Part B: Applied Biomaterials*, *67*(1), 655−665, An Official Journal of The Society for Biomaterials, The Japanese Society for Biomaterials, and The Australian Society for Biomaterials and the Korean Society for Biomaterials.

Barrere, F.V., van Blitterswijk, CA., De Groot, K., Layrolle, P. (2002b). Nucleation of biomimetic Ca−P coatings on Ti6Al4V from a SBF × 5 solution: influence of magnesium. Biomaterials, 23(10), 2211−2220.

Bauer, G., Nellesen, A., & Speck, T. (2010). Biological lattices in fast self-repair mechanisms in plants and the development of bio-inspired self-healing polymers. *WIT Trans. Ecol. Environ*, *138*, 453−459.

Bernhard, C. G. (1965). The insect corneal nipple array. A biological, broad-band impedance transformer that acts as an antireflection coating. *Acta Physiologica Scandinavica*, *63* (243), 1−79.

Bico, J., Marzolin, C., & Quéré, D. (1999). Pearl drops. *Europhysics Letters*, *47*(2), 220.

Bixler, G. D., & Bhushan, B. (2012). Bioinspired rice leaf and butterfly wing surface structures combining shark skin and lotus effects. *Soft matter*, *8*(44), 11271−11284.

Bixler, G. D., & Bhushan, B. (2013). Fluid drag reduction and efficient self-cleaning with rice leaf and butterfly wing bioinspired surfaces. *Nanoscale*, *5*(17), 7685−7710.

Blaiszik, B., Sottos, N., & White, S. (2008). Nanocapsules for self-healing materials. *Composites Science and Technology*, *68*(3−4), 978−986.

Bravo, J., Zhai, L., Wu, Z., Cohen, R. E., & Rubner, M. F. (2007). Transparent superhydrophobic films based on silica nanoparticles. *Langmuir: The ACS Journal of Surfaces and Colloids*, *23*(13), 7293−7298.

Cebeci, F. Ç., Wu, Z., Zhai, L., Cohen, R. E., & Rubner, M. F. (2006). Nanoporosity-driven superhydrophilicity: a means to create multifunctional antifogging coatings. *Langmuir: The ACS Journal of Surfaces and Colloids*, *22*(6), 2856−2862.

Cerman, Z., Striffler, B. F., & Barthlott, W. (2009). Dry in the water: the superhydrophobic water fern Salvinia−a model for biomimetic surfaces. *Functional Surfaces in Biology: Little Structures with Big Effects*, *1*, 97−111.

Chang, K.-C., Lu, H. I., Peng, C. W., & Lai, M. C. (2013). Nanocasting technique to prepare lotus-leaf-like superhydrophobic electroactive polyimide as advanced anticorrosive coatings. *ACS Applied Materials & Interfaces*, *5*(4), 1460–1467.

Chang, K.-C., Hsu, M. H., Lu, H. I., Lai, M. C., Liu, P. J., & Hsu, C. H. (2014). Room-temperature cured hydrophobic epoxy/graphene composites as corrosion inhibitor for cold-rolled steel. *Carbon*, *66*, 144–153.

Chen, K., & McCarthy, T. J. (2017). Environmental stimuli-responsive self-repairing waterbased superhydrophobic coatings. *RSC Advances*, 7(1), 543–550.

Chen, C. M., & Yang, S. (2014). Directed water shedding on high-aspect-ratio shape memory polymer micropillar arrays. *Advanced Materials*, *26*(8), 1283–1288.

Chen, C.-M., Chiang, C.-L., & Yang, S. (2015). Programming tilting angles in shape memory polymer Janus pillar arrays with unidirectional wetting against the tilting direction. *Langmuir: the ACS Journal of Surfaces and Colloids*, *31*(35), 9523–9526.

Chen, W., & McCarthy, T. J. (1999). Adsorption/migration of a perfluorohexylated fullerene from the bulk to the polymer/air interface. *Macromolecules*, *32*(7), 2342–2347.

Chen, W., Fadeev, A. Y., Hsieh, M. C., Öner, D., Youngblood, J., & McCarthy, T. J. (1999). Ultrahydrophobic and ultralyophobic surfaces: some comments and examples. *Langmuir: The ACS Journal of Surfaces and Colloids*, *15*(10), 3395–3399.

Chi, M.-H., Tsou, H. K., Chung, C. J., & He, J. L. (2013). Biomimetic hydroxyapatite grown on biomedical polymer coated with titanium dioxide interlayer to assist osteocompatible performance. *Thin Solid Films*, *549*, 98–102.

Chunder, A., Etcheverry, K., Londe, G., Cho, H. J., & Zhai, L. (2009). Conformal switchable superhydrophobic/hydrophilic surfaces for microscale flow control. *Colloids and Surfaces A: Physicochemical and Engineering Aspects*, *333*(1–3), 187–193.

Collins, C. M., & Safiuddin, M. (2022). Lotus-leaf-inspired biomimetic coatings: different types, key properties, and applications in infrastructures. *Infrastructures*, 7(4), 46.

Cook, J., & Gordon, J. (1964). A mechanism for the control of crack propagation in all-brittle systems. *Proceedings of the Royal Society of London. Series A: Mathematical and Physical Sciences*, *282*(1391), 508–520.

Currey, J., & Taylor, J. (1974). The mechanical behaviour of some molluscan hard tissues. *Journal of Zoology*, *173*(3), 395–406.

De Gennes., Brochard-Wyart, F., & Quéré, D. (2004). *Capillarity and wetting phenomena: Drops, bubbles, pearls, waves* (pp. 1–31). New York: Springer.

Del Bakhshayesh, A. R., Asadi, N., Alihemmati, A., Tayefi Nasrabadi, H., Montaseri, A., & Davaran, S. (2019). An overview of advanced biocompatible and biomimetic materials for creation of replacement structures in the musculoskeletal systems: focusing on cartilage tissue engineering. *Journal of Biological Engineering*, *13*, 1–21.

Deng, X., Mammen, L., Zhao, Y., Lellig, P., Müllen, K., Li, C., Butt, H. J., & Vollmer, D. (2011). Transparent, thermally stable and mechanically robust superhydrophobic surfaces made from porous silica capsules. *Advanced Materials*, *23*(26), 2962–2965.

Extrand, C. (2004). Criteria for ultralyophobic surfaces. *Langmuir: The ACS Journal of Surfaces and Colloids*, *20*(12), 5013–5018.

Fayyad, E. M., Almaadeed, M. A., & Jones, A. (2015). Encapsulation of tung oil for self-healing coatings in corrosion applications. *Science of Advanced Materials*, 7(12), 2628–2638.

Fu, Y., Yuan, C., & Bai, X. (2017). Marine drag reduction of shark skin inspired riblet surfaces. *Biosurface and Biotribology*, *3*(1), 11–24.

García-Huete, N., Cuevas, J. M., Laza Vilas, J. M., & León, L. M. (2015). Polymeric shape-memory micro-patterned surface for switching wettability with temperature. *Polymers*, 7(9), 1674–1688.

Geng, Z., & He, J. (2014). An effective method to significantly enhance the robustness and adhesion-to-substrate of high transmittance superamphiphobic silica thin films. *Journal of Materials Chemistry A*, *2*(39), 16601–16607.

Geng, Z., He, J., Xu, L., & Yao, L. (2013). Rational design and elaborate construction of surface nano-structures toward highly antireflective superamphiphobic coatings. *Journal of Materials Chemistry A*, *1*(31), 8721–8724.

Gordon, J., & Jeronimidis, G. (1980). Composites with high work of fracture. *Philosophical Transactions of the Royal Society of London. Series A, Mathematical and Physical Sciences*, *294*(1411), 545–550.

Gray-Munro, J. E., Seguin, C., & Strong, M. (2009). Influence of surface modification on the in vitro corrosion rate of magnesium alloy AZ31. *Journal of Biomedical Materials Research Part A*, *91*(1), 221–230, An Official Journal of The Society for Biomaterials, The Japanese Society for Biomaterials, and The Australian Society for Biomaterials and the Korean Society for Biomaterials.

Habibovic, P., Barrere, F., Van Blitterswijk, C. A., de Groot, K., & Layrolle, P. (2002). Biomimetic hydroxyapatite coating on metal implants. *Journal of the American Ceramic Society*, *85*(3), 517–522.

Hamodrakas, S. J., Willis, J. H., & Iconomidou, V. A. (2002). A structural model of the chitin-binding domain of cuticle proteins. *Insect Biochemistry and Molecular Biology*, *32* (11), 1577–1583.

Hansen, W. R., & Autumn, K. (2005). Evidence for self-cleaning in gecko setae. *Proceedings of the National Academy of Sciences*, *102*(2), 385–389.

Harvey, A. G., Hill, E. W., & Bayat, A. (2013). Designing implant surface topography for improved biocompatibility. *Expert Review of Medical Devices*, *10*(2), 257–267.

Herminghaus, S. (2000). Roughness-induced non-wetting. *Europhysics Letters*, *52*(2), 165.

Hikita, M., Tanaka, K., Nakamura, T., Kajiyama, T., & Takahara, A. (2005). Super-liquid-repellent surfaces prepared by colloidal silica nanoparticles covered with fluoroalkyl groups. *Langmuir: The ACS Journal of Surfaces and Colloids*, *21*(16), 7299–7302.

Hsieh, C.-T., Chen, W. Y., FL Wu, F. L., & Shen, Y. S. (2008). Fabrication and superhydrophobic behavior of fluorinated silica nanosphere arrays. *Journal of Adhesion Science and Technology*, *22*(3–4), 265–275.

Huang, L., McMillan, R. A., Apkarian, R. P., Pourdeyhimi, B., Conticello, V. P., & Chaikof, E. L. (2000). Generation of synthetic elastin-mimetic small diameter fibers and fiber networks. *Macromolecules*, *33*(8), 2989–2997.

Ionov, L., & Synytska, A. (2012). Self-healing superhydrophobic materials. *Physical Chemistry Chemical Physics*, *14*(30), 10497–10502.

Jackson, A., Vincent, J., & Turner, R. (1989). A physical model of nacre. *Composites Science and Technology*, *36*(3), 255–266.

Jackson, A., Vincent, J. F., & Turner, R. (1988). The mechanical design of nacre. *Proceedings of the Royal society of London. Series B. Biological sciences*, *234*(1277), 415–440.

Jeon, S., Jang, J. V., Youn, J. R., Jeong, J., Brenner, H., & Song, Y. S. (2013). Fullerene embedded shape memory nanolens array. *Scientific Reports*, *3*(1), 3269.

Keim, S., Brunner, J. G., Fabry, B., & Virtanen, S. (2011). Control of magnesium corrosion and biocompatibility with biomimetic coatings. *Journal of Biomedical Materials Research, Part B: Applied Biomaterials*, *96*(1), 84–90.

Kim, S. M., Jeon, H., Shin, S. H., Park, S. A., Jegal, J., Hwang, S. Y., Oh, D. X., & Park, J. (2018). Superior toughness and fast self-healing at room temperature engineered by transparent elastomers. *Advanced Materials*, *30*(1)1705145.

Kim, S. S., Gwak, S. J., & Kim, B. S. (2008). Orthotopic bone formation by implantation of apatite-coated poly (lactide-co-glycolide)/hydroxyapatite composite particulates and bone morphogenetic protein-2. *Journal of Biomedical Materials Research Part A*, *87*(1), 245–253, An Official Journal of The Society for Biomaterials, The Japanese Society for Biomaterials, and The Australian Society for Biomaterials and the Korean Society for Biomaterials.

Koju, N., Sikder, P., Ren, Y., Zhou, H., & Bhaduri, S. B. (2017). Biomimetic coating technology for orthopedic implants. *Current opinion in Chemical Engineering, 15*, 49–55.

Kokubo, T. (1998). Apatite formation on surfaces of ceramics, metals and polymers in body environment. *Acta Materialia, 46*(7), 2519–2527.

Kumar, A., & Gupta, A. K. (2015). Deformation and detachment of carbon tetra chloride droplet in the presence of different concentration of surfactant from solid substrate. *International Journal of Advanced Research in Engineering and Technology, 6*(7).

Lai, Y., Lin, Z, Huang, J., Sun, L., Chen, Z, & Lin, C. (2010). *Controllable construction of* ZnO/TiO_2 *patterning nanostructures by superhydrophilic/superhydrophobic templates. New Journal of Chemistry, 34*(1), 44–51.

Lee, D., Rubner, M. F., & Cohen, R. E. (2006). All-nanoparticle thin-film coatings. *Nano Letters, 6*(10), 2305–2312.

Law, K.-Y. (2022). Contact angle hysteresis on smooth/flat and rough surfaces. *Interpretation, Mechanism, and Origin. Accounts of Materials Research, 3*(1), 1–7.

Lee, S. M., Jung, I. D., & Ko, J. S. (2008). The effect of the surface wettability of nano-protrusions formed on network-type microstructures. *Journal of Micromechanics and Microengineering, 18*(12), 125007.

Li, L., Gao, J., & Wang, Y. (2004). Evaluation of cyto-toxicity and corrosion behavior of alkali-heat-treated magnesium in simulated body fluid. *Surface and Coatings Technology, 185*(1), 92–98.

Lim, H., Jung, D. H., Noh, J. H., Choi, G. R., & Kim, W. D. (2009). Simple nanofabrication of a superhydrophobic and transparent biomimetic surface. *Chinese Science Bulletin, 54*, 3613–3616.

Lin, Y.-W., & Tang, C. (2015). Electrochemical synthesis and deposition of surface-enhanced Raman scattering-active silver microstructures on a screen-printed carbon electrode. *The Journal of Physical Chemistry C, 119*(44), 24865–24874.

Liu, K., Yao, X., & Jiang, L. (2010a). Recent developments in bio-inspired special wettability. *Chemical Society Reviews, 39*(8), 3240–3255.

Liu, Y., Gao, H., Li, S., Han, Z., & Ren, L. (2018). Bioinspired platform with reversibly switchable wettability for transfer and storage of droplets. *Chemical Engineering Journal, 337*, 697–708.

Liu, Y., Wu, G., & de Groot, K. (2010b). Biomimetic coatings for bone tissue engineering of critical-sized defects. *Journal of the Royal Society Interface*, 7(suppl_5), S631–S647.

Lv, C., Wang, H., Liu, Z., Zhang, W., Wang, C., Tao, R., Li, M., & Zhu, Y. (2018). A sturdy self-cleaning and anti-corrosion superhydrophobic coating assembled by amino silicon oil modifying potassium titanate whisker-silica particles. *Applied Surface Science, 435*, 903–913.

Lv, T., Cheng, Z., Zhang, D., Zhang, E., Zhao, Q., Liu, Y., & Jiang, L. (2016). Superhydrophobic surface with shape memory micro/nanostructure and its application in rewritable chip for droplet storage. *ACS Nano, 10*(10), 9379–9386.

Lvov, Y., Ariga, K., Onda, M., Ichinose, I., & Kunitake, T. (1997). Alternate assembly of ordered multilayers of SiO_2 and other nanoparticles and polyions. *Langmuir: The ACS Journal of Surfaces and Colloids, 13*(23), 6195–6203.

Ma, J., Wong, H., Kong, L. B., & Peng, K. W. (2003). Biomimetic processing of nanocrystallite bioactive apatite coating on titanium. *Nanotechnology, 14*(6), 619.

Ma, M., Mao, Y., Gupta, M., Gleason, K. K., & Rutledge, G. C. (2005). Superhydrophobic fabrics produced by electrospinning and chemical vapor deposition. *Macromolecules, 38*(23), 9742–9748.

MacCallum, N., Wong, T. S., Kim, P., & Aizenberg, J. (2013). Fabrics coated with lubricated nanostructures display robust omniphobicity. *Nanotechnology, 25*(1), 014019.

Mahltig, B., & Böttcher, H. (2003). Modified silica sol coatings for water-repellent textiles. *Journal of Sol-Gel Science and Technology, 27*(1), 43–52.

Manca, M., Cannavale, A., De Marco, L., Arico, A. S., Cingolani, R., & Gigli, G. (2009). Durable superhydrophobic and antireflective surfaces by trimethylsilanized silica nanoparticles-based sol − gel processing. *Langmuir: The ACS Journal of Surfaces and Colloids*, *25*(11), 6357−6362.

Min, W.-L., Jiang, P., & Jiang, B. (2008). Large-scale assembly of colloidal nanoparticles and fabrication of periodic subwavelength structures. *Nanotechnology*, *19*(47), 475604.

Mistry, A. S., Pham, Q. P., Schouten, C., Yeh, T., Christenson, E. M., Mikos, A. G., & Jansen, J. A. (2010). In vivo bone biocompatibility and degradation of porous fumarate-based polymer/alumoxane nanocomposites for bone tissue engineering. *Journal of Biomedical Materials Research Part A*, *92*(2), 451−462, An Official Journal of The Society for Biomaterials, The Japanese Society for Biomaterials, and The Australian Society for Biomaterials and the Korean Society for Biomaterials.

Mizukoshi, T., Matsumoto, H., Minagawa, M., & Tanioka, A. (2007). Control over wettability of textured surfaces by electrospray deposition. *Journal of Applied Polymer Science*, *103*(6), 3811−3817.

Mohamed, A. M. A., Abdullah, A. M., & Younan, N. A. (2015). Corrosion behavior of superhydrophobic surfaces: A review. *Arabian Journal of Chemistry*, *8*(6), 749−765.

Monteiro, N. O., Oliveira, C., Silva, T. H., Martins, A., Fangueiro, J. F., Reis, R. L., & Neves, N. M. (2022). Biomimetic surface topography from the Rubus fruticosus leaf as a guidance of angiogenesis in tissue engineering applications. *ACS Biomaterials Science & Engineering*, *8*(7), 2943−2953.

Motornov, M., Sheparovych, R., Lupitskyy, R., MacWilliams, E., & Minko, S. (2008). Superhydrophobic surfaces generated from water-borne dispersions of hierarchically assembled nanoparticles coated with a reversibly switchable shell. *Advanced Materials*, *20*(1), 200−205.

Nakajima, A., Abe, K., Hashimoto, K., & Watanabe, T. (2000). Preparation of hard super-hydrophobic films with visible light transmission. *Thin Solid Films*, *376*(1−2), 140−143.

Nine, M. J., Cole, M. A., Johnson, L., & Tran, D. N. H. (2015). Robust superhydrophobic graphene-based composite coatings with self-cleaning and corrosion barrier properties. *ACS Applied Materials & Interfaces*, 7(51), 28482−28493.

Nosonovsky, M., & Bhushan, B. (2005). Roughness optimization for biomimetic superhydrophobic surfaces. *Microsystem Technologies*, *11*, 535−549.

Oyane, A., Uchida, M., Yokoyama, Y., Choong, C., Triffitt, J., & Ito, A. (2005). Simple surface modification of poly (ϵ-caprolactone) to induce its apatite-forming ability. *Journal of Biomedical Materials Research Part A*, *75*(1), 138−145, An Official Journal of The Society for Biomaterials, The Japanese Society for Biomaterials, and The Australian Society for Biomaterials and the Korean Society for Biomaterials.

Pollack, G. H. (2003). *Cells, gels and the engines of life: a fresh paradigm for cell function, IEEE EMBS Asian-pacific conference on biomedical engineering* (2003). IEEE.

Quéré, D., Lafuma, A., & Bico, J. (2003). Slippy and sticky microtextured solids. *Nanotechnology*, *14*(10), 1109.

Rahmany, M. B., & Van Dyke, M. (2013). Biomimetic approaches to modulate cellular adhesion in biomaterials: A review. *Acta Biomaterialia*, *9*(3), 5431−5437.

Rana, S., Döhler, D., Nia, A. S., Nasir, M., Beiner, M., & Binder, W. H. (2016). Macromol. Rapid Commun. 21/2016. *Macromolecular Rapid Communications*, *37*(21), 1709.

Rule, J. D., Sottos, N. R., & White, S. R. (2007). Effect of microcapsule size on the performance of self-healing polymers. *Polymer*, *48*(12), 3520−3529.

Sato, O., Kubo, S., & Gu, Z.-Z. (2009). Structural color films with lotus effects, superhydrophilicity, and tunable stop-bands. *Accounts of Chemical Research*, *42*(1), 1−10.

Schwartz, D., Steinberg, S., Israelachvili, J., & Zasadzinski, J. A. N. (1992). Growth of a self-assembled monolayer by fractal aggregation. *Physical Review Letters*, *69*(23), 3354.

Shang, H., Wang, Y., Limmer, S. J., Chou, T. P., & Takahashi, K. (2005). Optically transparent superhydrophobic silica-based films. *Thin Solid Films*, *472*(1–2), 37–43.

Sheen, Y.-C., Chang, W. H., Chen, W. C., Chang, Y. H., Huang, Y. C., & Chang, F. C. (2009). Non-fluorinated superamphiphobic surfaces through sol–gel processing of methyltriethoxysilane and tetraethoxysilane. *Materials Chemistry and Physics*, *114*(1), 63–68.

Sheikhpour, M., Barani, L., & Kasaeian, A. (2017). Biomimetics in drug delivery systems: A critical review. *Journal of Controlled Release*, *253*, 97–109.

Shirtcliffe, N., McHale, G., Newton, M. I., & Perry, C. C. (2003). Intrinsically superhydrophobic organosilica sol – gel foams. *Langmuir: The ACS Journal of Surfaces and Colloids*, *19*(14), 5626–5631.

Shirtcliffe, N. J., Aqil, S., Evans, C., McHale, G., Newton, M. I., Perry, C. C., & Roach, P. (2004). The use of high aspect ratio photoresist (SU-8) for super-hydrophobic pattern prototyping. *Journal of Micromechanics and Microengineering*, *14*(10), 1384.

Sittinger, M., Hutmacher, D. W., & Risbud, M. V. (2004). Current strategies for cell delivery in cartilage and bone regeneration. *Current Opinion in Biotechnology*, *15*(5), 411–418.

Soeno, T., Inokuchi, K., & Shiratori, S. (2004). Ultra-water-repellent surface: fabrication of complicated structure of SiO2 nanoparticles by electrostatic self-assembled films. *Applied Surface Science*, *237*(1–4), 539–543.

Sokolsky-Papkov, M., Agashi, K., Olaye, A., Shakesheff, K., & Domb, A. J. (2007). Polymer carriers for drug delivery in tissue engineering. *Advanced Drug Delivery Reviews*, *59*(4–5), 187–206.

Solga, A., Cerman, Z., Striffler, B. F., Spaeth, M., & Barthlott, W. (2007). The dream of staying clean: Lotus and biomimetic surfaces. *Bioinspiration & Biomimetics*, *2*(4), S126.

Song, W., Veiga, D. D., Custódio, C. A., & Mano, J. F. (2009). Bioinspired degradable substrates with extreme wettability properties. *Advanced Materials*, *21*(18), 1830–1834.

Song, W.-H., Jun, Y. K., Han, Y., & Hong, S. H. (2004). Biomimetic apatite coatings on micro-arc oxidized titania. *Biomaterials*, *25*(17), 3341–3349.

Staiger, M. P., Pietak, A. M., Huadmai, J., & Dias, G. (2006). Magnesium and its alloys as orthopedic biomaterials: A review. *Biomaterials*, *27*(9), 1728–1734.

Stojkovska, J., Zvicer, J., & Obradovic, B. (2020). Preclinical functional characterization methods of nanocomposite hydrogels containing silver nanoparticles for biomedical applications. *Applied Microbiology and Biotechnology*, *104*, 4643–4658.

Suárez-González, D., Barnhart, K., Migneco, F., Flanagan, C., Hollister, S. J., & Murphy, W. L. (2012). Controllable mineral coatings on PCL scaffolds as carriers for growth factor release. *Biomaterials*, *33*(2), 713–721.

Sun, C., Ge, L.-Q., & Gu, Z.-Z. (2007). Fabrication of super-hydrophobic film with dual-size roughness by silica sphere assembly. *Thin Solid Films*, *515*(11), 4686–4690.

Svagan, A. J., Azizi Samir, M. A., & Berglund, L. A. (2007). Biomimetic polysaccharide nanocomposites of high cellulose content and high toughness. *Biomacromolecules*, *8*(8), 2556–2563.

Tadanaga, K., Kitamuro, K., Matsuda, A., & Minami, T. (2003). Formation of superhydrophobic alumina coating films with high transparency on polymer substrates by the sol-gel method. *Journal of Sol-Gel Science and Technology*, *26*, 705–708.

Tadanaga, K., Morinaga, J., & Minami, T. (2000). Formation of superhydrophobic-superhydrophilic pattern on flowerlike alumina thin film by the sol-gel method. *Journal of Sol-Gel Science and Technology*, *19*, 211–214.

Tanvir, A., El-Gawady, Y. H., & Al-Maadeed, M. (2017). Cellulose nanofibers to assist the release of healing agents in epoxy coatings. *Progress in Organic Coatings*, *112*, 127–132.

Tian, P., & Guo, Z. (2019). Biomimetic Janus paper with controllable swelling for shape memory and energy conversion. *Journal of Bionic Engineering*, *16*, 1–12.

Tuteja, A., Choi, W., Ma, M., Mabry, J. M., Mazzella, S. A., Rutledge, G. C., McKinley, G. H., & Cohen, R. E. (2007). Designing superoleophobic surfaces. *SCIENCE*, *318* (5856), 1618–1622.

Vijayan P, P., & Al-Maadeed, M. A. S. (2016). *TiO_2 nanotubes and mesoporous silica as containers in self-healing epoxy coatings*. *Scientific Reports*, *6*(1), 1–9.

Vijayan P, P., Hany El-Gawady, Y. M., & Al-Maadeed, M. A. S. (2016). Halloysite nanotube as multifunctional component in epoxy protective coating. *Industrial & Engineering Chemistry Research*, *55*(42), 11186–11192.

Vijayan, P. P., & Puglia, D. (2019). Biomimetic multifunctional materials: A review. *Emergent Materials*, *2*(4), 391–415.

Vincent, J. F., & Wegst, U. G. (2004). Design and mechanical properties of insect cuticle. *Arthropod Structure & Development*, *33*(3), 187–199.

Vincent, J. F. (2009). Biomimetics—A review. *Proceedings of the institution of mechanical engineers, Part H: Journal of Engineering in Medicine*, *223*(8), 919–939.

Vogel, V., & Sheetz, M. (2006). Local force and geometry sensing regulate cell functions. *Nature Reviews. Molecular Cell Biology*, *7*(4), 265–275.

Walter, S., Flinn, B., & Mayer, G. (2007). Mechanisms of toughening of a natural rigid composite. *Materials Science and Engineering: C*, *27*(3), 570–574.

Wang, J., Sun, L., Zou, M., Gao, W., Liu, C., Shang, L., Gu, Z., Zhao, Y. (2017a). Bioinspired shape-memory graphene film with tunable wettability. Science advances, 3(6), Article e1700004.

Wang, N., Zhao, Y., & Jiang, L. (2008). Low-cost, thermoresponsive wettability of surfaces: Poly (N-isopropylacrylamide)/Polystyrene composite films prepared by electrospinning. *Macromolecular Rapid Communications*, *29*(6), 485–489.

Wang, W., Salazar, J., Vahabi, H., Joshi-Imre, A., Voit, WE., Kota, AK. (2017b). Metamorphic superomniphobic surfaces. Advanced Materials, 29(27), Article 1700295.

Wenzel, R. (1936). *Industrial & Engineering Chemistry Research*, *28*, 988.

Wenzel, R. N. (1949). Surface roughness and contact angle. *The Journal of Physical Chemistry*, *53*(9), 1466–1467.

Witte, F., Kaese, V., Haferkamp, H., Switzer, E., Meyer-Lindenberg, A., Wirth, C. J., & Windhagen, H. (2005). In vivo corrosion of four magnesium alloys and the associated bone response. *Biomaterials*, *26*(17), 3557–3563.

Wooh, S., Encinas, N., Vollmer, D., & Butt, H. J. (2017). Stable hydrophobic metal-oxide photocatalysts via grafting polydimethylsiloxane brush. *Advanced Materials*, *29* (16)1604637.

Wu, S., Liu, X., Yeung, K. W. K., Liu, C., & Yang, X. (2014). Biomimetic porous scaffolds for bone tissue engineering. *Materials Science and Engineering: R: Reports*, *80*, 1–36.

Wu, Z., Lee, D., Rubner, M. F., & Cohen, R. E. (2007). *Structural color in porous, superhydrophilic, and self-cleaning SiO_2/TiO_2 Bragg stacks*. *Small (Weinheim an der Bergstrasse, Germany)*, *3*(8), 1445–1451.

Xie, Q., Xu, J., Feng, L., Jiang, L., Tang, W., Luo, X., & Han, C. C. (2004). Facile creation of a super-amphiphobic coating surface with bionic microstructure. *Advanced Materials*, *16*(4), 302–305.

Xu, L., Gao, L., & He, J. (2012). Fabrication of visible/near-IR antireflective and superhydrophobic coatings from hydrophobically modified hollow silica nanoparticles and poly (methyl methacrylate). *RSC Advances*, *2*(33), 12764–12769.

Xue, C.-H., & Ma, J.-Z. (2013). Long-lived superhydrophobic surfaces. *Journal of Materials Chemistry A, 1*(13), 4146–4161.

Xue, C.-H., Jia, S. T., Zhang, J., & Tian, L. Q. (2009). Superhydrophobic surfaces on cotton textiles by complex coating of silica nanoparticles and hydrophobization. *Thin Solid Films, 517*(16), 4593–4598.

Yamanaka, M., Ishizaki, Y., Nakagawa, T., Taoka, A., & Fukumori, Y. (2013). Purification and characterization of coacervate-forming cuticular proteins from Papilio xuthus pupae. *Zoological Science, 30*(7), 534–542.

Yan, Y. Y., Gao, N., & Barthlott, W. (2011). Mimicking natural superhydrophobic surfaces and grasping the wetting process: A review on recent progress in preparing superhydrophobic surfaces. *Advances in Colloid and Interface Science, 169*(2), 80–105.

Yang, J., Jiao, Y. P., Cui, F. Z., Lee, I. S., Yin, Q. S., & Zhang, Y. (2008). Modification of degradation behavior of magnesium alloy by IBAD coating of calcium phosphate. *Surface and Coatings Technology, 202*(22–23), 5733–5736.

Yang, J., Zhang, Z., Xu, X., Zhu, X., Men, X., & Zhou, X. (2012). Superhydrophilic–superoleophobic coatings. *Journal of Materials Chemistry, 22*(7), 2834–2837.

Yang, X., Roach, H. I., Clarke, N. M. P., Howdle, S. M., Quirk, R., Shakesheff, K. M., & Oreffo, R. O. C. (2001). Human osteoprogenitor growth and differentiation on synthetic biodegradable structures after surface modification. *Bone, 29*(6), 523–531.

Yazdani, J., Ahmadian, E., Sharifi, S., Shahi, S., & Dizaj, S. M. (2018). A short view on nanohydroxyapatite as coating of dental implants. *Biomedicine & Pharmacotherapy, 105*, 553–557.

Yin, X., Liu, Z., Wang, D., Pei, X., Yu, B., & Zhou, F. (2015). Bioinspired self-healing organic materials: Chemical mechanisms and fabrications. *Journal of Bionic Engineering, 12*(1), 1–16.

Yu, S., Hariram, K. P., Kumar, R., Cheang, P., & Aik, K. K. (2005). In vitro apatite formation and its growth kinetics on hydroxyapatite/polyetheretherketone biocomposites. *Biomaterials, 26*(15), 2343–2352.

Yu, S., Guo, Z., & Liu, W. (2015). Biomimetic transparent and superhydrophobic coatings: from nature and beyond nature. *Chemical Communications, 51*(10), 1775–1794.

Zhang, D., Cheng, Z., & Liu, Y. (2019). Smart wetting control on shape memory polymer surfaces. *Chemistry—A European Journal, 25*(16), 3979–3992.

Zhang, Y., Venugopal, J., Huang, Z. M., Lim, C. T., & Ramakrishna, S. (2005). Characterization of the surface biocompatibility of the electrospun PCL-collagen nanofibers using fibroblasts. *Biomacromolecules, 6*(5), 2583–2589.

Zhang, Y., Tian, J., Zhong, J., & Shi, X. (2018). Thin nacre-biomimetic coating with super-anticorrosion performance. *ACS Nano, 12*(10), 10189–10200.

Zhang, Y., Zhang, G., & Wei, M. (2009). Controlling the biodegradation rate of magnesium using biomimetic apatite coating. *Journal of Biomedical Materials Research Part B: Applied Biomaterials, 89*(2), 408–414, An Official Journal of The Society for Biomaterials, The Japanese Society for Biomaterials, and The Australian Society for Biomaterials and the Korean Society for Biomaterials.

Zhao, G., Yuan, Y., Zhang, P., Zhou, T., Wang, H., Li, X., & Zhou, H. (2022). Effect of hardness gradient of laser bionic coupling unit on wear resistance of 6082 aluminum alloy. *Optics & Laser Technology, 153*, 108172.

Zhao, Y., Xiong, C., & Zhang, L. (2008). Frictional wear and thermal fatigue behaviours of biomimetic coupling materials for brake drums. *Journal of Bionic Engineering, 5*, 20–27.

Zheng, Y., Xiong, C., & Zhang, L. (2014). Formation of bone-like apatite on plasma-carboxylated poly (etheretherketone) surface. *Materials Letters, 126*, 147–150.

CHAPTER 10

Biomimetic coatings for tribocorrosion

Ruby Aslam[1] and Andreas Rosenkranz[2]
[1]School of Civil Engineering and Architecture, Chongqing University of Science and Technology, Chongqing, P.R. China
[2]Department of Chemical Engineering, Biotechnology and Materials, Universidad de Chile, Santiago, Chile

10.1 Introduction

Tribocorrosion is a complex process that can cause severe damage to applied materials used in many industrial applications (Celis et al., 2006; Landolt, 2006). This process involves the simultaneous action of mechanical and chemical wear, leading to material degradation and failure. There are several methods to mitigate tribocorrosion such as the use of coatings, lubricants, and surface treatments. While lubricants can be effective in reducing friction and wear, they can have limitations in tribocorrosion mitigation (Cao & Mischler, 2021). For instance, the degradation of lubricants can occur over time, which can reduce their effectiveness. Additionally, some lubricants can promote corrosion, particularly in the presence of certain chemicals or environments (Sun & Bailey, 2014). Surface treatments such as shot peening or electrochemical surface modification can be effective in mitigating tribocorrosion (Vella et al., 2023), but they also have other drawbacks such as being expensive and time-consuming thus limiting their practicality. Additionally, surface treatments can alter the surface properties of the material, which may affect its mechanical, chemical, or biological properties. Traditional coatings such as thermally sprayed coatings, plasma sprayed coatings, plasma electrolytic oxidation coatings, plasma vapor deposition (PVD) coatings, multilayered coatings, hard facings, and electrodeposited coatings have been used to protect materials from tribocorrosion by reducing friction and wear. However, these coatings tend to have limited effectiveness and durability.

Biomimetic coatings, in particular, offer a promising new approach to protect materials from tribocorrosion due to their enhanced mechanical, chemical, and biological properties (Yeh-Liu et al., 2020). Biomimetic coatings are

Smart Biomimetic Coatings
DOI: https://doi.org/10.1016/B978-0-443-21738-8.00010-2

materials that mimic the structure and properties of natural materials thus providing a superior performance and durability compared to traditional coatings (Antony et al., 2022).

This chapter will assess the existing state-of-the-art regarding tribocorrosion such as general and basic aspects and factors contributing to material degradation. The limitations of traditional coatings and the potential advantages of using biomimetic coatings will also be examined. The chapter further explores future directions of this research field. By the end of the chapter, readers will have a comprehensive understanding of the role that biomimetic coatings can play in tribocorrosion mitigation and the potential for these coatings to revolutionize the field of material science.

10.2 General aspects of tribocorrosion

Tribocorrosion is a field of study that combines tribology and corrosion and has attracted the interest of scientists and engineers working in a variety of research fields (Diomidis et al., 2010). This is because of its tangible impact on daily life and the associated monetary costs. It relates the permanent modification of a metal's subsurface layers caused by mechanical and chemical reactions as a result of friction in a corrosive environment (Landolt, 2006; Mischler, 2008). It resembles the process of material degradation brought by the interaction of wear and corrosion. The petrochemical and chemical, nuclear process, material handling, aerospace, maritime, culinary, automotive, and biomedical offshore industries are just a few of the industries that are impacted by tribocorrosion. The possible outcomes of tribocorrosion are material loss, decreased dependability, decreased durability, decreased energy efficiency, decreased safety performance, increased health risks, increased pollution, etc. It can harm restorative dentistry, prosthetics, and other equipment, which in turn can compromise life quality and general health (Diomidis et al., 2010).

10.2.1 Factors affecting tribocorrosion

The mechanics of the tribological contact, the properties of the contacting materials, and the physicochemical characteristics of the environment together affect tribocorrosion. These factors are closely related and may act synergistically or antagonistically, thus positively or negatively impacting on how well the tribological system functions. As tribocorrosion includes the integration of numerous subsystems, it is necessary to investigate it based on a system approach. Significant factors impacting tribocorrosion in a sliding contact under electrochemical control are illustrated in Fig. 10.1 (Mathew et al., 2009). These factors, including the type of material, the environment, the type and intensity of mechanical wear, and the presence of chemical species, can promote corrosion. For instance, materials with high hardness and low ductility are more susceptible to tribocorrosion, as materials that are exposed to high-stress environments or environments with high levels of corrosive species. The presence of abrasive particles or other debris can also increase the rate of mechanical wear, which can, in turn, increase the likelihood of tribocorrosion. Other factors that can affect tribocorrosion include the pH and temperature of the environment, the presence of oxygen or other oxidizing agents, and the presence of other chemical species that can promote corrosion. Some of the significant factors influencing this phenomenon are outlined in the following sections (Celis et al., 2006; Wood, 2007).

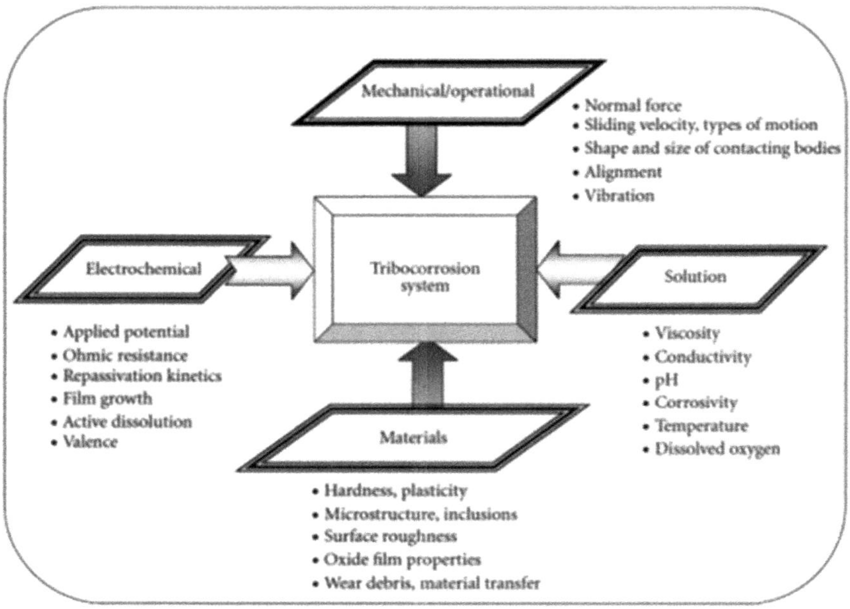

Figure 10.1 Summary of factors affecting tribocorrosion. *From Mathew, M. T., Srinivasa Pai, P., Pourzal, R., Fischer, A., & Wimmer, M. A. (2009). Significance of tribocorrosion in biomedical applications: overview and current status.* Advances in Tribology, *1–12. https://doi.org/10.1155/2009/250986.*

10.2.2 Materials properties

Material properties can have a significant impact on tribocorrosion. For instance, materials with high hardness and low ductility are more susceptible to tribocorrosion (Yaghoubi et al., 2022; Ponthiaux et al., 2012) because they are more prone to cracking and other forms of mechanical wear. Similarly, materials with low corrosion resistance are more susceptible to corrosion, which can exacerbate tribocorrosion (Yin et al., 2007). Other material properties that affect tribocorrosion include composition, microstructure, and surface finish of the material. For instance, materials with a high content of susceptible elements such as copper or zinc are more likely to undergo tribocorrosion. The microstructure of the material can influence tribocorrosion. Materials with a fine-grained microstructure are more resistant to tribocorrosion than those with a coarse-grained microstructure.

To prevent the charge transfer between the generally active bulk material and the corrosive environment, a wide variety of corrosion-resistant materials rely on a thin superficial oxide layer. Despite passivating the surface, this layer can be removed within tribological contacts by mechanical wear or impingement processes. Wherever the barrier film has been mechanically destroyed and removed, the charge transfer can occur at the interface without any resistance (Yoo et al., 2019).

The phase distribution, grain size, topography, and chemical composition of a material can have a significant impact on tribocorrosion. For instance, materials that have a bimodal grain size distribution, with both fine and coarse grains, are more susceptible to tribocorrosion than materials with a unimodal grain size distribution (Namus et al., 2021). This is because the presence of coarse grains can act as preferential sites for mechanical wear and corrosion. Similarly, materials that have a rough surface topography are more prone to tribocorrosion since they can trap wear particles and corrosion products, leading to increased damage (Allazadeh, 2009). The chemical composition also plays a crucial role regarding tribocorrosion. Materials with a high content of susceptible elements such as copper or zinc are more likely to undergo tribocorrosion. Finally, the phase distribution influences tribocorrosion. Materials with a high-volume fraction of hard, brittle phases may be more susceptible to cracking and other forms of mechanical wear.

10.2.3 Mechanical/operational parameters

The rate of tribocorrosion for a given metal-environment combination depends on the applied forces and the type of contact—sliding, fretting, rolling, or impact. Other factors include sliding speed, type of motion, shape and size of contacting bodies, alignment, and vibration. Other operational parameters that can affect tribocorrosion include temperature, humidity, and the presence of other chemical species that can promote corrosion.

10.2.4 Lubrication

The presence or absence of lubrication can significantly affect tribocorrosion. Lubricants can help to reduce friction and wear, but improper lubrication leads to increased mechanical wear and corrosion (Anaee & Abdulmajeed, 2016).

10.3 Testing approaches for tribocorrosion: standard procedures and best practices

Tribocorrosion testing lacks a proper, standardized test apparatus, which makes it challenging to compare results from different laboratories (Mathew et al., 2009). A tribometer rubs two surfaces against each other by producing relative motion that is either unidirectional (rotatory) or bidirectional (reciprocating). Electrochemical cells are used to record and control the electrochemical parameters. These cells normally consist of three electrodes: the reference electrode, the counter electrode, and the working electrode. The reference electrode employs the working electrode's steady, precisely defined potential to calculate the working electrode's potential. Reference electrodes include saturated calomel electrodes or silver/silver chloride electrodes (Ag/AgCl). The counter electrode, which is used to measure or regulate the current, is frequently made of inert materials like platinum, gold, or graphite. The electrodes are connected to a potentiostat to monitor the voltage between the reference electrode and the working electrode or the current between the counter electrode and the working electrode. A typical tribocorrosion test setup for a unidirectional tribometer using a ball-on-disk design is schematically depicted in Fig. 10.2A (López-Ortega et al., 2018). The test sequence, as depicted in Fig. 10.2B, was primarily divided into three phases: (1) the first stabilization period, (2) the sliding phase, and (3) the ultimate stabilization phase.

Tribocorrosion studies typically investigate the electrochemical behavior of surfaces prior to and throughout the tribological process to find out how wear influences the electrochemical response of materials exposed to certain corrosive media under established mechanical conditions. The electrochemical

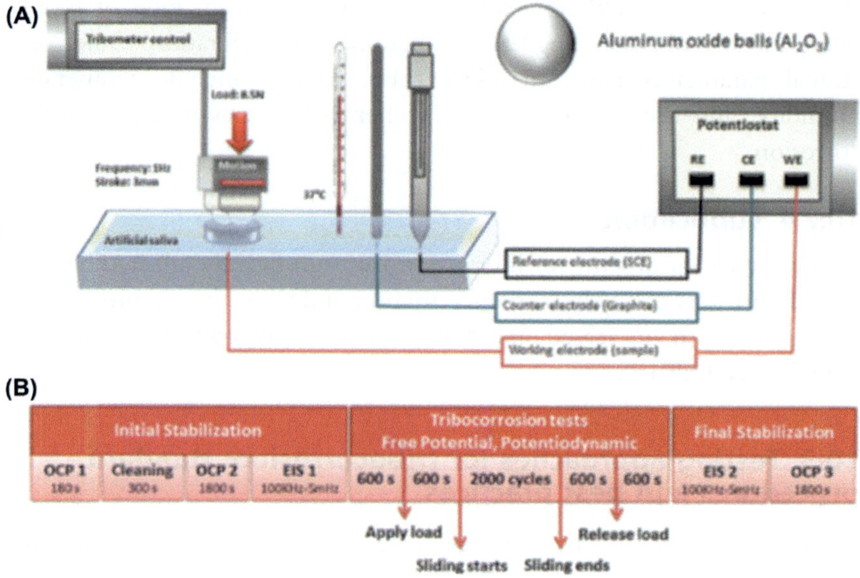

Figure 10.2 (A) Schematic illustration of the tribocorrosion setup. (B) Tribocorrosion protocol during free potential and potentiodynamic experiments. *From López-Ortega, A., Arana, J. L., & Bayón, R. (2018). Tribocorrosion of passive materials: A review on test procedures and standards.* International Journal of Corrosion, 2018.

methods that are most frequently used in tribocorrosion analysis include potentiodynamic and potentiostatic tests (da Silva Vieira Marques et al., 2016; Da et al., 2021), electrochemical impedance spectroscopy (Gonçalves et al., n.d.), open-circuit potential registration (OCP) (Ponthiaux et al., 2004), and electrochemical noise (EN) analysis. Many researchers also connect these measurements with a detailed analysis of the surface roughness (Hebbar et al., 2017; Visentin et al., 2019) and contact angle measurements (Acar et al., 1041; Çaha et al., 2021). Observing the morphology of worn areas (Sui et al., 2018; Wang et al., 2020; Zekonyte & Polcar, 2015) is also crucial for learning about the wear process.

Despite growing interest and improvements in electrochemical techniques, there was no standardised testing process for tribocorrosion evaluation until 2016. The only known standard was ASTM G119 (ASTM G119-09, 2016), which describes a process to determine how wear and corrosion react. However, to look into the flaws in the ASTM standard (Diomidis et al., 2009; Diomidis et al., 2010; Celis & Ponthiaux, 2012; Akonko et al., 2005), several techniques were developed to study the tribocorrosion behavior of passive materials. The ASTMG119 norm does not consider the total material loss of different components involved. According to the ASTM standard, material loss due to wear is measured using sliding tests at cathodic potentials, when corrosion is least prevalent. However, Diomidis et al. (Diomidis et al., 2010; Celis & Ponthiaux, 2012) clarified that in the absence of corrosion, the contribution of corrosion products to the mechanical response of the surface cannot be taken into account. Consequently, the material loss recorded may not accurately reflect the real conditions. Additionally, Akonko et al. (2005) showed how the wear volume varied by an order of magnitude due to the metal's sensitivity to hydrogen embrittlement and depending on the cathodic potential applied. Moreover, the standard does not take into account the galvanic couple created when sliding between the worn and unworn parts. In 2016 a new standard was established based on the test methods recommended by numerous researchers. While the new UNE 112086 (UNE 112086:2016, 2016) standard includes wear tests at open circuit potential, the ASTM (ASTM G119-09, 2016) standard considers wear testing under anodic and cathodic polarization. The technique outlined in the UNE standard to evaluate the ASTM standard's deficiencies can be utilized to identify and quantify the mechanical and electrochemical mechanisms causing material loss. Additionally, UNE standard can be utilized to identify the source of material loss in different worn areas, such as active regions and sections that are partially or fully repassivated within the track (Yan, 2013).

10.3.1 Biomimicry and biomimetic coatings—a new frontier in tribocorrosion research

Biomimicry is an approach that involves looking to nature for inspiration regarding the design of new products and technologies (Aziz & El Sherif, 2016). Biomimicry is an emerging field in corrosion control that gains more and more attention to develop new materials and coatings that can prevent or mitigate corrosion. By studying the ways how living organisms protect themselves against environmental damage, researchers can come up with new approaches to prevent corrosion that can be more effective and sustainable than traditional methods (Vazirinasab et al., 2018). One example of biomimicry in corrosion control is the use of proteins found in mussel adhesives to create coatings that are resistant to corrosion. Mussels can attach themselves to a wide range of surfaces, including metals, using a sticky adhesive that is composed of proteins that can withstand the harsh marine environment. Scientists have studied these proteins and developed synthetic versions that can be used to create coatings that are resistant to corrosion. Another example of biomimicry in corrosion control is the use of plant extracts to prevent corrosion. Some plants can produce compounds that can protect them from environmental stressors, including corrosion. Scientists explore the use of these compounds as natural corrosion inhibitors that can be applied to metal surfaces to prevent rust and other forms of corrosion. Overall, biomimicry offers a promising approach to developing new corrosion control products that are more effective, sustainable, and environment-friendly. By studying how nature has already solved the problem of corrosion, scientists and engineers can develop new materials and coatings that mimic these natural solutions and provide long-lasting protection for metal surfaces. Developing coatings with enhanced wear and corrosion properties has also aroused interest, and a great number of tribocorrosion studies have taken place over the last decade to evaluate the performance of coatings produced by different depositing techniques (HVOF, PVD, etc.) (Sun & Haruman, 2011; Obadele et al., 2014).

Superhydrophobic biomimetic coatings can be used to reduce tribocorrosion by repelling water and other liquids from metal surfaces. These coatings are inspired by the natural properties of certain plants and animals such as lotus leaves and geckos, which have evolved to repel water and other substances through the use of micro- and nanoscale structures on their surfaces. By mimicking these structures, biomimetic coatings can be applied to metal surfaces to reduce friction and wear and to prevent the build-up of moisture and other corrosive substances that can lead to tribocorrosion. Additionally, biomimetic coatings can reduce the need for lubricants, thus leading to less costly and more environment-friendly solutions. However, some strengths, weaknesses, opportunities, and threats need to be carefully analyzed to make sure that biomimetic coatings are sustainable bioproducts, as shown in Fig. 10.3.

10.3.2 Applications of biomimetic coatings in tribocorrosion—a literature review

To enhance the surface characteristics of biomedical implants, Marques et al. Marques et al. (2016) developed bioactive Ti-coatings doped with Ca, P, Si, and Ag generated by micro-arc oxidation and looked into the stability of the TiO_2 layer under wear and corrosion. The coating's microstructure and high Ca content both significantly increased its ability to withstand tribocorrosion for extended sliding time. Sui et al. created a titanium silicon carbide coating with a superhydrophobic carbon layer that exhibited self-lubricating abilities (Sui et al., 2009). The outcomes

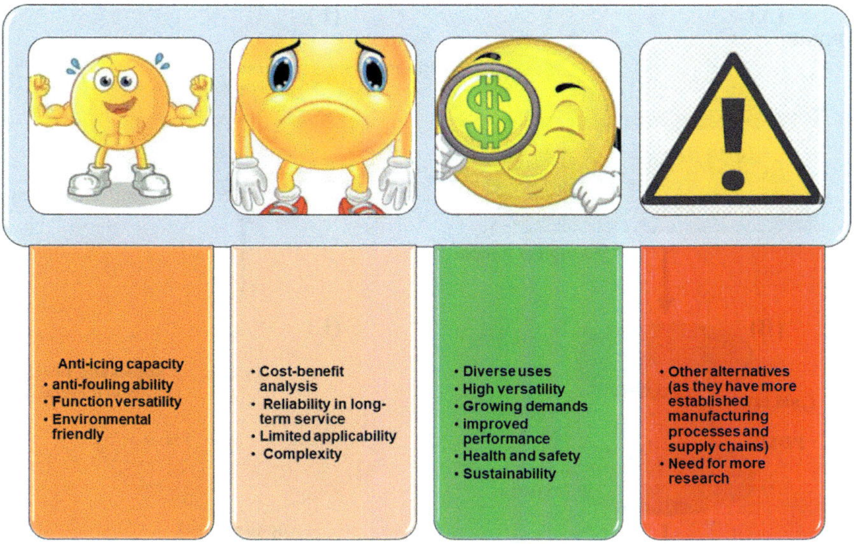

Figure 10.3 The SWOT (strengths, weaknesses, opportunities, and threats) of using biomimetic coatings as sustainable products.

highlight and confirm that the superhydrophobic carbon films maintained their superior low-friction and wear-resistant performance.

Wang et al. (2012) used natural lotus leaf templates to produce a diamond-like carbon (DLC) film that was hard (about 21 GPa), flexible, and superhydrophobic (with a contact angle of up to 160 degrees). Fig. 10.4 depicts the conceptual design for producing DLC films with bioinspired textures.

A ball-on-plate tribometer was used to examine the microtribological characteristics of the films Fig. 10.5. The textured nickel coatings (Ni(Lotus)) have been found to have poor wear resistance. As soon as the opposing ball started to rub on them, it was worn away. This went hand in hand with a steadily increasing coefficient of friction (reaching values of about 0.8). However, the antiwear properties of both the prepared DLC film with biomimicking microtextures, both modified with DLC(lotus)-PFPE and without PFPE DLC(lotus), as well as the as-prepared textured nickel coatings modified with PFPE Ni(lotus)-PFPE and Ni(Lotus)-PFPE, were significantly improved. At a load of 60 mN and a sliding velocity of 30 mm/s, they can continue to function as a useful lubricating layer for more than 3600 seconds.

Rahmawan et al. fabricated SiO_x-DLC nanocomposites by replica molding of poly(dimethylsiloxane) (PDMS) micropillars followed by a thin, and hard covering of SiO_x-DLC on its top (Rahmawan et al., 2010). In another study,

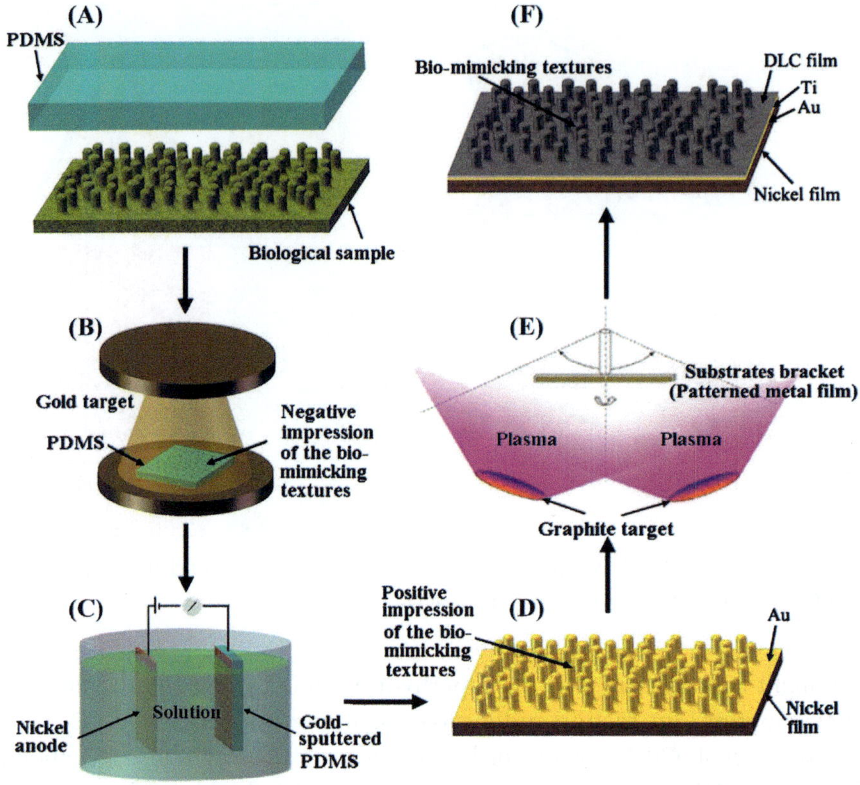

Figure 10.4 Schematic diagram of creating DLC films with biomimicking textures. (A) A poly(dimethylsiloxane) (PDMS) film is used to replicate the microtextures of the biological sample. (B) A thin layer of gold is sputtered on the textured PDMS film to provide a conductive surface. (C) A metallic layer is electrodeposited on the top of the PDMS film before (D) the PDMS film is peeled off to obtain a metallic layer with positive impression of the biomimicking textures. (E) A thin hard DLC film was deposited on the top of the metallic layer resulting in (F) the final DLC film with the biomimicking textures. *From Wang, Y., Wang, L., Wang, S., Wood, R. J. K., & Xue, Q. (2012). From natural lotus leaf to highly hard-flexible diamond-like carbon surface with superhydrophobic and good tribological performance.* Surface and Coatings Technology, *206(8–9), 2258–2264. https://doi.org/10.1016/j.surfcoat.2011.10.001.*

Cui et al. (2019) developed a nanocrystalline TiZrN-graded coating using a DC reactive magnetron sputtering. X-ray diffraction (XRD), Transmission electron microscope (TEM), and Electron Probe Microanalyzer (EPMA) were used to characterize the coating's microstructure and composition. In Hank's solution with and without 25% calf serum, the electrochemical corrosion and biotribocorrosion behavior of the coated titanium alloy was studied under

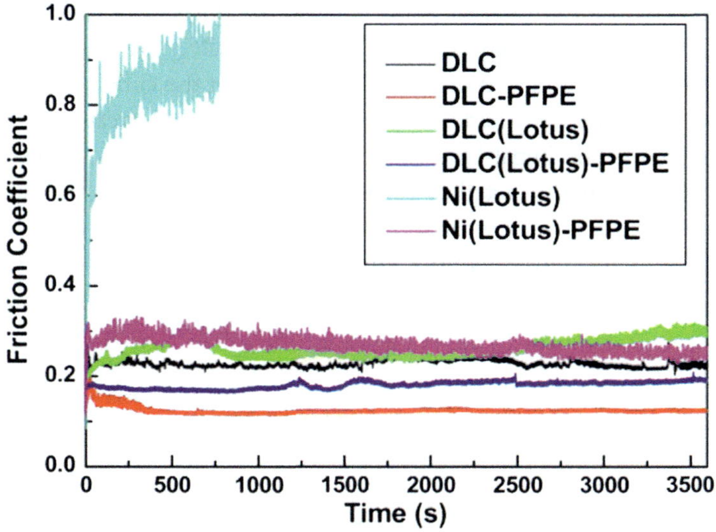

Figure 10.5 Variation in the temporal coefficient of fiction using a normal load of 60 mN and a sliding velocity of 30 mm/s. *From Wang, Y., Wang, L., Wang, S., Wood, R. J. K., & Xue, Q. (2012). From natural lotus leaf to highly hard-flexible diamond-like carbon surface with superhydrophobic and good tribological performance.* Surface and Coatings Technology, *206(8–9), 2258–2264. https://doi.org/10.1016/j.surfcoat.2011.10.001.*

OCP and applied potentials of 0.15 ± 0.25 V. The volumetric wear rates of TiZrN coating were as low as about 10^{-7} mm^3/Nm at OCP and applied potentials environments, which is 40%–60% lower than those of TiN coating. The Zr component is crucial to improve the mechanical and chemical characteristics of the TiN coating. When it comes to surface modification of Ti alloy artificial joints, which are subjected to heavy loads and severe wear, nanocrystalline TiZrN coating is a good option.

The tribological characteristics of carbon fiber-reinforced polyphenylene sulphide (PPS) composite covering in water were studied by Xu et al. (2005). The findings showed that under water lubrication, PPS composite coatings had superior tribological capabilities over pure PPS coating. In this regard, water was essential for cooling and washing. The friction and wear characteristics of spray-welded alloyed wear-resistant coating in oilfield wastewater were investigated by Wang et al. (2004). They concluded that using the right coating thickness can help to significantly increase the resulting wear resistance.

In a recent study (Beliardouh et al., 2022), radio frequency magnetron sputtering was used to deposit a multilayer coating made of alternating bilayers of $(ZrN/Ta)_n$ over Ti-6Al-4 V alloy. The tribocorrosion performance was guaranteed by the top layer of ZrN, whereas the ductility originated from the Ta interfacial layer. By dip coating on commercially pure titanium (Cp-Ti), Celik et al. (2023) produced duplex coatings utilizing the cuticle of the Japanese jewel beetle (*Chrysochroa rajah*) to offer protection against wear and corrosion. Chitin served as the initial layer of the duplex coated surfaces, while layers of TiO_2, SiC, and h-BN acted as second layers. According to the findings of the wear tests, the lowest wear rate on a surface coated with chitin and TiO_2 was $0.12 \pm 0.011 \times 10^{-3}$ mm^3/Nm in a dry environment and $0.28 \pm 0.017 \times 10^{-3}$ mm^3/Nm in Simulated Body Fluid (SBF) solution (Fig. 10.6).

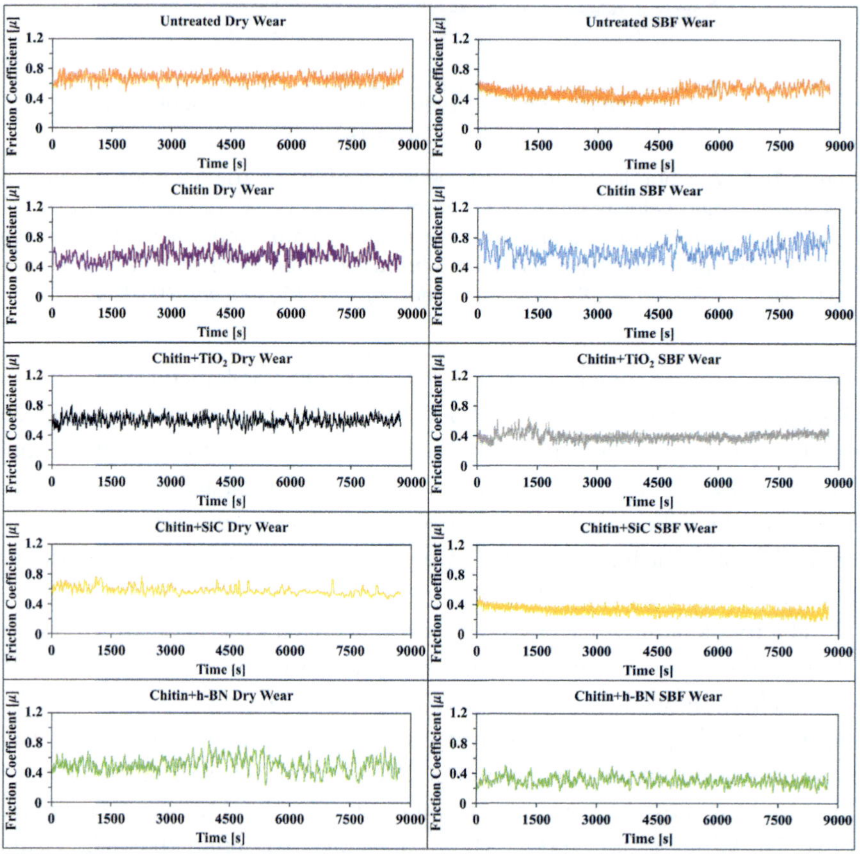

Figure 10.6 Friction coefficient-time graphs of untreated, chitin and duplex coated samples dry and SBF solution. *From Çelik, A., Atik, B., Uzun, Y., Bozkurt, Y. B., & Kovacı, H. (2023). Wear and corrosion properties of CP-titanium coated with chitin–ceramic nanocomposites.* Materials Chemistry and Physics, 303. *https://doi.org/10.1016/j.matchemphys.2023.127801.*

Additionally, the surface coated with chitin and TiO_2 had the maximum surface hardness, measuring 4 ± 0.28 GPa. The chitin + TiO_2 duplex coated surface exhibited the best resistance in tribocorrosion tests conducted in SBF solution.

10.4 Mechanism of action

Biomimetic coatings can prevent tribocorrosion in several ways. First, these coatings can form a protective barrier on the surface, which can help to avoid the penetration of corrosive agents thus reducing the rate of corrosion. Second, they can be designed to be self-healing, which implies that they can repair themselves when damaged, further improving their durability and longevity. Third, biomimetic coatings can be designed to mimic the properties of natural materials. For instance, some biomimetic coatings can mimic the surface structure of shark skin, which reduces drag and friction in water. Other coatings can mimic the self-cleaning properties of lotus leaves, which repel water and prevent the build-up of contaminants. Additionally, some coatings can incorporate particles or fibers that have been shown to improve wear resistance and reduce corrosion. These particles can be made from natural materials, such as cellulose or chitin, or from synthetic materials, such as carbon nanotubes or graphene. Furthermore, biomimetic coatings can be designed to be multifunctional, thus improving the wear and corrosion resistance simultaneously. This can be achieved by incorporating nanoparticles or other materials that can form a dense, protective layer on the surface of the material.

10.5 Conclusions and future perspective

Tribocorrosion is a hazardous type of corrosion since it degrades the material's surface before failure suddenly occurs. The methods currently employed to estimate the contributions of mechanical and electrochemical processes to the overall material loss in passive materials are inadequate. To extend the useful life of these materials in applications where passive materials are unsuitable due to their higher costs and inferior mechanical properties, a deeper understanding of the tribocorrosion degradation mechanism of the active metals and alloys is necessary. Biomimetic coatings are important in tribocorrosion since they can significantly improve the wear and corrosion resistance. The strength, self-cleaning ability, and superhydrophobicity of biomimetic coatings are their major characteristics. Biomimetic coatings can help to reduce friction and minimize wear, which can improve the efficiency of mechanical systems and reduce energy consumption. While biomimetic coatings have many advantages in tribocorrosion, there are also some limitations. One limitation is that these coatings can be difficult and expensive to produce, as they require specialized equipment and processes. There is a need for more research to determine the most effective methods for producing and applying biomimetic coatings. The detailed analysis of the microstructure and composition of biomimetic coatings could help researchers to better understand how these coatings interact with the underlying material and how they respond to mechanical wear and corrosion. Further, researchers can also explore the use of computational modeling and simulation to better understand the underlying mechanisms of tribocorrosion and to design new coatings with an enhanced performance. Finally, scientists are also suggested to study the environmental impact of biomimetic coatings, including their potential toxicity and their ability to biodegrade. This aspect is important to ensure that these coatings are safe and suitable for use in a wide range of applications. By combining these approaches, many exciting new developments in the field of biomimetic coatings for preventing triobocorrosion in the years to come are expected to be seen. In conclusion, biomimetic coatings may have significant positive effects on the economy and the environment due to their resilience, unique qualities, superhydrophobicity, and ability to clean and repair themselves.

References

Acar, M., Kovacı, H., & Çelik, A. (2022). Investigation of corrosion and tribocorrosion behavior of boron doped and graphene oxide doped TiO_2 nanotubes produced on. Cp-Ti. *Materials Today Communications*, *1041*, 104182.

Akonko, S., Li, D. Y., & Ziomek-Moroz, M. (2005). Effects of cathodic protection on corrosive wear of 304 stainless steel. *Tribology Letters*, *18*(3), 405–410. Available from https://doi.org/10.1007/s11249-004-3205-1.

Allazadeh, M. R. (2009). Formation of defects in the steel microstructure during solidification and their effects on the steel material properties. *Journal of ASTM International*, *6* (5), 1–12.

Anaee, Rana Afif Majed, & Abdulmajeed, Majid Hameed (2016). *Tribocorrosion*. InTech. Available from https://doi.org/10.5772/63657.

Antony, Sherin, Anju, T. R., & Thomas, Bejoy (2022). *Nature-inspired biomimetic polymeric materials and their applications* (pp. 1–31). Springer Science and Business Media LLC. Available from https://doi.org/10.1007/978-981-16-6603-2_50-1.

Aziz, M. S., & El Sherif, A. Y. (2016). Biomimicry as an approach for bio-inspired structure with the aid of compu tation. *Alexandria Engineering Journal*, *55*(1), 707–714. Available from https://doi.org/10.1016/j.aej.2015.10.015, http://www.elsevier.com/wps/find/journaldescription.cws_home/724292/description#description.

Beliardouh, N. E., Ramoul, C. E., Nouveau, C., Kaleli, E. H., & Montagne, A. (2022). Thin solid films synthesis and tribocorrosion performances of multilayer (Ta/ZrN)*n* coatings. *Thin Solid Films, 749.*

Çaha, I., Alves, A. C., Chirico, C., Pinto, A. M., Tsipas, S., Gordo, E., & Toptan, F. (2021). Improved tribocorrosion behavior on bio-functionalized β-type titanium alloy by the pillar effect given by TiN reinforcements. *Surface and Coatings Technology, 415.* Available from https://doi.org/10.1016/j.surfcoat.2021.127122, http://www.journals.elsevier.com/surface-and-coatings-technology/.

Cao, Shoufan, & Mischler, Stefano (2021). A lubricated tribocorrosion model incorporating surface roughness. *Biotribology, 26,* 100181. Available from https://doi.org/10.1016/j.biotri.2021.100181.

Çelik, A., Atik, B., Uzun, Y., Bozkurt, Y. B., & Kovacı, H. (2023). Wear and corrosion properties of CP-titanium coated with chitin—ceramic nanocomposites. *Materials Chemistry and Physics, 303.* Available from https://doi.org/10.1016/j.matchemphys.2023.127801, http://www.journals.elsevier.com/materials-chemistry-and-physics.

Celis, J.-P., & Ponthiaux, P.- (2012). ISBN: 978-1-907975-20-2 *Testing tribocorrosion of passivatingmaterials supporting research and industrial innovation.* Handbook: Maney Publishing.

Celis, J. P., Ponthiaux, P., & Wenger, F. (2006). Tribo-corrosion of materials: Interplay between chemical, electrochemical, and mechanical reactivity of surfaces. *Wear, 261* (9), 939—946. Available from https://doi.org/10.1016/j.wear.2006.03.027.

Cui, W., Cheng, J., & Liu, Z. (2019). Bio-tribocorrosion behavior of a nanocrystalline TiZrN coating on biomedical titanium alloy. *Surface and Coatings Technology, 369,* 79—86. Available from https://doi.org/10.1016/j.surfcoat.2019.04.036, http://www.journals.elsevier.com/surface-and-coatings-technology/.

da Silva Vieira Marques, I., Alfaro, M. F., Saito, M. T., da Cruz, N. C., Takoudis, C., Landers, R., Mesquita, M. F., Nociti, F. H., Mathew, M. T., Sukotjo, C., & Barão, V. A. R. (2016). Biomimetic coatings enhance tribocorrosion behavior and cell responses of commercially pure titanium surfaces. *Biointerphases, 11*(3). Available from https://doi.org/10.1116/1.4960654, http://scitation.aip.org/content/avs/journal/bip.

Da, B., Yaxuan, L., Vasu, A. T., Yongxin, G., Hao, T., Yongwu, Z., & Yongguang, W. (2021). Improving tribocorrosion performance of chemically bonded ceramic phosphate coating reinforced by GO-ZnO. *Ceramics International, 47*(11), 15722—15731. Available from https://doi.org/10.1016/j.ceramint.2021.02.143, https://www.journals.elsevier.com/ceramics-international.

Diomidis, N., Celis, J. P., Ponthiaux, P., & Wenger, F. (2010). Tribocorrosion of stainless steel in sulfuric acid: Identification of corrosion-wear components and effect of contact area. *Wear, 269*(1—2), 93—103. Available from https://doi.org/10.1016/j.wear.2010.03.010.

Diomidis, N., Celis, J. P., Ponthiaux, P., & Wenger, F. (2009). A methodology for the assessment of the tribocorrosion of passivating metallic materials. *Lubrication Science, 21* (2), 53—67. Available from https://doi.org/10.1002/ls.73Belgium, http://www3.interscience.wiley.com/cgi-bin/fulltext/122267601/PDFSTART.

Gonçalves, V. R. M., Çaha, I., Alves, A. C., Toptan, F., & Rocha, L. A. (2022). Improved tribocorrosion behavior obtained by in-situ precipitation of Ti2C in Ti-Nb alloy. *Metals, 12.*

Hebbar, R. S., Isloor, A. M., & Ismail, A. F. (2017). *Contact angle measurements* Elsevier Inc., India*Membrane Characterization* (pp. 219—255). Elsevier Inc., India. Available from http://www.sciencedirect.com/science/book/9780444637765, https://doi.org/10.1016/B978-0-444-63776-5.00012-7.

Landolt, D. (2006). Electrochemical and materials aspects of tribocorrosion systems. *Journal of Physics D: Applied Physics, 39*(15), 3121—3127. Available from https://doi.org/10.1088/0022-3727/39/15/S01.

López-Ortega, A., Arana, J.L., & Bayón, R. (2018). Tribocorrosion of passive materials: A review on test procedures and standards. *International Journal of Corrosion, 2018.*

Marques, I. S. V., Alfaro, M. F., Saito, M. T., Cruz, N. C., C.T.R., Landers, Mesquita, M. F., Junior, F. H. N., Mathew, M. T., Sukotjo, C., & Barão, V. A. R. (2016). Biomimetic coatings enhance tribocorrosion behavior and cell responses of commercially pure titanium surfaces. *Biointerphases, 11*, 031008.

Mathew, M. T., Srinivasa Pai, P., Pourzal, R., Fischer, A., & Wimmer, M. A. (2009). Significance of tribocorrosion in biomedical applications: Overview and current status. *Advances in Tribology, 2009*, 1–12. Available from https://doi.org/10.1155/2009/250986.

Mischler, S. (2008). Triboelectrochemical techniques and interpretation methods in tribocorrosion: A comparative evaluation. *Tribology International, 41*(7), 573–583. Available from https://doi.org/10.1016/j.triboint.2007.11.003.

Namus, R., Rainforth, W. M., Huang, Y., & Langdon, T. G. (2021). Effect of grain size and crystallographic structure on the corrosion and tribocorrosion behaviour of a CoCrMo biomedical grade alloy in simulated body fluid. *Wear, 478–479.* Available from https://doi.org/10.1016/j.wear.2021.203884, https://www.journals.elsevier.com/wear.

Obadele, B. A., Lepule, M. L., Andrews, A., & Olubambi, P. A. (2014). Tribocorrosion characteristics of laser deposited Ti-Ni-ZrO2 composite coatings on AISI 316 stainless steel. *Tribology International, 78*, 160–167. Available from https://doi.org/10.1016/j.triboint.2014.05.011.

Ponthiaux, P., Wenger, F., Drees, D., & Celis, J. P. (2004). Electrochemical techniques for studying tribocorrosion processes. *Wear, 256*(5), 459–468. Available from https://doi.org/10.1016/S0043-1648(03)00556-8.

Ponthiaux, Pierre, Wenger, Franois, & Pierre, Jean (2012). *Tribocorrosion: material behaviour under combined conditions of corrosion and mechanical loading.* InTech. Available from https://doi.org/10.5772/35634.

Rahmawan, Y., Moon, M. W., Kim, K. S., Lee, K. R., & Suh, K. Y. (2010). *Langmuir: the ACS Journal of Surfaces and Colloids, 26.*

(2016). *Standard guide for determining synergism between wear and corrosio.* ASTM International.

Sui, X., Xu, R., Liu, J., Zhang, S., Wu, Y., Yang, J., & Hao, J. (2018). Tailoring the Tribocorrosion and Antifouling Performance of (Cr, Cu)-GLC Coatings for Marine Application. American Chemical Society, China. *ACS Applied Materials and Interfaces, 10*(42), 36531–36539. Available from https://doi.org/10.1021/acsami.8b12359, http://pubs.acs.org/journal/aamick.

Sui, J., Zhang, J., Ren, S., Rinke, M., Lu, J., & Jia, J. (2009). Carbon coating with combined super-hydrophobic and self-lubricating properties on titanium silicon carbide. *Carbon, 47*(3), 629–634.

Sun, Y., & Bailey, R. (2014). Improvement in tribocorrosion behavior of 304 stainless steel by surface mechanical attrition treatment. Elsevier, United Kingdom. *Surface and Coatings Technology, 253*, 284–291. Available from https://doi.org/10.1016/j.surfcoat.2014.05.057, http://www.journals.elsevier.com/surface-and-coatings-technology/.

Sun, Y., & Haruman, E. (2011). Tribocorrosion behaviour of low temperature plasma carburised 316L stainless steel in 0.5M NaCl solution. *Corrosion Science, 53*(12), 4131–4140. Available from https://doi.org/10.1016/j.corsci.2011.08.021.

UNE 112086:2016. (2016). Ensayos de tribocorrosión en materiales pasivos.

Vazirinasab, E., Jafari, R., & Momen, G. (2018). Application of superhydrophobic coatings as a corrosion barrier: A review. Elsevier B.V., Canada. *Surface and Coatings Technology, 341*, 40–56. Available from https://doi.org/10.1016/j.surfcoat.2017.11.053, http://www.journals.elsevier.com/surface-and-coatings-technology/.

Vella, K. A., Buhagiar, J., Cassar, G., Pizzuto, M. M., Bonnici, L., Chen, J., Zhang, X., Huang, Z., & Zammit, A. (2023). The effect of a duplex surface treatment on the corrosion and tribocorrosion characteristics of additively manufactured Ti-6Al-4V.

Materials, *16*(5). Available from https://doi.org/10.3390/ma16052098, http://www.mdpi.com/journal/materials.

Visentin, F., Galenda, A., Fabrizio, M., Battiston, S., Brianese, N., Gerbasi, R., Zin, V., & El Habra, N. (2019). Assessment of synergistic effects of LP-MOCVD TiO_2 and Ti surface finish for dental implant purposes. *Applied Surface Science*, *490*, 568–579. Available from http://www.journals.elsevier.com/applied-surface-science/, https://doi.org/10.1016/j.apsusc.2019.06.067.

Wang, H. X., Sui, Y. K., & Zhang, J. Z. (2004). Friction and wear behaviors of sucker rod and tubing string in the presence of oil-field wastewater as the lubricating medium. *Mocaxue Xuebao/Tribology*, *24*(5), 467–470.

Wang, Y., Wang, L., Wang, S., Wood, R. J. K., & Xue, Q. (2012). From natural lotus leaf to highly hard-flexible diamond-like carbon surface with superhydrophobic and good tribological performance. *Surface and Coatings Technology*, *206*(8–9), 2258–2264. Available from https://doi.org/10.1016/j.surfcoat.2011.10.001.

Wang, Y., Zhang, J., Zhou, S., Wang, Y., Wang, C., Wang, Y., Sui, Y., Lan, J., & Xue, Q. (2020). Improvement in the tribocorrosion performance of CrCN coating by multilayered design for marine protective application. *Applied Surface Science*, *528*, 147061.

Wood, R. J. K. (2007). Tribo-corrosion of coatings: A review. *Journal of Physics D: Applied Physics*, *40*(18), 5502–5521. Available from https://doi.org/10.1088/0022-3727/40/18/S10.

Xu, H. Y., Chen, J. M., Zhou, H. D., & Feng, Z. Z. (2005). Tribological behavior of poly(phenylene sulphide) coating and carbon fiber reinforced composites coating under dry sliding and water lubrication. *Mocaxue Xuebao/Tribology*, *25*(5), 416–420.

Yaghoubi, A., Mirsalehi, S. E., & Jamali, A. (2022). Investigation on microstructure, mechanical properties and tribological behavior of AlZnMgCu1.5-T6/zirconia surface nanocomposites developed by FSP. *Journal of Materials Research and Technology*, *20*, 397–414. Available from https://doi.org/10.1016/j.jmrt.2022.07.093, http://www.elsevier.com/journals/journal-of-materials-research-and-technology/2238-7854.

Yan, Y. (2013). *Bio-tribocorrosion in biomaterials and medical implants*. Elsevier, 2013.

Yeh-Liu, Li-Kai, Hsu, Sheng-Yu, Chen a, Po-Yu, Lee, Jyh-Wei, & Duh, Jenq-Gong (2020). Improvement of CrMoN/SiNx coatings on mechanical and high temperature tribological properties through biomimetic laminated structure design. *Surface and Coatings Technology*, *393*.

Yin, S., Li, D. Y., & Bouchard, R. (2007). Effects of the strain rate of prior deformation on the wear-corrosion synergy of carbon steel. *Wear*, *263*(1–6), 801–807. Available from https://doi.org/10.1016/j.wear.2007.01.058.

Yoo, Y. S. J., Lim, H., Emery, J., & Kacher, J. (2019). Relating microstructure to defect behavior in AA6061 using a combined computational and multiscale electron microscopy approach. *Acta Materialia Inc, United States Acta Materialia*, *174*, 81–91. Available from https://doi.org/10.1016/j.actamat.2019.05.033, http://www.journals.elsevier.com/acta-materialia/.

Zekonyte, J., & Polcar, T. (2015). Friction force microscopy analysis of self-adaptive W-S-C coatings: Nanoscale friction and wear. *ACS Applied Materials and Interfaces*, 7(38), 21056–21064. Available from https://doi.org/10.1021/acsami.5b05546, http://pubs.acs.org/journal/aamick.

CHAPTER 11

Biomimetic antimicrobial coatings

Nasreena Lone
School of Allied Healthcare & Sciences, JAIN (Deemed-to-be University), Bangalore, Karnataka, India

11.1 Introduction

11.1.1 Microbial infestation on surfaces

Microbial infestation starts with the physical adsorption of organic molecules, exopolysaccharides, proteins, and glycoproteins, involving a hierarchical colonization process to prepare a conditioning biofilm for the primary settlement of microorganisms (Marić & Vraneš, 2007; Zardus et al., 2008). Such conditioning of the surfaces can be quickly prompted in the presence of moisture. This conditioning film serves as the initial stage in the complex process of surface microbial contamination, leading to the transmission of infectious diseases, product spoilage, equipment failure, compromised water treatment and underwater engineered structures, and other aquaculture-related equipment (Bekele et al., 2018; Boudarel et al., 2018; Gotz, 2002). In the case of underwater engineered systems, the severity of this initial microbial infestation pays the way for subsequent deposition, accumulation, and growth of micro- and macroorganisms, which proves economically and ecologically detrimental (Fusetani, 2004; Ludyansky, 1991). The reader is advised to go through the antifouling chapter of this book for detailed information about biofouling and related material.

Microbial contamination on wet surfaces is a persistent concern due to the potential for the growth and proliferation of pathogenic microorganisms. The presence of moisture creates an ideal environment for microbial colonization, providing a continuous source of water and nutrients. Under medical settings, such pathogenic contamination and propagation can prove extremely dangerous for several reasons. Such infestation and consistent microfouling degrades medical equipment performance, poses a high risk of healthcare-associated infections imposing potential complications or even proving fatal, and can even create insecticide-resistant

Smart Biomimetic Coatings
DOI: https://doi.org/10.1016/B978-0-443-21738-8.00011-4

microbial strains over time (Cangui-Panchi et al., 2022; Dadi et al., 2021; Lode, 2009; Medis et al., 2023). Thus understanding the dynamics and implications of microbial infestation on wet surfaces is crucial for implementing effective control measures and minimizing the associated risks. This chapter provides an overview of the dynamics and impacts of microbial infestation on wet surfaces and highlights current strategies for prevention, detection, and control of microbial contamination on wet surfaces, emphasizing the importance of regular monitoring and effective disinfection practices, with a focus on the biomimetic antimicrobial mitigation techniques.

11.1.2 Microbial biofilm formation

The representative illustration of biofilm formation is depicted in Fig. 11.1. The hierarchical colonization starts from conditioning the surfaces with moisture proximity. Conditioning is followed by the secretion of sticky extracellular polymeric substances that help the microorganisms to adhere to potential surfaces preparing a biofilm gel matrix. The continuous process involves microbial adhesion, detachment, and proliferation of the adhered microbes to thriven colonies (Landini et al., 2010; Marić & Vraneš, 2007). The adhesion and detachment processes counterbalance each other, ultimately creating a stable biofilm, often termed primary colonization. Planktonic adhesion on the substrates is regulated by a sequence of physicochemical interactions orchestrated by "quorum sensing," which

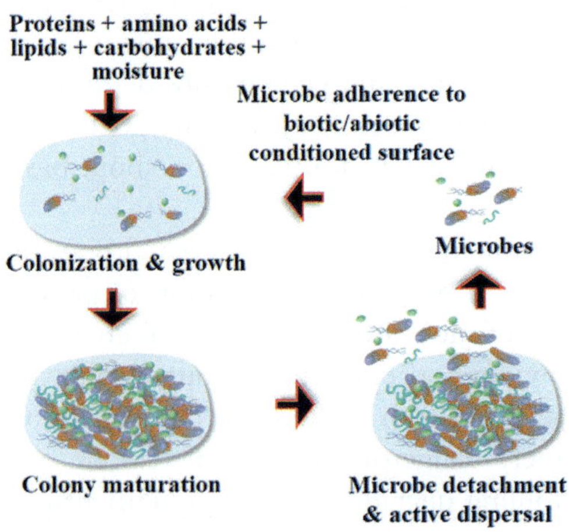

Figure 11.1 Schematic illustration of the microbial biofilm formation on biotic and abiotic surfaces.

is basically an intercellular signaling system involving the cell density-dependent recognition of specific low-molecular-weight compounds (Chambers et al., 2006; Cooksey & Wigglesworth-Cooksey, 1995; Yebra et al., 2004; Zardus et al., 2008). In biofouling, the intricate presence of microbial biofilms goes beyond mere facilitation; it assumes a pivotal role in mediating and influencing the adhesion and settlement of subsequent fouling populations. Furthermore, the cooperative behavior among the bacterial biofilm community is orchestrated through cell-cell communication. This elaborate enactment aids in their collective resistance against antimicrobial attacks and various environmental threats. Notably, within the context of biofouling, several prominent bacterial species have been identified, including *Pseudomonas aeruginosa*, *Pseudomonas fluorescens*, *Bacillus cereus*, *Escherichia coli*, and *Staphylococcus aureus* each contributing to the complex interplay of biofilm dynamics and fouling processes, further highlighting the multifaceted nature of this ecological interaction(Gotz, 2002; Mah et al., 2003; Medis et al., 2023; Rodriguez-Emmenegger et al., 2014).

Under optimum conditions, successful biofilm formation and upscaling engender the creation of a highly conducive and habitable environment that facilitates secondary colonization, wherein multicellular species firmly fixate within the biofilm matrix. This sequential progression encompasses primary colonization, followed by subsequent secondary colonization and macrofoulant accumulation stages, each exhibiting remarkable resilience against conventional toxicants and antimicrobial formulations, rendering them challenging to combat. Notably, the phases of stable microbial colonization and macrofoulant accumulation within this intricate process tend to assume a predominantly irreversible nature perpetuating the biofouling process, thereby underscoring their long-lasting impact (Zardus et al., 2008). Consequently, the formation of bacterial biofilms stands as the pivotal precursor and prominent stage in the intricate phenomenon of biofouling, highlighting its significance in prevention and mitigation strategies.

11.1.3 Factors affecting microbial biofilm formation

The complex phenomenon of microbial biofilm formation and maturation entails a multifaceted, ever-evolving, and uninterrupted process intricately influenced by a multitude of physical, chemical, and biological parameters. The foulant colonization on substrates is subject to a myriad of impelling factors that collectively guide its dynamics and outcomes.

These parameters encompass a broad spectrum, including, but not limited to, temperature, pH, water flow, and salinity, along with the physicochemical nature of the substrate and foulant (charge, substrate surface energy, wettability, roughness, and porosity). Within this complex framework, the hydrophobicity and hydrophilicity of both the substrates and the foulants act as crucial factors, exerting their distinctive influences and dictating the preferential interactions that govern adhesion dynamics (Callow & Fletcher, 1994; Lindner, 1992; MAKI et al., 1989). The unique interplay between the physicochemical properties of the substrate and the foulant further contributes to the intricate substrate–foulant interrelationship, shaping the colonization patterns that manifest in fouling complications. A comprehensive representation of the intricate thermodynamic interactions that govern the phenomenon of spontaneous cell adhesion was expertly crafted by Van Oss Van Oss et al. (1991). He encapsulated the multifaceted interplay of Gibbs free energy (ΔG) by taking into account various contributing factors like electrostatic interactions (ΔG^{E}), van der Waals interactions (ΔG^{W}), acid-base interactions (ΔG^{AB}), and the cumulative effect of these interactions, manifesting as the total Gibbs free energy (ΔG^{T}), as they collectively influence and shape the process of bacterial adhesion.

11.1.4 Consequences of microbial biofilm formation

The bacterial infestation and colonization lead to severe healthcare-related infections which can often prove fatal (Cangui-Panchi et al., 2022; Hofer, 2022; Medis et al., 2023; Patel et al., 2005). Given that the microbial biofilm is primarily responsible for facilitating the adhesion and subsequent accumulation of fouling organisms, its presence bears significant and far-reaching implications for the marine industry, exerting adverse effects on both economic and ecological fronts. The prevention of fouling and the maintenance of various aquatic engineered structures, including, but not limited to, ships, coastal infrastructure, aquacultural facilities, and biomedical equipment, necessitate substantial financial investments, amounting to billions of dollars each year on a global scale. Micro- and macroorganism accumulation elicits a range of adverse effects, including the insidious biocorrosion of metallic surfaces, generates surface roughness, surface biodeterioration, clogs heat exchangers, knocks out underwater sensors, compromising the efficiency of biomedical equipment, and subjects severe aftermaths to ship industry (Chambers et al., 2006; Cooksey & Wigglesworth-Cooksey, 1995;

Gittens et al., 2013; Larsen et al., 2003). From an ecological standpoint, biofouling contributes to species alienation as well. Introducing nonnative invasive species into ecosystems engenders a profound perturbation that disrupts the delicate equilibrium of the original ecological framework and emerges as the predominant conduit of species alienation which, in extreme cases, causes the outright extinction of native species (Larsen et al., 2003). The biofouling chapter of this book covers this in detail. This insightful information accentuates the criticality of conducting thorough investigations and explorations into biofilm prevention and mitigation, focusing on unveiling effective strategies to address this complex phenomenon.

11.2 Antimicrobial strategies

In essence, antimicrobial coatings can be described as chemical formulations strategically employed to impede the adhesion and proliferation of microorganisms on various surfaces. Notably, these coatings should exhibit exceptional durability, enabling them to retain their performance even when subjected to regular and repeated exposure to water and rigorous cleaning protocols. Despite the predominant emphasis on antibacterial capabilities within the antimicrobial coatings, it is essential to acknowledge the inescapable significance of viruses on various surfaces, as highlighted by the ongoing COVID-19 pandemic, which has propelled the combat strategies to the forefront (Mallakpour et al., 2021; Sawai & Yoshikawa, 2004). Antimicrobial coatings typically consist of integrated potent active agents that exert inhibitory effects on the growth and viability of microorganisms, thus presenting a pragmatic tool for bolstering hygiene standards, curbing infection rates, promoting public health, and subduing the subsequent attachment and accumulation of macroorganisms. Commonly used agents include silver, copper, zinc, and quaternary ammonium compounds. These substances interfere with microbial cell membranes, disrupt metabolic pathways, and hinder vital cellular processes, leading to the inactivation or death of pathogens (Dizaj et al., 2014; He et al., 2021; Sawai & Yoshikawa, 2004; Sawai, 2003). Furthermore, some coatings incorporate nanoparticles or nanoscale structures with antimicrobial properties, enabling prolonged and efficient pathogen control (Cloutier et al., 2015; Ding et al., 2018; Hofer, 2022; Khan & Shakoor, 2023).

Through extensive research, scientists have explored various approaches aimed at combating bacterial transmission and inhibiting biofilm formation. Two primary strategies have emerged from these endeavors. The first approach entails the implementation of surface-bound active antimicrobials and biocidal coatings designed to actively eliminate or reduce microbial attachment. This is achieved through the adept utilization of nanomaterials, chemical modifications, and micro- and nanostructuring techniques. The second strategy revolves around developing passive pathogen-repellent surfaces, which serve as a passive deterrent mechanism against the attachment and subsequent colonization of harmful pathogens (Cangui-Panchi et al., 2022; Rajaramon et al., 2023; Rather et al., 2021; Roy et al., 2018). These approaches have significantly contributed to advancing preventive measures against bacterial transmission and mitigating the formation of persistent biofilms. Some of these commonly employed antimicrobial coating strategies are briefly mentioned for the reader and illustrated in Fig. 11.2. However, the major portion of this chapter will emphasize the biomimetic antimicrobial coating approaches detailing the technological developments, action mechanisms, and challenges. It is essential to note that the selection of antimicrobial coating strategies depends on the specific application, the target microorganisms, and the desired durability and effectiveness of the coating.

11.2.1 Surface-bound/biocide-loaded antimicrobial coatings

The surface-bound antimicrobials approach encompasses a sophisticated methodology wherein antimicrobial agents are meticulously incorporated directly into the very composition of the coating material, thereby engendering the creation of an impervious and resilient layer(s) that envelops the surface. By virtue of their specialized properties and interactions, these antimicrobial agents effectively disrupt the vital functions and structural integrity of microorganisms, curtailing their ability to colonize and propagate on the coated surface, thereby significantly mitigating the lurking risk of contamination. Often classified as biocidal-loaded coatings and distinguished by their unique composition, these formulations harbor a distinctive array of ingredients meticulously selected for their remarkable tendency to directly exterminate microorganisms or hinder their growth (Lejars et al., 2012; Nurioglu et al., 2015). Crucially, the efficacy of biocidal coatings is often contingent upon the intricately orchestrated and regulated release of these potent agents, ensuring a sustained and enduring shield against microbial incursions. By employing advanced techniques to precisely control the diffusion and gradual liberation of biocidal agents, these coatings can effectively extend their antimicrobial protection over extended periods, rendering them indispensable tools in safeguarding

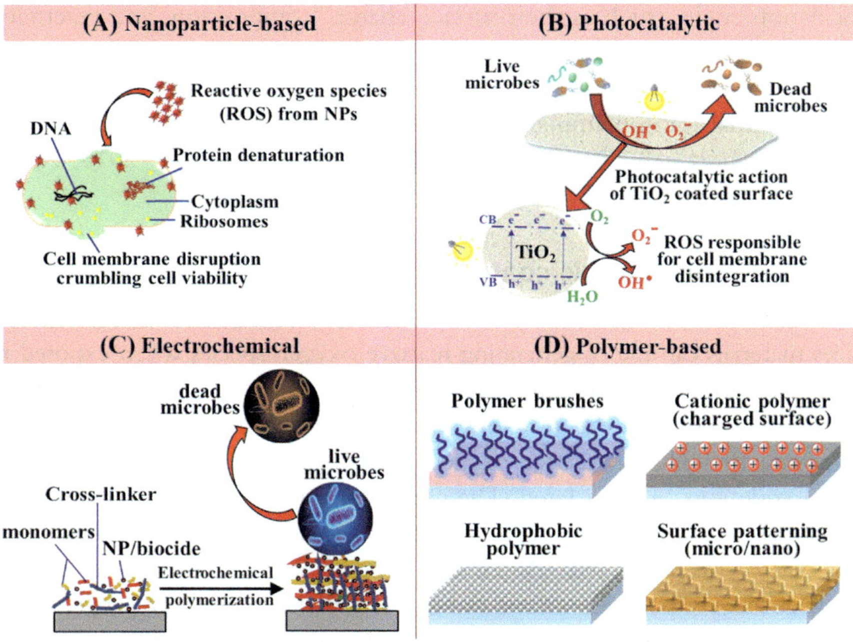

Figure 11.2 Types of antibacterial coatings: (A) nanoparticle armored coatings: reactive oxygen species (ROSs) generated interact with the microbial cells disintegrating cell membrane and other molecules, causing microbial death. (B) Photocatalytic action of TiO_2-coated surface generates ROSs that can decompose a wide range of microorganisms. This mechanism operates due to the strong redox ability of TiO_2. (C) Electrochemical polymerization/deposition aids in mitigating microbes on the surface. (D) Different polymer-based antimicrobial approaches.

against microbial contamination and preserving hygiene across a diverse range of applications.

11.2.2 Nanotechnology-based coatings

Nanotechnology-based coatings represent a cutting-edge paradigm wherein the seamless integration of nanomaterials into coating formulations confers exceptional antimicrobial attributes. These nanoparticles, characterized by their diminutive size and vast surface area, harbor distinctive physicochemical properties that endow them with unparalleled antimicrobial efficacy. The heightened antimicrobial performance of nanomaterials arises from their ability to engage in intricate interactions at the nanoscale level, allowing for enhanced surface contact and interaction with microbial entities. Moreover, the unique physicochemical properties of nanoparticles, such as their surface charge, composition, and reactivity, contribute to their ability to disrupt the vital functions and structural integrity of microorganisms, thereby impeding their growth and curtailing the potential for contamination (Ahmed et al., 2020; Azizi-Lalabadi et al., 2019; Dizaj et al., 2014; Durdu et al., 2023; Galvão et al., 2018; Xiong et al., 2019; Yildiz et al., 2023).

11.2.3 Photocatalytic coatings

Photocatalytic coatings comprise a sophisticated antimicrobial strategy that utilizes materials capable of generating reactive oxygen species when exposed to light, such as titanium dioxide (TiO_2). These coatings have the unique ability to initiate photocatalytic reactions when subjected to light energy. Upon exposure to sunlight, reactive oxygen species, such as hydroxyl radicals and superoxide ions, are generated. The generated reactive oxygen species exhibit a robust and indiscriminate capacity to degrade and destroy the essential components of microbial cells (Auten & Davis, 2009; Di Credico et al., 2015). This effectively neutralizes their viability and makes them highly effective in neutralizing and annihilating microorganisms on the coated surface (He et al., 2021; Koshani et al., 2021; Lundin et al., 2014; Ma et al., 2020).

11.2.4 Electrochemical coatings

Leveraging the potent force of electrical potential, these coatings orchestrate a symphony of antimicrobial effects that reverberate throughout the coated surface. Through the controlled release of ions or the initiation of intricate electrochemical reactions directly on the coated surface, these coatings navigate the delicate terrain of microbial cell functions, expertly disrupting their essential processes and impeding their ability to flourish and propagate (Jafari et al., 2023; Lee et al., 2020; Lichter et al., 2009; Wang et al., 2018).

11.3 Biomimetic antimicrobial coatings

Biomimetic antimicrobial coatings represent an innovative and nature-inspired approach. Drawing inspiration from the intricate designs and mechanisms found in nature, these coatings mimic and harness the remarkable antimicrobial properties exhibited by certain organisms and their biochemical systems. By emulating the structural features, surface characteristics, and molecular compositions of natural antimicrobial agents, biomimetic coatings strive to recreate the formidable defense mechanisms observed in nature. By incorporating biomolecules, peptides, or bioactive compounds, these coatings effectively combat microbial threats by disrupting essential microbial functions, inhibiting adhesion, and impeding the growth and proliferation of microorganisms. These coatings are meticulously engineered to replicate the structural and functional characteristics of the natural defense mechanisms observed in living organisms (Chee & Brown, 2020; Chen, Duan et al., 2021; Ergene et al., 2018; Oopath et al., 2023; Yang, Liang et al., 2022; Zhao et al., 2019). Through careful design and fabrication, these coatings aim to create surfaces that mimic nature's self-sterilizing properties and effectively deter microbial adhesion, colonization, and subsequent growth. The biomimetic approach capitalizes on the inherent efficacy and selectivity of natural antimicrobial systems, providing a promising avenue for developing advanced coatings that offer enhanced antimicrobial protection, reduced environmental impact, and improved biocompatibility in various applications, ranging from healthcare settings to food processing facilities (Charlot et al., 2009; Chen, Duan et al., 2021; Moerman, 2014; Michalska et al., 2018). By unlocking the secrets of nature's antimicrobial prowess, biomimetic antimicrobial coatings hold immense potential in revolutionizing the field of antimicrobial technology and driving innovation towards safer and more sustainable solutions for creating a safer and healthier future by effectively mitigating the risks of microbial pathogens.

11.3.1 Peptide-based coating

Peptide-based coatings fall under the bioactive category, representing a fascinating research and development area in materials science and biotechnology. These coatings are inspired by the natural properties and functions of peptides, which are short chains of amino acids found in living organisms and can exhibit inherent antimicrobial activity. Peptides have attracted significant attention due to their versatility and ability to mimic various biological processes. One of the key advantages of peptide-based biomimetic coatings is their ability to provide functionalization at the nanoscale level. The peptide coatings can exhibit enhanced biocompatibility, antimicrobial activity, cell adhesion, and controlled release of bioactive molecules. These properties make them highly versatile and applicable in various fields, including biomedical engineering, tissue engineering, drug delivery systems, and surface modification of implants or medical devices (Atefyekta et al., 2021; Cardoso et al., 2021; Carmona-Ribeiro & Carrasco, 2014; Chen, Gao et al., 2021; Drexelius & Neundorf, 2021; Gan et al., 2021; Kazemzadeh-Narbat et al., 2021; Negut et al., 2022; Sakala & Reches, 2018; Thapa et al., 2021; Yan et al., 2021; Ye et al., 2021; Yuan et al., 2021). These functional coatings can incorporate synthetic or naturally occurring antimicrobial peptides that mimic those found in organisms such as insects, amphibians, or plants (Seyfi et al., 2020). These peptides can disrupt microbial cell membranes or interfere with essential cellular processes, effectively inhibiting microbial growth, as illustrated in Fig. 11.3. This approach allows researchers to harness the unique nature of peptides and apply them to create functional coatings tailored with antimicrobial properties, achieved via solid-phase peptide synthesis, peptide ligation, peptide self-assembly (Carmona-Ribeiro & Carrasco, 2014; Jeong et al., 2018; Stillger & Müller, 2022; Su et al., 2020; Townsend et al., 2017; Yu et al., 2021), etc.

Biomimicking of peptides is a complex process involving several key steps. Specific peptides with desired properties are identified for a particular application, such as biocompatibility, adhesion, self-assembly, antimicrobial activity, or cell adhesion and growth promotion (Gonzales et al., 2023; Gu et al., 2017; Novick & Dordick, 2002). Researchers optimize and modify the peptide sequences based on molecular structure and interactions to enhance desired functionalities. The selected peptides are tailored and

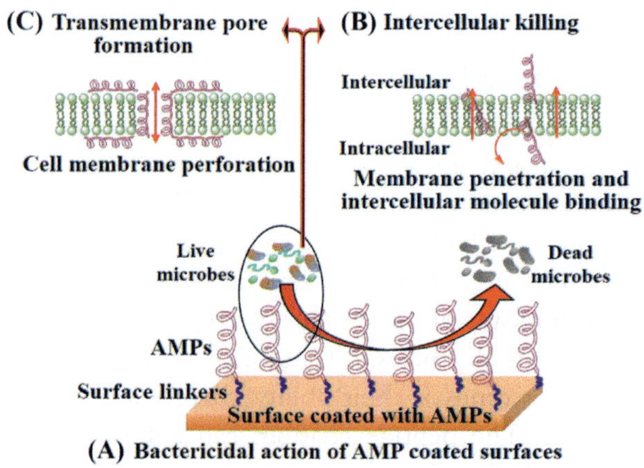

Figure 11.3 (A) Illustration of bactericidal action of peptide-based coatings. Possible modes of action are also depicted: (B) AMPs penetrate the cell membrane and bind with intercellular molecules disrupting their integration, and (C) depicts the membrane perforation.

incorporated into a coating matrix or surface. Techniques like chemical conjugation, physical adsorption, or covalent immobilization achieve the desired alterations. The selection of an appropriate technique is contingent upon the precise requirements and the surface in question, as their unique characteristics necessitate a tailored approach to modification. The resulting peptide-based biomimetic coatings exhibit a range of intriguing properties. For example, they can enhance biocompatibility or improve interactions with biological systems, such as cells and tissues (Li et al., 2023; Moussa et al., 2019; Xie et al., 2022). These coatings can also possess self-cleaning properties, similar to the lotus leaf, due to their ability to repel water and prevent the adhesion of dirt or contaminants. Additionally, peptide-based coatings can exhibit antimicrobial activity, inhibiting the growth of bacteria or other harmful microorganisms on surfaces (Carmona-Ribeiro & Carrasco, 2014; Fichman et al., 2021; Hasan et al., 2020; Xiao et al., 2020; Yu et al., 2021). The applications of peptide-based biomimetic coatings are diverse and expanding rapidly. Examples of applications include biomedical implants, drug delivery systems, biosensors, antimicrobial surfaces, tissue engineering scaffolds, medical equipment, ceramics, and metal surfaces. The coating process can be achieved through methods such as dip coating, spray coating, or electrostatic deposition, depending on the specific requirements and characteristics of the substrate (Cardoso et al., 2021; Drexelius & Neundorf, 2021; Fichman et al., 2021; Hasan et al., 2020; Kazemzadeh-Narbat et al., 2021; Negut et al., 2022; Shi et al., 2020; Thapa et al., 2021; Ye et al., 2021; Yu et al., 2021; Yuan et al., 2021).

11.3.2 Enzyme-based coatings

Enzymes play a crucial role in the defense mechanisms of many organisms by breaking down microbial cell walls or interfering with their metabolic processes. In biomimetic enzyme-based coatings, scientists aim to mimic the catalytic capabilities of enzymes by integrating them into coating materials. Biomimetic coatings can incorporate desired enzymes with antimicrobial properties, such as lysozyme or lactoferrin, to create coatings that can actively degrade microbial cells and prevent their proliferation (Efremenko et al., 2023; Grover et al., 2013; Olsen et al., 2007; Thallinger et al., 2013). The enzymes are meticulously identified and engineered to exhibit remarkable selectivity and efficiency, allowing for precise catalysis of target reactions. This can be achieved via physical entrapment, covalent immobilization, or encapsulation techniques. Enzyme-based coatings can operate under mild conditions and facilitate the catalyst's regeneration and recycling, enhancing sustainability (Hu et al., 2016; Ivanova et al., 2015; Pangule et al., 2010; Seijsing et al., 2020; Vaterrodt et al., 2016). As the understanding of enzyme functionalities and the development of enzyme engineering techniques advance, the possibilities for biomimetic enzyme-based coatings continue to expand, opening up new avenues for innovation and scientific advancement.

11.3.3 Surface patterning

Surface patterning is a technique that involves creating micro- or nano-scale patterns on the coating surface to mimic the natural surface features observed in organisms, like insect wings, shark skin, butterflies, geckos, or carapace of *Cancer pagurus*, etc. In these organisms, the surfaces have inherent high-density nanopillars, nanogrooves, or nanowrinkles that create a hostile environment for microorganisms predominantly determined by their physical structure (Hansen & Autumn, 2005; Hasan et al., 2019; Ivanova et al., 2012; Kelleher et al., 2016; Pogodin et al., 2013; Sakamoto et al., 2014; Watson, Cribb, et al., 2015; Wen et al., 2014). By replicating the topographical features found in nature, such as these hierarchical structures on insect wings or the rough surfaces of certain plant leaves, surface patterning coatings can effectively prevent the attachment and growth of microbes. Micro/nanoarray structures in insect wings, like the cicada, induce mechanical stress on the microbial cell membrane and eventually deform and rupture it. This mechno-bactericidal activity of micro- and nano-sequenced patterning of surfaces also instills the hydrophilic/hydrophobic/superhydrophobic character to the surface altering its water contact angle and consequently aiding in preventing microbial adherence (Alameda et al., 2022; Hanson et al., 2015; Hawi et al., 2022; Jiang et al., 2021; Valiei et al., 2020). This mechanism has been demonstrated to operate against a series of bacteria. The proposed mechanism for the mechanical lysis of microbial cells is believed to be intricately linked to several key parameters, including the nanopillar density, elasticity, height, aspect ratio, and wettability (Bandara et al., 2017; Pogodin et al., 2013; Watson et al., 2017). Extensive research literature exists to substantiate this notion, elucidating the interplay between these factors and their influence on the efficacy of the mechanical lysis process (Fig. 11.4).

Nanopillar height and density have been related to the stress induced on bacterial membranes. Inspired by cicada wings, Elena et al. reported an

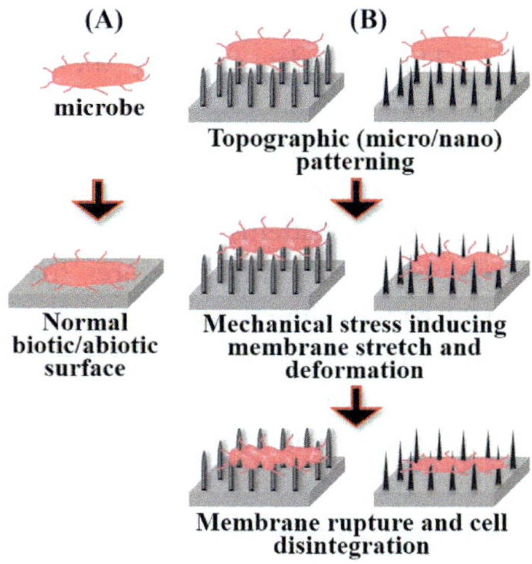

Figure 11.4 Illustration of topographic micro/nanopatterning for efficient bactericidal application. (A) Microbial adsorption on normal biotic/abiotic surface. (B) The microbial cell disintegration due to the induced mechanical stress on the cell membrane, which eventually causes its rupture.

ideal nanopillar height (320 nm) capable of killing *P. aeruginosa* (95%) and *S. aureus* (83%) on the surface. High aspect ratio nanoprotrusions protrusions of *Diplacodes bipunctata* wings have also been found to exhibit bactericidal activity against different strains. Similarly, nanogroove and nanowrinkle geometry of shark skin and crab carapace, respectively, have been investigated, as well, and have been found to disrupt microbe cell adherence entirely. Studies have shown that nanowrinkle geometry in crab carapace presents a hierarchical arrangement of smaller and larger ridges. Such hierarchical structure engineering of multiple length scales can emerge as another approach to designing nature-inspired antimicrobial surfaces. For example, incorporating nanoscale features on microscale patterns or macroscopic structures can enhance the surface's antibacterial properties. This multiscale approach can provide additional contact points and increase the chances of bacterial deformation or penetration, leading to improved antimicrobial efficacy (Hanson et al., 2015; Hawi et al., 2022; Valiei et al., 2020).

The fundamental principle behind biomimetic surface patterning techniques lies in replicating or modifying natural surface structures to create artificial surfaces with equivalent qualities. Antimicrobial techniques using biomimetic surface patterning entail numerous crucial phases. First, researchers analyze and comprehend the features and underlying mechanisms of natural antimicrobial surfaces. This includes studying the topography, chemical makeup, and other elements contributing to their antimicrobial properties. The intended surface patterns are then recreated on synthetic materials using cutting-edge production techniques, including lithography, laser ablation, or electrochemical etching. These patterns can range from regular arrays of microstructures to complex hierarchical structures that resemble those in nature. The selection of pattern dimensions and spacing is critical in determining the antimicrobial efficacy of the resulting surface. Furthermore, the surface patterns can alter the hydrophobicity or hydrophilicity of the material, affecting the wetting properties and reducing the moisture availability for microbial growth. Additionally, by modulating fluid dynamics and surface interactions, the patterns can enhance the shedding or removal of microbes. Biomimetic surface patterning techniques can even integrate chemical cues inspired by the assimilation of natural antimicrobial agents, like peptides, enzymes, or other bioactive molecules, into the surface coating or modification. Such chemical cues inhibit microbial growth or disrupt their adherence and biofilm formation. The resulting biomimetic surface patterning approach offers several benefits. First, the surface patterns disrupt the attachment and colonization of microbial cells by physically impeding their movement or inhibiting their adhesion to the surface. This disruption prevents the formation of biofilms, which are often associated with persistent infections. Second, the antimicrobial agents integrated into the surface coating or modified surface chemistry contribute to the overall effectiveness of the technique. This harmonious interplay of physical disruptions and chemical interventions helps to fortify the surface against microbes (Elbourne et al., 2017; Erkoc & Ulucan-Karnak, 2021; Fürstner et al., 2005; Huang & Liu, 2022; Kaur & Liu, 2016; Lee et al., 2023; Michalska et al., 2018; Mohd et al., 2023; Szilágyi et al., 2013; Tripathy et al., 2017; Wang et al., 2020).

Biomimetic surface patterning antimicrobial techniques find applications in various fields, including healthcare, food industry, and water treatment. For example, in healthcare settings, these techniques can be applied to medical devices, implants, and hospital surfaces to prevent the colonization and transmission of harmful pathogens. In the food industry, antimicrobial surfaces can inhibit the growth of bacteria on food packaging or processing equipment, reducing the risk of contamination. In water treatment, these techniques can aid in developing self-cleaning surfaces or filters that prevent biofouling and microbial growth (Moerman, 2014; Koshani et al., 2021; Mérian & Goddard, 2012; Pérez et al., 2022).

11.3.4 Bioinspired materials

Biomimetic antimicrobial coatings also employ bioinspired materials that exhibit inherent antimicrobial properties. For example, researchers have developed coatings incorporating materials like nanoparticles or proteins, which possess potent antimicrobial activity. Marine organisms, such as certain fish or marine plants, possess antimicrobial properties that help them thrive in aquatic environments. Scientific reports and studies have extensively explored surface patterning and nanoparticle incorporation in biomimetic coatings. One prominent approach in biomimetic coatings is the incorporation of nanoparticles, like carbon-based (graphene oxide), TiO-based, and particularly silver-based nanoparticles. Nanoparticles can disrupt microbial cell membranes and interfere with essential cellular processes. These nanoparticles are either embedded or immobilized within the coating matrix, enabling a controlled release over time or inducing surface patterning (Glinel et al., 2012; Gonzales et al., 2023; Katiyar et al., 2021; Lee et al., 2023; Oopath et al., 2023; Zhang et al., 2022).

One highly sophisticated biomimetic inspiration comes from the adhesive nature of mussel proteins. Mussels, displaying a remarkable tenacity in adhering to diverse surfaces, even amidst the harsh and relentless conditions prevalent in marine environments, owe their adhesion prowess to the adhesive proteins secreted by their extraordinary byssal threads (Chen, Gao et al., 2021; Cheng et al., 2017; Fichman et al., 2021; Gan et al., 2019; Manolakis & Azhar, 2020; Tian et al., 2020; Xiao et al., 2020). The development and fabrication of cutting-edge mussel-inspired biomimetic antimicrobial coatings necessitate the integration of key elements reminiscent of mussel adhesive proteins, with particular emphasis on including the remarkable catechol groups found therein. Catechol groups are intriguing due to their aromatic ring and two hydroxyl groups. The unique adhesive nature of mussel proteins is attributed to the hydroxyl moieties because of their potential interactions with various organic and inorganic surfaces. Scientists utilize multiple strategies to incorporate catechol groups into the coating materials to create mussel-inspired antimicrobial coatings. This may entail synthesizing artificial analogs of mussel adhesive proteins or modifying existing polymers by introducing catechol functional groups creating environmentally benign, durable, and robust protective formulations (Sedõ et al., 2013; Sousa & Mano, 2017; Yang, Liang et al., 2022; Ye et al., 2011; Zhang, Wang et al., 2020; Zhang, Wu et al., 2020) (Fig. 11.5).

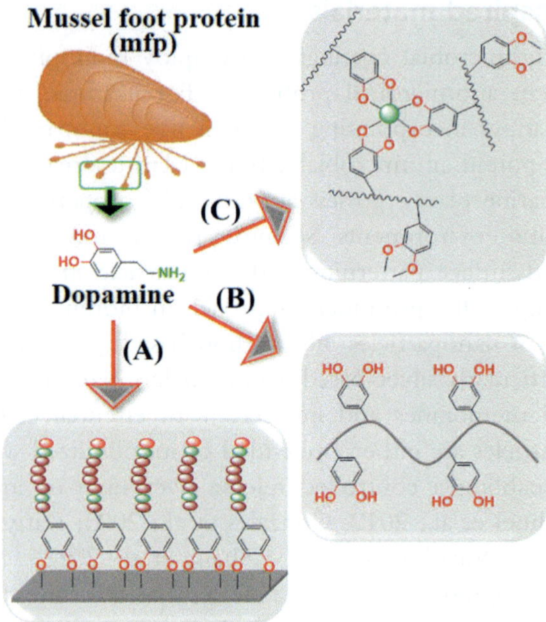

Figure 11.5 Image depicting dopamine in mussel foot proteins. Various possible routes/mechanisms to prepare mimicked polymer systems are also given. (A) Peptide mimicking with dopamine anchors, (B) dopamine functionalized polymerization, (C) metal ion/NP coordination and cross-linking of catechol-functionalized polymers.

The antimicrobial properties of mussel-inspired biomimetic coatings arise from the multitude of intricate operative mechanisms working in synergy. First, the catechol groups can bind to the microbial cell surface, disrupting the integrity of the cell membrane and inducing cell death. This direct contact acts as a physical barrier, impeding the growth and proliferation of microorganisms. Additionally, the catechol groups facilitate immobilizing antimicrobial agents or nanoparticles onto the coating surface. These agents can include antimicrobial peptides, silver nanoparticles, or other bioactive molecules with established antimicrobial properties. The coatings ensure a sustained release by immobilizing these agents, enhancing their long-term effectiveness against microbial colonization. Furthermore, mussel-inspired biomimetic coatings possess inherent resistance to biofilm formation. Biofilms are complex communities of microorganisms encased in a protective matrix, posing significant challenges in antimicrobial treatments. The adhesive nature of the catechol-containing coatings hinders microbial attachment and disrupts the formation of the extracellular matrix, thereby preventing biofilm formation (Huang et al., 2017; Liu et al., 2018; Lyu et al., 2019; Rao et al., 2022; Wang et al., 2021; Ye et al., 2011).

The applications of mussel-inspired biomimetic antimicrobial coatings are vast and transcend boundaries across multiple fields. In the healthcare sector, these coatings can be employed on medical devices, implants, or wound dressings to prevent microbial infections and biofilm formation. There are numerous research publications available that highlight the use of mussel-inspired formulations. For example, an intriguing study using catechol-based hydrogels for wound healing was reported by Liang et al. The research demonstrated the excellent antimicrobial activity of the cross-linked hydrogel with exemplary self-healing and biocompatibility. With their diverse applications in healthcare, food safety, and water treatment, these coatings offer innovative solutions to combat microbial colonization and infections, contributing to improved public health and safety.

11.3.5 Self-cleaning coatings

Self-cleaning biomimetic coatings represent a fascinating and pioneering approach to antimicrobial strategies, taking inspiration from the remarkable self-cleaning abilities observed in various organisms. It provides an ingenious approach to surface engineering aimed at repelling contaminants and facilitating the removal of microbial species from the coated surfaces. These coatings are designed to capitalize on the extraordinary hydrophobic or superhydrophobic properties to prevent the adhesion of microorganisms and other contaminants. By leveraging the principles of surface energy and interfacial interactions, self-cleaning coatings create an environment that actively repels water and particles, enabling the effortless removal of dirt, debris, and microbes through natural cleaning mechanisms, including rainfall. These coatings impart a high degree of water repellency through astute manipulation of the surface characteristics and chemical composition. Building upon the concept of hydrophobicity, superhydrophobic coatings take the repellency to an even greater extent. These coatings exhibit an exceptionally high contact angle, impel water droplets to assume nearly perfect spherical shapes, and exhibit exceptional mobility. Consequently, the droplets engage in a sweeping ballet, effectively dislodging and whisking away any contaminants on the surface, including microorganisms, thereby maintaining a clean and sanitized surface (Chauhan et al., 2019; Chermahini et al., 2018; Fürstner et al., 2005; Lundin et al., 2014; Ma et al., 2020), depicted in Fig. 11.6.

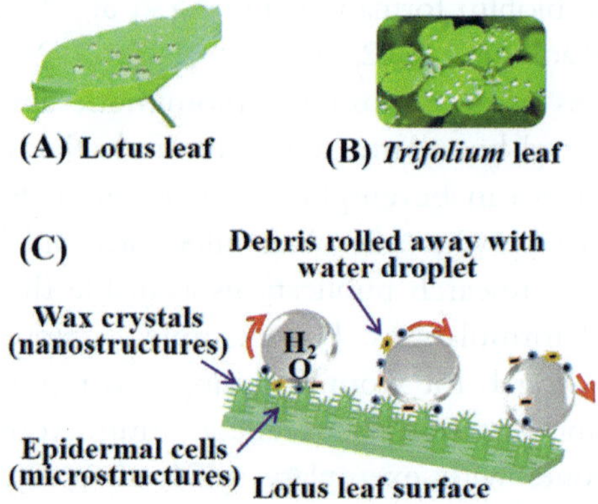

Figure 11.6 Water droplets rolled off the (A) lotus leaf and (B) Trifolium leaf surfaces. Part (C) illustrates the hierarchical micro- and nanostructural arrangement on the lotus leaf surface that renders it hydrophobic and can clean off debris by rolling water droplets.

Microorganisms, including bacteria and fungi, often require a moist environment for growth and attachment. However, the hydrophobic or superhydrophobic surfaces repel water, inhibiting the formation of a conducive environment for microbial colonization. This discourages their attachment and proliferation, minimizing contamination risks, biofilm formation, and subsequent infections. By repelling water and particles, self-cleaning coatings enable easy cleaning through natural processes like rainfall, minimizing the accumulation of microbes on the surface. This self-cleaning action significantly reduces the need for manual cleaning or harsh cleaning agents, offering an environmentally friendly and cost-effective solution (Bayer, 2020; Bhushan, Jung, et al., 2009; Bhushan, Koch, et al., 2009; Celik et al., 2023; Chan et al., 2021; Konar et al., 2020; Park et al., 2010; Shirtcliffe et al., 2011; Wang et al., 2022; Zhang, Wang et al., 2013). The "gold standard" for understanding the epidermal topography of natural superhydrophobic and self-cleaning surfaces and engineering synthetic analogs is the lotus leaf, frequently used as a reference point for comparison and in-depth understanding. Inspired by the lotus effect, these coatings replicate micro- and nanoscale structures and hydrophobic properties found in nature. By recreating these surface characteristics, self-cleaning coatings prevent the attachment of microorganisms and unwanted substances. These structures can be engineered using techniques such as micro- and nano-lithography, chemical vapor deposition, or self-assembly methods. The resulting surface topography comprising tiny protrusions, ridges, or roughened textures, creates air pockets and reduces the contact area between the coating and contaminants. As a result, water droplets and particles are unable to adhere to the surface, simply rolling off due to the low surface energy and the air trapped within the micro- and nanofeatures (Cheng et al., 2006; Collins & Safiuddin, 2022; Kim et al., 2018; Koch et al., 2009; Li et al., 2019; Solga et al., 2007; Watson et al., 2017; Watson, Green, et al., 2015; Yamamoto et al., 2015).

The self-cleaning properties of these coatings have significant implications in various industries and applications. In healthcare settings, for instance, self-cleaning coatings on medical equipment and surfaces can reduce the risk of nosocomial infections and cross-contamination. In architectural and infrastructure applications, self-cleaning coatings can help maintain the cleanliness and esthetics of buildings, bridges, and other structures. Moreover, in the food industry, these coatings can aid in ensuring hygienic conditions by minimizing the accumulation of contaminants on processing equipment and surfaces (Pérez et al., 2022; Ruzi et al., 2022). They provide an efficient and sustainable means of maintaining clean surfaces, reducing the need for frequent and intensive cleaning procedures, and promoting overall hygiene in diverse settings.

11.3.6 Biomimetic hybrid coatings

Biomimetic antimicrobial coatings can also be created by combining different methods and materials with complementary antimicrobial properties. These materials include polymers, ceramics, metals, nanoparticles, or biological components such as peptides, proteins, or DNA. The choice of materials is driven by the desired functionalities and properties achieved in the coating, such as enhanced mechanical strength, improved biocompatibility, or tailored surface interactions. For example, a coating may combine a hydrophobic material to repel water and inhibit microbial adhesion, along with a material that releases antimicrobial compounds to actively combat microbial growth. Another example of achieving synergy is by mixing nanoparticles with a polymer matrix. Incorporating nanoparticles can enhance the mechanical strength or impart antimicrobial properties to the coating while integrating polymers can provide flexibility and durability. Biomimetic hybrid coatings can mimic the self-cleaning abilities of lotus leaves and gecko feet to repel contaminants, replicate antireflective properties of insect eyes and butterfly wings to enhance optical performance and reduce glare, or imitate hierarchical structures found in shark skin or plant surfaces to reduce friction, improving hydrophobicity, or increasing durability (Cheng et al., 2019; Coll Ferrer et al., 2012; Galvão et al., 2018; Kanehashi et al., 2014; Li et al., 2021; Liao et al., 2020; Ye et al., 2021; Zhang & Seeger, 2013).

The applications of biomimetic hybrid coatings span a wide range of fields. In biomedicine, these coatings can be utilized for tissue engineering scaffolds, implants, or drug delivery systems, offering enhanced biocompatibility and controlled release properties. In the energy sector, they can be applied to solar cells, fuel cells, or batteries, improving performance and stability. In sensing and diagnostics, biomimetic hybrid coatings can also create sensitive and selective surfaces for detecting biomolecules or environmental pollutants (Manabe et al., 2014; Peng et al., 2022). Hence, by carefully designing the mixed composition and structure, researchers can achieve coatings with superior properties that surpass those of individual components. With their broad applications in biomedicine, energy, sensing, and beyond, biomimetic hybrid coatings hold tremendous potential for advancing various technological fields and addressing complex challenges.

11.4 Biomimetic antimicrobial coatings—challenges

Despite the promising potential of biomimetic antimicrobial coatings, several challenges must be addressed for their successful implementation (Bastarrachea et al., 2015; Bhatia & Narain, 2010; Cloutier et al., 2015; Moerman, 2014; Linklater & Ivanova, 2023; Maréchal & Hellio, 2009; Sarker et al., 2022; Viswanathan et al., 2006). Some of the key challenges associated with biomimetic antimicrobial coatings are discussed in the following sections.

11.4.1 Scalability and cost-effectiveness

Developing biomimetic antimicrobial coatings that are scalable and cost-effective for large-scale production can be challenging. The synthesis or extraction of biomimetic compounds and incorporation of complex structures or materials may involve intricate and costly processes. Achieving cost-effective production methods without compromising performance is a significant hurdle.

11.4.2 Durability and longevity

Biomimetic coatings must retain antimicrobial efficacy over extended periods, especially in applications requiring continuous protection. Ensuring the durability and longevity of these coatings is crucial for their practical use in real-world applications. Factors such as mechanical wear, exposure to diverse environmental conditions, and chemical interactions can affect the stability and effectiveness of the coatings. Thus evaluating the performance of these coatings in diverse environments and understanding their limitations is crucial for their practical application.

11.4.3 Biocompatibility and adhesion

Biomimetic coatings must be compatible with various substrates, including metals, polymers, and ceramics. Achieving strong adhesion between the coating and the substrate is crucial to prevent delamination or degradation of the coating over time. Ensuring good adhesion across different substrate materials can be challenging. As biomimetic coatings are intended for use in various applications, including healthcare and consumer products, ensuring their biocompatibility and safety is essential (Galvão et al., 2018; Rao et al., 2022; Xie et al., 2022).

11.4.4 Specificity and selectivity

Biomimetic coatings should possess antimicrobial activity against target pathogens while sparing beneficial microorganisms. Achieving the desired specificity and selectivity can be complex, as microbial populations can vary widely, and different pathogens may exhibit varying susceptibility to antimicrobial agents. Ensuring the coatings effectively target harmful microbes while preserving the natural microbiota is a critical consideration.

11.4.5 Resistance development

Microorganisms have a remarkable ability to adapt and develop resistance to antimicrobial agents over time. This poses a challenge, as prolonged exposure to the same antimicrobial mechanisms could potentially lead to the development of microbial resistance. Strategies to mitigate the risk of resistance development, such as combining multiple antimicrobial approaches or periodically altering the antimicrobial mechanisms, need to be considered. A multiple antimicrobial approach is adopting a multifaceted antimicrobial strategy combining multiple action mechanisms. The likelihood of resistance development can be minimized by targeting microorganisms through different pathways, such as disrupting cell membranes, interfering with metabolic processes, or inhibiting DNA replication. The utilization of synergistic combinations of antimicrobial agents with distinct modes of action can further enhance the effectiveness of the coatings and reduce the selective pressure for resistance development. Another strategy involves periodically altering the antimicrobial mechanisms employed by the coatings. By periodically changing the type or concentration of antimicrobial agents, microorganisms are less likely to develop resistance due to the transient nature of the exposure. Furthermore, continuous monitoring and surveillance of microbial populations in contact with biomimetic coatings are essential to detect early signs of resistance emergence (Bhatia & Narain, 2010; Cloutier et al., 2015; Moerman, 2014; Linklater & Ivanova, 2023; Maréchal & Hellio, 2009; Medis et al., 2023).

11.4.6 Regulatory considerations and safety

Before biomimetic antimicrobial coatings can be widely implemented, they must undergo rigorous testing to ensure their safety and compliance with regulatory standards. These coatings need to demonstrate their effectiveness in inhibiting microbial growth without causing harm to humans, animals, or the environment. Addressing potential toxicity concerns and meeting regulatory requirements is essential for their successful adoption (Kazemzadeh-Narbat et al., 2021; Muhammad et al., 2020). Addressing these challenges requires interdisciplinary collaboration between scientists, engineers, industry experts, and regulatory bodies. Continued research and development efforts are needed to optimize biomimetic antimicrobial coatings, enhance their performance, and address the practical hurdles that limit their widespread implementation for diverse applications, ranging from healthcare and consumer products to infrastructure and environmental protection.

11.5 Future directions

Antimicrobial coatings have emerged as a promising technology for combatting the spread of pathogens on various surfaces. In healthcare or general, the preliminary strategy to tackle the development and proliferation of bacterial biofilms involves cleaning and sterilization. Thus microbial biofilms and related infections are vital in clinical settings. The field of biomimetic antimicrobial coatings continues to evolve, driven by ongoing research and technological advancements. By leveraging the power of biomimicry, scientists and engineers are exploring innovative solutions to combat microbial threats, reduce the risk of contamination, and promote better health and hygiene in various industries and settings (Khan & Shakoor, 2023; Ramasamy & Lee, 2016; Roy et al., 2023; Yang, Zhang et al., 2022). Each biomimetic antimicrobial coating approach discussed in this chapter aims to emulate nature's antimicrobial strategies and adapt them for practical applications. Future endeavors include the development of multifunctional coatings with enhanced antimicrobial properties, increased durability, and reduced toxicity. Integrating innovative and self-healing materials could further improve the efficacy and longevity of such coatings. Additionally, exploring sustainable and eco-friendly alternatives to conventional antimicrobial agents will be crucial to minimize environmental impacts.

References

Ahmed, F. Y., Aly, U. F., Abd El-Baky, R. M., & Waly, N. G. F. M. (2020). Comparative study of antibacterial effects of titanium dioxide nanoparticles alone and in combination with antibiotics on MDR *pseudomonas aeruginosa* strains. *International Journal of Nanomedicine*, *15*, 3393–3404. Available from https://doi.org/10.2147/IJN.S246310, https://www.dovepress.com/getfile.php?fileID = 58116.

Alameda, M. T., Osorio, M. R., Pedraz, P., & Rodríguez, I. (2022). Mechano-dynamic analysis of the bactericidal activity of bioinspired moth-eye nanopatterned surfaces. *Advanced Materials Interfaces*, *9*(23). Available from https://doi.org/10.1002/admi.202200608, http://onlinelibrary.wiley.com/journal/10.1002/(ISSN)2196-7350.

Atefyekta, S., Blomstrand, E., Rajasekharan, A. K., Svensson, S., Trobos, M., Hong, J., Webster, T. J., Thomsen, P., & Andersson, M. (2021). Antimicrobial peptide-functionalized mesoporous hydrogels. *ACS Biomaterials Science and Engineering*, 7(4), 1693–1702. Available from https://doi.org/10.1021/acsbiomaterials.1c00029, http://pubs.acs.org/journal/abseba.

Auten, R. L., & Davis, J. M. (2009). Oxygen toxicity and reactive oxygen species: The devil is in the details. *Pediatric Research*, *66*(2), 121–127. Available from https://doi.org/10.1203/PDR.0b013e3181a9eafb.

Azizi-Lalabadi, M., Ehsani, A., Divband, B., & Alizadeh-Sani, M. (2019). Antimicrobial activity of titanium dioxide and zinc oxide nanoparticles supported in 4A zeolite and evaluation the morphological characteristic. *Scientific Reports*, *9*(1). Available from https://doi.org/10.1038/s41598-019-54025-0, http://www.nature.com/srep/index.html.

Bandara, Chaturanga D., Singh, Sanjleena, Afara, Isaac O., Wolff, Annalena, Tesfamichael, Tuquabo, Ostrikov, Kostya, & Oloyede, Adekunle (2017). Bactericidal effects of natural nanotopography of dragonfly wing on *Escherichia coli*. *ACS Applied Materials & Interfaces*, *9*(8), 6746–6760. Available from https://doi.org/10.1021/acsami.6b13666.

Bastarrachea, L. J., Denis-Rohr, A., & Goddard, J. M. (2015). Antimicrobial food equipment coatings: Applications and challenges. *Annual Review of Food Science and Technology*, *6*, 97–118. Available from https://doi.org/10.1146/annurev-food-022814-015453, http://www.annualreviews.org/journal/food.

Bayer, I. S. (2020). Superhydrophobic coatings from ecofriendly materials and processes: A review. *Advanced Materials Interfaces*, 7(13). Available from https://doi.org/10.1002/admi.202000095, http://onlinelibrary.wiley.com/journal/10.1002/(ISSN)2196-7350.

Bekele, S. T., Abay, G. K., Gelaw, B., & Tessema, B. (2018). Bacterial biofilms; Links to pathogenesis and résistance mechanism. *Preprints*. Available from https://doi.org/10.20944/preprints201807.0598.v1.

Bhatia, R., & Narain, J. P. (2010). The growing challenge of antimicrobial resistance in the South-East Asia region – Are we losing the battle? *Indian Journal of Medical Research, 132* (11), 482–486. Available from http://icmr.nic.in/ijmr/2010/november/editorial3.pdf, India.

Bhushan, B., Jung, Y. C., & Koch, K. (2009). Micro-, nano- and hierarchical structures for superhydrophobicity, self-cleaning and low adhesion. *Philosophical Transactions of the Royal Society A: Mathematical, Physical and Engineering Sciences, 367*(1894), 1631–1672. Available from https://doi.org/10.1098/rsta.2009.0014, http://rsta.royalsocietypublishing.org/content/367/1894/1631.full.pdf.

Bhushan, B., Koch, K., & Jung, Y. C. (2009). Fabrication and characterization of the hierarchical structure for superhydrophobicity and self-cleaning. *Ultramicroscopy, 109*(8), 1029–1034. Available from https://doi.org/10.1016/j.ultramic.2009.03.030.

Boudarel, H., Mathias, J. D., Blaysat, B., & Grédiac, M. (2018). Towards standardized mechanical characterization of microbial biofilms: analysis and critical review. *npj Biofilms and Microbiomes, 4*(1). Available from https://doi.org/10.1038/s41522-018-0062-5, https://www.nature.com/npjbiofilms/.

Callow, M. E., & Fletcher, R. L. (1994). The influence of low surface energy materials on bioadhesion – A review. *International Biodeterioration and Biodegradation, 34*(3–4), 333–348. Available from https://doi.org/10.1016/0964-8305(94)90092-2.

Cangui-Panchi, Sandra Pamela, Ñacato-Toapanta, Anahí Lizbeth, Enríquez-Martínez, Leonardo Joshué, Reyes, Jorge, Garzon-Chavez, Daniel, & Machado, António (2022). Biofilm-forming microorganisms causing hospital-acquired infections from intravenous catheter: A systematic review. *Current Research in Microbial Sciences, 3*, 100175. Available from https://doi.org/10.1016/j.crmicr.2022.100175.

Cardoso, P., Glossop, H., Meikle, T. G., Aburto-Medina, A., Conn, C. E., Sarojini, V., & Valery, C. (2021). Molecular engineering of antimicrobial peptides: Microbial targets, peptide motifs and translation opportunities. *Biophysical Reviews, 13*(1), 35–69. Available from https://doi.org/10.1007/s12551-021-00784-y, http://www.springer.com/life + sciences/biochemistry + %26 + biophysics/journal/12551.

Carmona-Ribeiro, A. M., & Carrasco, L. Dd. M. (2014). Novel formulations for antimicrobial peptides. *International Journal of Molecular Sciences, 15*(10), 18040–18083. Available from https://doi.org/10.3390/ijms151018040, http://www.mdpi.com/1422-0067/15/10/18267/pdf.

Celik, N., Sahin, F., Ozel, S. S., Sezer, G., Gunaltay, N., Ruzi, M., & Onses, M. S. (2023). Self-healing of biocompatible superhydrophobic coatings: The interplay of the size and loading of particles. *Langmuir: The ACS Journal of Surfaces and Colloids, 39*(9), 3194–3203. Available from https://doi.org/10.1021/acs.langmuir.2c02795, http://pubs.acs.org/journal/langd5.

Chambers, L. D., Stokes, K. R., Walsh, F. C., & Wood, R. J. K. (2006). Modern approaches to marine antifouling coatings. *Surface and Coatings Technology, 201*(6), 3642–3652. Available from https://doi.org/10.1016/j.surfcoat.2006.08.129, http://www.journals.elsevier.com/surface-and-coatings-technology/.

Chan, Y., Wu, X. H., Chieng, B. W., Ibrahim, N. A., & Then, Y. Y. (2021). Superhydrophobic nanocoatings as intervention against biofilm-associated bacterial infections. *Nanomaterials, 11*(4). Available from https://doi.org/10.3390/nano11041046, https://www.mdpi.com/2079-4991/11/4/1046/pdf.

Charlot, A., Sciannaméa, V., Lenoir, S., Faure, E., Jérôme, R., Jérôme, C., Van De Weerdt, C., Martial, J., Archambeau, C., Willet, N., Duwez, A. S., Fustin, C. A., & Detrembleur, C. (2009). All-in-one strategy for the fabrication of antimicrobial biomimetic films on stainless steel. *Journal of Materials Chemistry, 19*(24), 4117–4125. Available from https://doi.org/10.1039/b820832h.

Chauhan, P., Kumar, A., & Bhushan, B. (2019). Self-cleaning, stain-resistant and antibacterial superhydrophobic cotton fabric prepared by simple immersion technique.

Journal of Colloid and Interface Science, *535*, 66–74. Available from https://doi.org/10.1016/j.jcis.2018.09.087, http://www.elsevier.com/inca/publications/store/6/2/2/8/6/1/index.htt.

Chee, E., & Brown, A. C. (2020). Biomimetic antimicrobial material strategies for combating antibiotic resistant bacteria. *Biomaterials Science*, *8*(4), 1089–1100. Available from https://doi.org/10.1039/c9bm01393h, http://pubs.rsc.org/en/journals/journal/bm.

Cheng, Q., Guo, X., Hao, X., Shi, Z., Zhu, S., & Cui, Z. (2019). Fabrication of robust antibacterial coatings based on an organic-inorganic hybrid system. *ACS Applied Materials and Interfaces*, *11*(45), 42607–42615. Available from https://doi.org/10.1021/acsami.9b15031, http://pubs.acs.org/journal/aamick.

Cheng, Y. T., Rodak, D. E., Wong, C. A., & Hayden, C. A. (2006). Effects of micro- and nano-structures on the self-cleaning behaviour of lotus leaves. *Nanotechnology*, *17* (5), 1359–1362. Available from https://doi.org/10.1088/0957-4484/17/5/032.

Cheng, Hao, Yue, Kan, Kazemzadeh-Narbat, Mehdi, Liu, Yanhui, Khalilpour, Akbar, Li, Bingyun, Zhang, Yu. Shrike, Annabi, Nasim, & Khademhosseini, Ali (2017). Mussel-inspired multifunctional hydrogel coating for prevention of infections and enhanced osteogenesis. *ACS Applied Materials & Interfaces*, *9*(13), 11428–11439. Available from https://doi.org/10.1021/acsami.6b16779.

Chen, Liren, Duan, Yanyi, Cui, Mei, Huang, Renliang, Su, Rongxin, Qi, Wei, & He, Zhimin (2021). Biomimetic surface coatings for marine antifouling: Natural antifoulants, synthetic polymers and surface microtopography. *Science of the Total Environment*, *766*, 144469. Available from https://doi.org/10.1016/j.scitotenv.2020.144469.

Chen, X., Gao, Y., Wang, Y., & Pan, G. (2021). Mussel-inspired peptide mimicking: An emerging strategy for surface bioengineering of medical implants. *Smart Materials in Medicine*, *2*, 26–37. Available from https://doi.org/10.1016/j.smaim.2020.10.005, http://www.keaipublishing.com/en/journals/smart-materials-in-medicine/.

Chermahini, Siavash Hosseinpour, Ostad-Ali-Askari, Kaveh, Eslamian, Saeid, & Singh, Vijay P. (2018). Recent progress in self-cleaning materials with different suitable applications. *American Journal of Engineering and Applied Sciences*, *11*(2), 560–573. Available from https://doi.org/10.3844/ajeassp.2018.560.573.

Cloutier, M., Mantovani, D., & Rosei, F. (2015). Antibacterial coatings: Challenges, perspectives, and opportunities. *Trends in Biotechnology*, *33*(11), 637–652. Available from https://doi.org/10.1016/j.tibtech.2015.09.002, http://www.elsevier.com/locate/tibtech.

Coll Ferrer, M. Carme, Hickok, Noreen J., Eckmann, David M., & Composto, Russell J. (2012). Antibacterial biomimetic hybrid films. *Soft Matter*, *8*(8), 2423. Available from https://doi.org/10.1039/c2sm06969e.

Collins, Christopher M., & Safiuddin, Md (2022). Lotus-leaf-inspired biomimetic coatings: Different types, key properties, and applications in infrastructures. *Infrastructures*, 7(4), 46. Available from https://doi.org/10.3390/infrastructures7040046.

Cooksey, K. E., & Wigglesworth-Cooksey, B. (1995). Adhesion of bacteria and diatoms to surfaces in the sea: A review. *Aquatic Microbial Ecology*, *9*(1), 87–96. Available from https://doi.org/10.3354/ame009087.

Di Credico, B., Bellobono, I. R., D'Arienzo, M., Fumagalli, D., Redaelli, M., Scotti, R., & Morazzoni, F. (2015). Efficacy of the reactive oxygen species generated by immobilized Tio_2 in the photocatalytic degradation of diclofenac. *International Journal of Photoenergy*, *2015*, 1–13. Available from https://doi.org/10.1155/2015/919217.

Dadi, N. C. T., Radochová, B., Vargová, J., & Bujdáková, H. (2021). Impact of healthcare-associated infections connected to medical devices—An update. *Microorganisms*, *9*(11). Available from https://doi.org/10.3390/microorganisms9112332, https://www.mdpi.com/2076-2607/9/11/2332/pdf.

Ding, Xiaokang, Duan, Shun, Ding, Xuejia, Liu, Runhui, & Xu, Fu-Jian (2018). Versatile antibacterial materials: An emerging arsenal for combatting bacterial pathogens.

Advanced Functional Materials, *28*(40), 1802140. Available from https://doi.org/10.1002/adfm.201802140.

Dizaj, S. M., Lotfipour, F., Barzegar-Jalali, M., Zarrintan, M. H., & Adibkia, K. (2014). Antimicrobial activity of the metals and metal oxide nanoparticles. *Materials Science and Engineering C*, *44*, 278–284. Available from https://doi.org/10.1016/j.msec.2014.08.031.

Drexelius, Marco G., & Neundorf, Ines (2021). Application of antimicrobial peptides on biomedical implants: Three ways to pursue peptide coatings. *International Journal of Molecular Sciences*, *22*(24), 13212. Available from https://doi.org/10.3390/ijms222413212.

Durdu, S., Yalçin, E., Altinkök, A., & Çavuşoğlu, K. (2023). Characterization and investigation of electrochemical and biological properties of antibacterial silver nanoparticle-deposited TiO2 nanotube array surfaces. *Scientific Reports*, *13*(4699), 1–13. Available from https://doi.org/10.1038/s41598-023-31937-6, https://www.nature.com/srep/.

Efremenko, Elena, Stepanov, Nikolay, Aslanli, Aysel, Lyagin, Ilya, Senko, Olga, & Maslova, Olga (2023). Combination of enzymes with materials to give them antimicrobial features: Modern trends and perspectives. *Journal of Functional Biomaterials*, *14*(2), 64. Available from https://doi.org/10.3390/jfb14020064.

Elbourne, A., Crawford, R. J., & Ivanova, E. P. (2017). Nano-structured antimicrobial surfaces: From nature to synthetic analogues. *Journal of Colloid and Interface Science*, *508*, 603–616. Available from https://doi.org/10.1016/j.jcis.2017.07.021, http://www.elsevier.com/inca/publications/store/6/2/2/8/6/1/index.htt.

Ergene, C., Yasuhara, K., & Palermo, E. F. (2018). Biomimetic antimicrobial polymers: Recent advances in molecular design. *Polymer Chemistry*, *9*(18), 2407–2427. Available from https://doi.org/10.1039/c8py00012c, http://pubs.rsc.org/en/journals/journal/py.

Erkoc, P., & Ulucan-Karnak, F. (2021). Nanotechnology-based antimicrobial and antiviral surface coating strategies. *Prosthesis*, *3*(1), 25–52. Available from https://doi.org/10.3390/prosthesis3010005, http://www.mdpi.com/journal/prosthesis.

Fichman, G., Andrews, C., Patel, N. L., & Schneider, J. P. (2021). Antibacterial gel coatings inspired by the cryptic function of a mussel byssal peptide. *Advanced Materials*, *33*(40). Available from https://doi.org/10.1002/adma.202103677, http://onlinelibrary.wiley.com/journal/10.1002/(ISSN)1521-4095.

Fusetani, N. (2004). Biofouling and antifouling. *Natural Product Reports*, *21*(1), 94–104. Available from https://doi.org/10.1039/b302231p.

Fürstner, R., Barthlott, W., Neinhuis, C., & Walzel, P. (2005). Wetting and self-cleaning properties of artificial superhydrophobic surfaces. *Langmuir: the ACS Journal of Surfaces and Colloids*, *21*(3), 956–961. Available from https://doi.org/10.1021/la0401011.

Galvão, Carolina, Sanches, Luccas, Mathiazzi, Beatriz, Ribeiro, Rodrigo, Petri, Denise, & Carmona-Ribeiro, Ana (2018). Antimicrobial coatings from hybrid nanoparticles of biocompatible and antimicrobial polymers. *International Journal of Molecular Sciences*, *19*(10), 2965. Available from https://doi.org/10.3390/ijms19102965.

Gan, B. H., Gaynord, J., Rowe, S. M., Deingruber, T., & Spring, D. R. (2021). The multifaceted nature of antimicrobial peptides: Current synthetic chemistry approaches and future directions. *Chemical Society Reviews*, *50*(13), 7820–7880. Available from https://doi.org/10.1039/d0cs00729c, http://pubs.rsc.org/en/journals/journal/cs.

Gan, D., Xu, T., Xing, W., Ge, X., Fang, L., Wang, K., Ren, F., & Lu, X. (2019). Mussel-inspired contact-active antibacterial hydrogel with high cell affinity, toughness, and recoverability. *Advanced Functional Materials*, *29*(1). Available from https://doi.org/10.1002/adfm.201805964, http://onlinelibrary.wiley.com/journal/10.1002/(ISSN)1616-3028.

Gittens, J. E., Smith, T. J., Suleiman, R., & Akid, R. (2013). Current and emerging environmentally-friendly systems for fouling control in the marine environment. *Biotechnology Advances*, *31*(8), 1738–1753. Available from https://doi.org/10.1016/j.biotechadv.2013.09.002.

Glinel, K., Thebault, P., Humblot, V., Pradier, C. M., & Jouenne, T. (2012). Antibacterial surfaces developed from bio-inspired approaches. *Acta Biomaterialia*, *8*(5), 1670–1684. Available from https://doi.org/10.1016/j.actbio.2012.01.011, http://www.journals.elsevier.com/acta-biomaterialia.

Gonzales, R. R., Kumagai, K., Yang, Z., Yang, Y., Shigemura, K., & Matsuyama, H. (2023). Simple bio-inspired coating of ureteral stent for protein and bacterial fouling and calcium encrustation control. *Journal of Biomedical Materials Research – Part B Applied Biomaterials*, *111*(8), 1511–1522. Available from https://doi.org/10.1002/jbm.b.35250, http://onlinelibrary.wiley.com/journal/10.1002/(ISSN)1552-4965.

Gotz, Friedrich (2002). Staphylococcus and biofilms. *Molecular Microbiology*, *43*(6), 1367–1378. Available from https://doi.org/10.1046/j.1365-2958.2002.02827.x.

Grover, N., Dinu, C. Z., Kane, R. S., & Dordick, J. S. (2013). Enzyme-based formulations for decontamination: Current state and perspectives. *Applied Microbiology and Biotechnology*, *97*(8), 3293–3300. Available from https://doi.org/10.1007/s00253-013-4797-x.

Gu, Jin, Su, Yajuan, Liu, Peng, Li, Peng, & Yang, Peng (2017). An environmentally benign antimicrobial coating based on a protein supramolecular assembly. *ACS Applied Materials & Interfaces*, *9*(1), 198–210. Available from https://doi.org/10.1021/acsami.6b13552.

Hansen, W. R., & Autumn, K. (2005). Evidence for self-cleaning in gecko setae. *Proceedings of the National Academy of Sciences of the United States of America. 00278424.*, *102*(2), 385–389. Available from https://doi.org/10.1073/pnas.0408304102.

Hanson, Lindsey, Zhao, Wenting, Lou, Hsin-Ya, Lin, Ziliang Carter, Lee, Seok Woo, Chowdary, Praveen, Cui, Yi, & Cui, Bianxiao (2015). Vertical nanopillars for in situ probing of nuclear mechanics in adherent cells. *Nature Nanotechnology*, *10*(6), 554–562. Available from https://doi.org/10.1038/nnano.2015.88.

Hasan, Abshar, Lee, Kyueui, Tewari, Kunal, Pandey, Lalit M., Messersmith, Phillip B., Faulds, Karen, Maclean, Michelle, & Lau, King Hang Aaron (2020). Surface design for immobilization of an antimicrobial peptide mimic for efficient anti-biofouling. *Chemistry – A European Journal*, *26*(26), 5789–5793. Available from https://doi.org/10.1002/chem.202000746.

Hasan, J., Roy, A., Chatterjee, K., & Yarlagadda, P. K. D. V. (2019). Mimicking Insect Wings: The Roadmap to Bioinspiration. *ACS Biomaterials Science and Engineering*, *5*(7), 3139–3160. Available from https://doi.org/10.1021/acsbiomaterials.9b00217, http://pubs.acs.org/journal/abseba.

Hawi, Sara, Goel, Saurav, Kumar, Vinod, Pearce, Oliver, Ayre, Wayne Nishio, & Ivanova, Elena P. (2022). Critical review of nanopillar-based mechanobactericidal systems. *ACS Applied Nano Materials*, *5*(1), 1–17. Available from https://doi.org/10.1021/acsanm.1c03045.

He, Juhua, Kumar, Ashutosh, Khan, Musharib, & Lo, Irene M. C. (2021). Critical review of photocatalytic disinfection of bacteria: From noble metals- and carbon nanomaterials-TiO_2 composites to challenges of water characteristics and strategic solutions. *Science of the Total Environment*, *758*, 143953. Available from https://doi.org/10.1016/j.scitotenv.2020.143953.

Hofer, U. (2022). Implants to defeat bacterial infection, Nature Research, undefined*Nature Reviews. Microbiology*, *20*(2), 64. Available from https://doi.org/10.1038/s41579-021-00675-9, http://www.nature.com/nrmicro/index.html.

Huang, X., Bao, X., Liu, Y., Wang, Z., & Hu, Q. (2017). Catechol-functional chitosan/silver nanoparticle composite as a highly effective antibacterial agent with species-specific mechanisms. *Scientific Reports*, 7(1). Available from https://doi.org/10.1038/s41598-017-02008-4, http://www.nature.com/srep/index.html.

Huang, Lin, & Liu, Chuan-Jun (2022). Progress for the development of antibacterial surface based on surface modification technology. *Supramolecular Materials*, *1*, 100008. Available from https://doi.org/10.1016/j.supmat.2022.100008.

Hu, Y., Liang, B., Fang, L., Ma, G., Yang, G., Zhu, Q., Chen, S., & Ye, X. (2016). Antifouling zwitterionic coating via electrochemically mediated atom transfer radical polymerization on enzyme-based glucose sensors for long-time stability in 37°C serum. *Langmuir: The ACS Journal of Surfaces and Colloids*, *32*(45), 11763–11770. Available from https://doi.org/10.1021/acs.langmuir.6b03016, http://pubs.acs.org/journal/langd5.

Ivanova, K., Fernandes, M. M., Mendoza, E., & Tzanov, T. (2015). Enzyme multilayer coatings inhibit *Pseudomonas aeruginosa* biofilm formation on urinary catheters. *Applied Microbiology and Biotechnology*, *99*(10), 4373–4385. Available from https://doi.org/10.1007/s00253-015-6378-7, http://link.springer.de/link/service/journals/00253/index.htm.

Ivanova, E. P., Hasan, J., Webb, H. K., Truong, V. K., Watson, G. S., Watson, J. A., Baulin, V. A., Pogodin, S., Wang, J. Y., Tobin, M. J., Löbbe, C., & Crawford, R. J. (2012). Natural bactericidal surfaces: Mechanical rupture of pseudomonas aeruginosa cells by cicada wings. *Small (Weinheim an der Bergstrasse, Germany)*, *8*(16), 2489–2494. Available from https://doi.org/10.1002/smll.201200528.

Jafari, Behnaz, Lacerda, Carla M. R., & Botte, Gerardine G. (2023). Facile electrochemical preparation of hydrophobic antibacterial fabrics using reduced graphene oxide/silver nanoparticles. *ChemElectroChem*, *10*(6). Available from https://doi.org/10.1002/celc.202201111.

Jeong, G. M., Seong, H., Im, S. G., Sung, B. H., Kim, S. C., & Jeong, K. J. (2018). Coating of an antimicrobial peptide on solid substrate via initiated chemical vapor deposition. *Journal of Industrial and Engineering Chemistry*, *58*, 51–56. Available from https://doi.org/10.1016/j.jiec.2017.09.006, http://www.sciencedirect.com/science/journal/1226086X.

Jiang, R., Yi, Y., Hao, L., Chen, Y., Tian, L., Dou, H., Zhao, J., Ming, W., & Ren, L. (2021). Thermoresponsive nanostructures: From mechano-bactericidal action to bacteria release. *ACS Applied Materials and Interfaces*, *13*(51), 60865–60877. Available from https://doi.org/10.1021/acsami.1c16487, http://pubs.acs.org/journal/aamick.

Kanehashi, S., Oyagi, H., Lu, R., & Miyakoshi, T. (2014). Development of bio-based hybrid resin, from natural lacquer. *Progress in Organic Coatings*, 77(1), 24–29. Available from https://doi.org/10.1016/j.porgcoat.2013.07.013.

Katiyar, N. K., Goel, G., Hawi, S., & Goel, S. (2021). Nature-inspired materials: Emerging trends and prospects. *NPG Asia Materials*, *13*(1). Available from https://doi.org/10.1038/s41427-021-00322-y, http://www.nature.com/am/index.html.

Kaur, R., & Liu, S. (2016). Antibacterial surface design – Contact kill. *Progress in Surface Science*, *91*(3), 136–153. Available from https://doi.org/10.1016/j.progsurf.2016.09.001.

Kazemzadeh-Narbat, Mehdi, Cheng, Hao, Chabok, Rosa, Alvarez, Mario Moisés, de la Fuente-Nunez, Cesar, Phillips, K. Scott, & Khademhosseini, Ali (2021). Strategies for antimicrobial peptide coatings on medical devices: a review and regulatory science perspective. *Critical Reviews in Biotechnology*, *41*(1), 94–120. Available from https://doi.org/10.1080/07388551.2020.1828810.

Kelleher, S. M., Habimana, O., Lawler, J., O'reilly, B., Daniels, S., Casey, E., & Cowley, A. (2016). Cicada Wing surface topography: An investigation into the bactericidal properties of nanostructural features. *ACS Applied Materials and Interfaces*, *8*(24), 14966–14974. Available from https://doi.org/10.1021/acsami.5b08309, http://pubs.acs.org/journal/aamick.

Khan, Shakeel Ahmad, & Shakoor, Adnan (2023). Recent strategies and future recommendations for the fabrication of antimicrobial, antibiofilm, and antibiofouling biomaterials. *International Journal of Nanomedicine, 18*, 3377–3405. Available from https://doi.org/10.2147/IJN.S406078.

Kim, Woochan, Kim, Daun, Park, Sunho, Lee, Dohyeon, Hyun, Hoon, & Kim, Jangho (2018). Engineering lotus leaf-inspired micro- and nanostructures for the manipulation of functional engineering platforms. *Journal of Industrial and Engineering Chemistry, 61*, 39–52. Available from https://doi.org/10.1016/j.jiec.2017.11.045.

Koch, Kerstin, Bhushan, Bharat, Jung, Yong Chae, & Barthlott, Wilhelm (2009). Fabrication of artificial Lotus leaves and significance of hierarchical structure for superhydrophobicity and low adhesion. *Soft Matter, 5*(7), 1386. Available from https://doi.org/10.1039/b818940d.

Konar, Mouli, Roy, Bappaditya, & Govindaraju, Thimmaiah (2020). Molecular architectonics-guided fabrication of superhydrophobic and self-cleaning materials. *Advanced Materials Interfaces*, 7(11), 2000246. Available from https://doi.org/10.1002/admi.202000246.

Koshani, Roya, Zhang, Jingbin, van de Ven, Theo G. M., Lu, Xiaonan, & Wang, Yixiang (2021). Modified hairy nanocrystalline cellulose as photobactericidal nanofillers for food packaging application. *ACS Sustainable Chemistry & Engineering, 9*(31), 10513–10523. Available from https://doi.org/10.1021/acssuschemeng.1c02289.

Landini, P., Antoniani, D., Burgess, J. G., & Nijland, R. (2010). Molecular mechanisms of compounds affecting bacterial biofilm formation and dispersal. *Applied Microbiology and Biotechnology, 86*(3), 813–823. Available from https://doi.org/10.1007/s00253-010-2468-8.

Larsen, D. K., Wagner, I., Gustavson, K., Forbes, V. E., & Lund, T. (2003). Long-term effect of sea-nine on natural coastal phytoplankton communities assessed by pollution induced community tolerance. *Aquatic Toxicology, 62*(1), 35–44. Available from https://doi.org/10.1016/S0166-445X(02)00065-6.

Lee, M. S., Hussein, H. R., Chang, S. W., Chang, C. Y., Lin, Y. Y., Chien, Y., Yang, Y. P., Kiew, L. V., Chen, C. Y., Chiou, S. H., & Chang, C. C. (2023). Nature-inspired surface structures design for antimicrobial applications. *International Journal of Molecular Sciences, 24*(2). Available from https://doi.org/10.3390/ijms24021348. http://www.mdpi.com/journal/ijms.

Lee, C. L., Lin, T. S., Hwang, L. C., Kuo, C. H., Huang, X. H., Chen, Y. C., Ou, S. F., Ma, C. H., Chen, S. T., Hsueh, Y. H., & Wu, C. H. (2020). Electrochemical synthesis of a composite coating with antibacterial ability on NiTi alloy. *Progress in Organic Coatings, 146*. Available from https://doi.org/10.1016/j.porgcoat.2020.105711, http://www.elsevier.com/locate/porgcoat.

Lejars, M., Margaillan, A., & Bressy, C. (2012). Fouling release coatings: A nontoxic alternative to biocidal antifouling coatings. *Chemical Reviews, 112*(8), 4347–4390. Available from https://doi.org/10.1021/cr200350v.

Liao, Y., Zhang, Y., Blum, N. T., Lin, J., & Huang, P. (2020). Biomimetic hybrid membrane-based nanoplatforms: Synthesis, properties and biomedical applications. *Nanoscale Horizons, 5*(9), 1293–1302. Available from https://doi.org/10.1039/d0nh00267d, http://www.rsc.org/journals-books-databases/about-journals/nanoscale-horizons/?id = 8277.

Lichter, J. A., Van Vlietpa, K. J., & Rubner, M. F. (2009). Design of antibacterial surfaces and interfaces: Polyelectrolyte multilayers as a multifunctional platform. *Macromolecules, 42*(22), 8573–8586. Available from https://doi.org/10.1021/ma901356s, http://pubs.acs.org/doi/pdfplus/10.1021/ma901356s, United States.

Lindner, E. (1992). A low surface free energy approach in the control of marine biofouling. *Biofouling, 6*(2), 193–205. Available from https://doi.org/10.1080/08927019209386222.

Linklater, Denver, & Ivanova, Elena P. (2023). Challenges to the design and testing of antimicrobial nanostructured surfaces. *Microbiology Australia, 44*(2), 79–82. Available from https://doi.org/10.1071/ma23023.

Liu, M., Liu, T., Chen, X., Yang, J., Deng, J., He, W., Zhang, X., Lei, Q., Hu, X., Luo, G., & Wu, J. (2018). Nano-silver-incorporated biomimetic polydopamine coating on a thermoplastic polyurethane porous nanocomposite as an efficient antibacterial wound dressing. *Journal of Nanobiotechnology*, *16*(1). Available from https://doi.org/10.1186/s12951-018-0416-4, http://www.jnanobiotechnology.com/start.asp.

Li, N., Cui, W., Cong, P., Tang, J., Guan, Y., Huang, C., Liu, Y., Yu, C., Yang, R., & Zhang, X. (2021). Biomimetic inorganic-organic hybrid nanoparticles from magnesium-substituted amorphous calcium phosphate clusters and polyacrylic acid molecules. *Bioactive Materials*, *6*(8), 2303–2314. Available from https://doi.org/10.1016/j.bioactmat.2021.01.005, http://www.keaipublishing.com/en/journals/bioactive-materials/.

Li, G., Lai, Z., & Shan, A. (2023). Advances of antimicrobial peptide-based biomaterials for the treatment of bacterial infections. *Advanced Science*, *10*(11). Available from https://doi.org/10.1002/advs.202206602, http://onlinelibrary.wiley.com/journal/10.1002/(ISSN)2198-3844.

Li, X., Li, J., Peng, Z., & Chen, S. (2019). Spontaneous dewetting of a hydrophobic micro-structured surface. *Journal of Physics Condensed Matter*, *31*(29). Available from https://doi.org/10.1088/1361-648X/ab1998, https://iopscience.iop.org/article/10.1088/1361-648X/10.1088/1361-648X/ab1998/pdf.

Lode, H. M. (2009). Clinical impact of antibiotic-resistant Gram-positive pathogens. *Clinical Microbiology and Infection*, *15*(3), 212–217. Available from https://doi.org/10.1111/j.1469-0691.2009.02738.x, http://onlinelibrary.wiley.com/journal/10.1111/(ISSN)1469-0691.

Ludyansky, M. L. (1991). Algal fouling in cooling water systems. *Biofouling*, *3*(1), 13–21. Available from https://doi.org/10.1080/08927019109378158.

Lundin, J. G., Giles, S. L., Cozzens, R. F., & Wynne, J. H. (2014). Self-cleaning photocatalytic polyurethane coatings containing modified C60 fullerene additives. *Coatings*, *4*(3), 614–629. Available from https://doi.org/10.3390/coatings4030614, https://res.mdpi.com/coatings/coatings-04-00614/article_deploy/coatings-04-00614.pdf?filename = &attachment = 1.

Lyu, Q., Hsueh, N., & Chai, C. L. L. (2019). The chemistry of bioinspired catechol (amine)-based coatings. *ACS Biomaterials Science and Engineering*, *5*(6), 2708–2724. Available from https://doi.org/10.1021/acsbiomaterials.9b00281, http://pubs.acs.org/journal/abseba.

Mah, T. F., Pitts, B., Pellock, B., Walker, G. C., Stewart, P. S., & O'Toole, G. A. (2003). A genetic basis for *Pseudomonas aeruginosa* biofilm antibiotic resistance. *Nature*, *426*(6964), 306–310. Available from https://doi.org/10.1038/nature02122.

Maki, J. S., Rittschof, D., Schmidt, A. R., Snyder, A. G., & Mitchell, R. (1989). Factors controlling attachment of bryozoan larvae: A comparison of bacterial films and unfilmed surfaces. *The Biological Bulletin*, 177(2), 295–302. Available from https://doi.org/10.2307/1541944.

Mallakpour, S., Azadi, E., & Hussain, C. M. (2021). Recent breakthroughs of antibacterial and antiviral protective polymeric materials during COVID-19 pandemic and after pandemic: Coating, packaging, and textile applications. *Current Opinion in Colloid and Interface Science*, *55*. Available from https://doi.org/10.1016/j.cocis.2021.101480, http://www.elsevier.com/inca/publications/store/6/2/0/0/5/3.

Manabe, K., Nishizawa, S., Kyung, K. H., & Shiratori, S. (2014). Optical phenomena and antifrosting property on biomimetics slippery fluid-infused antireflective films via layer-by-layer comparison with superhydrophobic and antireflective films. *ACS Applied Materials and Interfaces*, *6*(16), 13985–13993. Available from https://doi.org/10.1021/am503352x, http://pubs.acs.org/journal/aamick.

Manolakis, Ioannis, & Azhar, Usaid (2020). Recent advances in mussel-inspired synthetic polymers as marine antifouling coatings. *Coatings*, *10*(7), 653. Available from https://doi.org/10.3390/coatings10070653.

Marić, S., & Vraneš, J. (2007). Characteristics and significance of microbial biofilm formation. *Periodicum Biologorum*, *109*(2), 115–121.

Maréchal, J. P., & Hellio, C. (2009). Challenges for the development of new non-toxic antifouling solutions. *International Journal of Molecular Sciences*, *10*(11), 4623–4637. Available from https://doi.org/10.3390/ijms10114623Martinique, http://www.mdpi.com/1422-0067/10/11/4623/pdf.

Ma, W., Li, Y., Zhang, M., Gao, S., Cui, J., Huang, C., & Fu, G. (2020). Biomimetic durable multifunctional self-cleaning nanofibrous membrane with outstanding oil/water separation, photodegradation of organic contaminants, and antibacterial performances. *ACS Applied Materials and Interfaces*, *12*(31), 34999–35010. Available from https://doi.org/10.1021/acsami.0c09059, http://pubs.acs.org/journal/aamick.

Medis, S., Dissanayake, T., Kottahachchi, J., Namali, D., Gunasekara, S., Wijesinghe, G., Dilrukshi, N., & Weerasekera, M. (2023). Biofilm formation and antibiotic resistance among Coagulase Negative Staphylococcus species isolated from central venous catheters of intensive care unit patients. *Indian Journal of Medical Microbiology*, *42*, 71–76. Available from https://doi.org/10.1016/j.ijmmb.2022.10.007, https://www.sciencedirect.com/journal/indian-journal-of-medical-microbiology/issues.

Michalska, M., Gambacorta, F., Divan, R., Aranson, I. S., Sokolov, A., Noirot, P., & Laible, P. D. (2018). Tuning antimicrobial properties of biomimetic nanopatterned surfaces. *Nanoscale*, *10*(14), 6639–6650. Available from https://doi.org/10.1039/c8nr00439k, http://pubs.rsc.org/en/journals/journal/nr.

Moerman, F. (2014). Antimicrobial materials, coatings and biomimetic surfaces with modified microtography to control microbial fouling of product contact surfaces within food processing equipment: legislation, requirements, effectiveness, and challenges. *Journal of Hygienic Engineering and Design*.

Mohd, Ghulam, Majid, Kowsar, & Lone, Saifullah (2023). Synergetic role of nano-/microscale structures of the Trifolium leaf surface for self-cleaning properties. *Langmuir: the ACS Journal of Surfaces and Colloids*, *39*(17), 6178–6187. Available from https://doi.org/10.1021/acs.langmuir.3c00317.

Moussa, D. G., Fok, A., & Aparicio, C. (2019). Hydrophobic and antimicrobial dentin: A peptide-based 2-tier protective system for dental resin composite restorations. *Acta Biomaterialia*, *88*, 251–265. Available from https://doi.org/10.1016/j.actbio.2019.02.007, http://www.journals.elsevier.com/acta-biomaterialia.

Muhammad, M. H., Idris, A. L., Fan, X., Guo, Y., Yu, Y., Jin, X., Qiu, J., Guan, X., & Huang, T. (2020). Beyond risk: Bacterial biofilms and their regulating approaches. *Frontiers in Microbiology*, *11*. Available from https://doi.org/10.3389/fmicb.2020.00928, https://www.frontiersin.org/journals/microbiology#.

Mérian, T., & Goddard, J. M. (2012). Advances in nonfouling materials: Perspectives for the food industry. *Journal of Agricultural and Food Chemistry*, *60*(12), 2943–2957. Available from https://doi.org/10.1021/jf204741p.

Negut, Irina, Bita, Bogdan, & Groza, Andreea (2022). Polymeric coatings and antimicrobial peptides as efficient systems for treating implantable medical devices associated-infections. *Polymers*, *14*(8), 1611. Available from https://doi.org/10.3390/polym14081611.

Novick, S. J., & Dordick, J. S. (2002). Protein-containing hydrophobic coatings and films. *Biomaterials*, *23*(2), 441–448. Available from https://doi.org/10.1016/S0142-9612(01)00123-5.

Nurioglu, A. G., Esteves, A. C. C., & De With, G. (2015). Non-toxic, non-biocide-release antifouling coatings based on molecular structure design for marine applications. *Journal of*

Materials Chemistry B, 3(32), 6547–6570. Available from https://doi.org/10.1039/c5tb00232j, http://pubs.rsc.org/en/journals/journalissues/tb.

Olsen, S. M., Pedersen, L. T., Laursen, M. H., Kiil, S., & Dam-Johansen, K. (2007). Enzyme-based antifouling coatings: A review. *Biofouling, 23*(5), 369–383. Available from https://doi.org/10.1080/08927010701566384.

Oopath, S. V., Baji, A., Abtahi, M., Luu, T. Q., Vasilev, K., & Truong, V. K. (2023). Nature-inspired biomimetic surfaces for controlling bacterial attachment and biofilm development. *Advanced Materials Interfaces, 10*(4). Available from https://doi.org/10.1002/admi.202201425, http://onlinelibrary.wiley.com/journal/10.1002/(ISSN)2196-7350.

Pangule, R. C., Brooks, S. J., Dinu, C. Z., Bale, S. S., Salmon, S. L., Zhu, G., Metzger, D. W., Kane, R. S., & Dordick, J. S. (2010). Antistaphylococcal nanocomposite films based on enzyme – Nanotube conjugates. *ACS Nano, 4*(7), 3993–4000. Available from https://doi.org/10.1021/nn100932t.

Park, S. G., Moon, J. H., Lee, S. K., Shim, J., & Yang, S. M. (2010). Bioinspired holographically featured superhydrophobic and supersticky nanostructured materials. *Langmuir: The ACS Journal of Surfaces and Colloids, 26*(3), 1468–1472. Available from https://doi.org/10.1021/la9035826, http://pubs.acs.org/doi/pdfplus/10.1021/la9035826, South Korea.

Patel, R., Osmon, D.R., & Hanssen, A.D. (2005). The diagnosis of prosthetic joint infection: Current techniques and emerging technologies. Clinical Orthopaedics and Related Research, 437, 55–58.

Peng, J., Wu, L., Zhang, H., Wang, B., Si, Y., Jin, S., & Zhu, H. (2022). Research progress on eco-friendly superhydrophobic materials in environment, energy and biology. *Chemical Communications, 58*(80), 11201–11219. Available from https://doi.org/10.1039/d2cc03899d, http://pubs.rsc.org/en/journals/journal/cc.

Pogodin, S., Hasan, J., Baulin, V. A., Webb, H. K., Truong, V. K., Phong Nguyen, T. H., Boshkovikj, V., Fluke, C. J., Watson, G. S., Watson, J. A., Crawford, R. J., & Ivanova, E. P. (2013). Biophysical model of bacterial cell interactions with nanopatterned cicada wing surfaces. *Biophysical Journal, 104*(4), 835–840. Available from https://doi.org/10.1016/j.bpj.2012.12.046.

Pérez, Hugo, Vargas, Gregorio, & Silva, Rodolfo (2022). Use of nanotechnology to mitigate biofouling in stainless steel devices used in food processing, healthcare, and marine environments. *Toxics, 10*(1), 35. Available from https://doi.org/10.3390/toxics10010035.

Rajaramon, S., David, H., Sajeevan, A., Shanmugam, K., Sriramulu, H., Dandela, R., & Solomon, A. P. (2023). Multi-functional approach in the design of smart surfaces to mitigate bacterial infections: a review. *Frontiers in Cellular and Infection Microbiology, 13.* Available from https://doi.org/10.3389/fcimb.2023.1139026, http://www.frontiersin.org/Cellular_and_Infection_Microbiology/archive.

Ramasamy, M., & Lee, J. (2016). Recent nanotechnology approaches for prevention and treatment of biofilm-associated infections on medical devices. *BioMed Research International, 2016.* Available from https://doi.org/10.1155/2016/1851242, http://www.hindawi.com/journals/biomed/.

Rao, K. M., Narayanan, K. B., Uthappa, U. T., Park, P. H., Choi, I., & Han, S. S. (2022). Tissue adhesive, self-healing, biocompatible, hemostasis, and antibacterial properties of fungal-derived carboxymethyl chitosan-polydopamine hydrogels. *Pharmaceutics, 14* (5). Available from https://doi.org/10.3390/pharmaceutics14051028, https://www.mdpi.com/1999-4923/14/5/1028/pdf?version = 1652179664.

Rather, M. A., Gupta, K., & Mandal, M. (2021). Microbial biofilm: Formation, architecture, antibiotic resistance, and control strategies. *Brazilian Journal of Microbiology, 52*(4), 1701–1718. Available from https://doi.org/10.1007/s42770-021-00624-x, https://link.springer.com/journal/42770.

Rodriguez-Emmenegger, Cesar, Decker, Antje, Surman, František, Preuss, Corinna M., Sedláková, Zdeňka, Zydziak, Nicolas, Barner-Kowollik, Christopher, Schwartz, Thomas, & Barner, Leonie (2014). Suppressing *Pseudomonas aeruginosa* adhesion via non-fouling polymer brushes. *RSC Advances*, *4*(110), 64781–64790. Available from https://doi.org/10.1039/c4ra12663g.

Roy, S., Hasan, I., & Guo, B. (2023). Recent advances in nanoparticle-mediated antibacterial applications. *Coordination Chemistry Reviews*, *482*. Available from https://doi.org/10.1016/j.ccr.2023.215075, http://www.journals.elsevier.com/coordination-chemistry-reviews/.

Roy, R., Tiwari, M., Donelli, G., & Tiwari, V. (2018). Strategies for combating bacterial biofilms: A focus on anti-biofilm agents and their mechanisms of action. *Virulence*, *9*(1), 522–554. Available from https://doi.org/10.1080/21505594.2017.1313372, http://www.tandfonline.com/loi/kvir20.

Ruzi, Mahmut, Celik, Nusret, & Serdar Onses, M. (2022). Superhydrophobic coatings for food packaging applications: A review. *Food Packaging and Shelf Life*, *32*, 100823. Available from https://doi.org/10.1016/j.fpsl.2022.100823.

Sakala, G. P., & Reches, M. (2018). Peptide-based approaches to fight biofouling. *Advanced Materials Interfaces*, *5*(18). Available from https://doi.org/10.1002/admi.201800073, http://onlinelibrary.wiley.com/journal/10.1002/(ISSN)2196-7350.

Sakamoto, A., Terui, Y., Horie, C., Fukui, T., Masuzawa, T., Sugawara, S., Shigeta, K., Shigeta, T., Igarashi, K., & Kashiwagi, K. (2014). Antibacterial effects of protruding and recessed shark skin micropatterned surfaces of polyacrylate plate with a shallow groove. *FEMS Microbiology Letters*, *361*(1), 10–16. Available from https://doi.org/10.1111/1574-6968.12604, http://femsle.oxfordjournals.org/.

Sarker, A., Mondal, S. C., Ahmmed, R., Rana, J., Waheda Rahman Ansary, M., & Bilal, M. (2022). *Prospects and challenges of polymer nanocomposites for innovative food packaging* Elsevier, South Korea*Smart polymer nanocomposites: design, synthesis, functionalization, properties, and applications* (pp. 355–377). South Korea: Elsevier. Available from https://www.sciencedirect.com/book/9780323916110, 10.1016/B978-0-323-91611-0.00021-9.

Sawai, J. (2003). Quantitative evaluation of antibacterial activities of metallic oxide powders (ZnO, MgO and CaO) by conductimetric assay. *Journal of Microbiological Methods*, *54*(2), 177–182. Available from https://doi.org/10.1016/S0167-7012(03)00037-X, http://www.elsevier.com/locate/jmicmeth.

Sawai, J., & Yoshikawa, T. (2004). Quantitative evaluation of antifungal activity of metallic oxide powders (MgO, CaO and ZnO) by an indirect conductimetric assay. *Journal of Applied Microbiology*, *96*(4), 803–809. Available from https://doi.org/10.1111/j.1365-2672.2004.02234.x, https://academic.oup.com/jambio.

Sedõ, J., Saiz-Poseu, J., Busqué, F., & Ruiz-Molina, D. (2013). Catechol-based biomimetic functional materials. *Advanced Materials*, *25*(5), 653–701. Available from https://doi.org/10.1002/adma.201202343.

Seijsing, F., Nilebäck, L., Öhman, O., Pasupuleti, R., Ståhl, C., Seijsing, J., & Hedhammar, M. (2020). Recombinant spider silk coatings functionalized with enzymes targeting bacteria and biofilms. *MicrobiologyOpen*, *9*(4). Available from https://doi.org/10.1002/mbo3.993, http://onlinelibrary.wiley.com/journal/10.1002/(ISSN)2045-8827.

Seyfi, R., Kahaki, F. A., Ebrahimi, T., Montazersaheb, S., Eyvazi, S., Babaeipour, V., & Tarhriz, V. (2020). Antimicrobial peptides (AMPs): Roles, functions and mechanism of action. *International Journal of Peptide Research and Therapeutics*, *26*(3), 1451–1463. Available from https://doi.org/10.1007/s10989-019-09946-9, http://www.springer-online.com/sgw/cda/frontpage/0,11855,4-40109-70-35677487-0,00.html.

Shirtcliffe, N. J., McHale, G., & I. Newton, M. (2011). The superhydrophobicity of polymer surfaces: Recent developments. *Journal of Polymer Science, Part B: Polymer Physics, 49*(17), 1203–1217. Available from https://doi.org/10.1002/polb.22286.

Shi, Chang, Chen, Xi, Zhang, Zhuying, Chen, Qihao, Shi, Dongjian, & Kaneko, Daisaku (2020). Mussel inspired bio-adhesive with multi-interactions for tissue repair. *Journal of Biomaterials Science, Polymer Edition, 31*(4), 491–503. Available from https://doi.org/10.1080/09205063.2019.1702276.

Solga, A., Cerman, Z., Striffler, B.F., Spaeth, M., & Barthlott, W. (2007). The dream of staying clean: Lotus and biomimetic surfaces. *Bioinspiration & Biomimetics, 2*, S126–S134. Available from https://doi.org/10.1088/1748-3182/2/4/S02.

Sousa, M. P., & Mano, J. F. (2017). Cell-adhesive bioinspired and catechol-based multilayer freestanding membranes for bone tissue engineering. *Biomimetics, 2*(4). Available from https://doi.org/10.3390/biomimetics2040019, https://res.mdpi.com/d_attachment/biomimetics/biomimetics-02-00019/article_deploy/biomimetics-02-00019-v2.pdf.

Stillger, L., & Müller, D. (2022). Peptide-coating combating antimicrobial contaminations: a review of covalent immobilization strategies for industrial applications. *Journal of Materials Science, 57*(24), 10863–10885. Available from https://doi.org/10.1007/s10853-022-07266-w, http://www.springer.com/journal/10853.

Su, C., Hu, Y., Song, Q., Ye, Y., Gao, L., Li, P., & Ye, T. (2020). Initiated chemical vapor deposition of graded polymer coatings enabling antibacterial, antifouling, and biocompatible surfaces. *ACS Applied Materials and Interfaces, 12*(16), 18978–18986. Available from https://doi.org/10.1021/acsami.9b22611, http://pubs.acs.org/journal/aamick.

Szilágyi, Imre Miklós, Teucher, Georg, Härkönen, Emma, Färm, Elina, Hatanpää, Timo, Nikitin, Timur, Khriachtchev, Leonid, Räsänen, Markku, Ritala, Mikko, & Leskelä, Markku (2013). Programming nanostructured soft biological surfaces by atomic layer deposition. *Nanotechnology, 24*(24), 245701. Available from https://doi.org/10.1088/0957-4484/24/24/245701.

Thallinger, B., Prasetyo, E. N., Nyanhongo, G. S., & Guebitz, G. M. (2013). Antimicrobial enzymes: An emerging strategy to fight microbes and microbial biofilms. *Biotechnology Journal, 8*(1), 97–109. Available from https://doi.org/10.1002/biot.201200313.

Thapa, R. K., Diep, D. B., & Tønnesen, H. H. (2021). Nanomedicine-based antimicrobial peptide delivery for bacterial infections: Recent advances and future prospects. *Journal of Pharmaceutical Investigation, 51*(4), 377–398. Available from https://doi.org/10.1007/s40005-021-00525-z, http://www.springer.com/biomed/journal/40005.

Tian, J., Yang, G., Huang, H., Liu, M., Liu, L., Zhang, X., & Wei, Y. (2020). Recent progress and development for the fabrication of antibacterial materials through mussel-inspired chemistry. *Journal of Environmental Chemical Engineering, 8*(6). Available from https://doi.org/10.1016/j.jece.2020.104383, http://www.journals.elsevier.com/journal-of-environmental-chemical-engineering/.

Townsend, L., Williams, R. L., Anuforom, O., Berwick, M. R., Halstead, F., Hughes, E., Stamboulis, A., Oppenheim, B., Gough, J., Grover, L., Scott, R. A. H., Webber, M., Peacock, A. F. A., Belli, A., Logan, A., & De Cogan, F. (2017). Antimicrobial peptide coatings for hydroxyapatite: Electrostatic and covalent attachment of antimicrobial peptides to surfaces. *Journal of the Royal Society Interface, 14*(126). Available from https://doi.org/10.1098/rsif.2016.0657, http://rsif.royalsocietypublishing.org/content/royinterface/14/126/20160657.full.pdf.

Tripathy, A., Sen, P., Su, B., & Briscoe, W. H. (2017). Natural and bioinspired nanostructured bactericidal surfaces. *Advances in Colloid and Interface Science, 248*, 85–104. Available from https://doi.org/10.1016/j.cis.2017.07.030.

Valiei, A., Lin, N., Bryche, J. F., McKay, G., Canva, M., Charette, P. G., Nguyen, D., Moraes, C., & Tufenkji, N. (2020). Hydrophilic mechano-bactericidal nanopillars require external forces to rapidly kill bacteria. *Nano Letters*, *20*(8), 5720–5727. Available from https://doi.org/10.1021/acs.nanolett.0c01343, http://pubs.acs.org/journal/nalefd.

Van Oss, C. J., Good, R. J., & Chaudhury, M. K. (1991). *Theory of adhesive forces across interfaces. Fundamentals of adhesion* (pp. 153–172). Springer. Available from https://doi.org/10.1007/978-1-4899-2073-7_4.

Vaterrodt, A., Thallinger, B., Daumann, K., Koch, D., Guebitz, G. M., & Ulbricht, M. (2016). Antifouling and Antibacterial multifunctional polyzwitterion/enzyme coating on silicone catheter material prepared by electrostatic layer-by-layer assembly. *Langmuir: The ACS Journal of Surfaces and Colloids*, *32*(5), 1347–1359. Available from https://doi.org/10.1021/acs.langmuir.5b04303, http://pubs.acs.org/journal/langd5.

Viswanathan, V., Laha, T., Balani, K., Agarwal, A., & Seal, S. (2006). Challenges and advances in nanocomposite processing techniques. *Materials Science and Engineering R: Reports*, *54*(5-6), 121–285. Available from https://doi.org/10.1016/j.mser.2006.11.002.

Wang, L., Guo, X., Zhang, H., Liu, Y., Wang, Y., Liu, K., Liang, H., & Ming, W. (2022). Recent advances in superhydrophobic and antibacterial coatings for biomedical materials. *Coatings*, *12*(10). Available from https://doi.org/10.3390/coatings12101469, http://www.mdpi.com/journal/coatings.

Wang, Tao, Huang, Lei, Liu, Yuzhi, Li, Xingxing, Liu, Chunhua, Handschuh-Wang, Stephan, Xu, Yang, Zhao, Ying, & Tang, Yongbing (2020). Robust biomimetic hierarchical diamond architecture with a self-cleaning, antibacterial, and antibiofouling surface. *ACS Applied Materials & Interfaces*, *12*(21), 24432–24441. Available from https://doi.org/10.1021/acsami.0c02460.

Wang, L. S., Xu, S., Gopal, S., Kim, E., Kim, D., Brier, M., Solanki, K., & Dordick, J. S. (2021). Facile fabrication of antibacterial and antiviral perhydrolase-polydopamine composite coatings. *Scientific Reports*, *11*(1). Available from https://doi.org/10.1038/s41598-021-91925-6, http://www.nature.com/srep/index.html.

Wang, Y., Yan, L., Cheng, R., Muhtar, M., Shan, X., Xiang, Y., & Cui, W. (2018). Multifunctional HA/Cu nano-coatings on titanium using PPy coordination and doping: Via pulse electrochemical polymerization. *Biomaterials Science*, *6*(3), 575–585. Available from https://doi.org/10.1039/c7bm01104k, http://pubs.rsc.org/en/journals/journal/bm.

Watson, G. S., Cribb, B. W., Schwarzkopf, L., & Watson, J. A. (2015). Contaminant adhesion (aerial/ground biofouling) on the skin of a gecko. *Journal of the Royal Society Interface*, *12*(108). Available from https://doi.org/10.1098/rsif.2015.0318, http://rsif.royalsocietypublishing.org/content/royinterface/12/108/20150318.full.pdf.

Watson, G. S., Green, D. W., Cribb, B. W., Brown, C. L., Meritt, C. R., Tobin, M. J., Vongsvivut, J., Sun, M., Liang, A. P., & Watson, J. A. (2017). Insect analogue to the lotus leaf: A planthopper wing membrane incorporating a low-adhesion, nonwetting, superhydrophobic, bactericidal, and biocompatible surface. *ACS Applied Materials and Interfaces*, *9*(28), 24381–24392. Available from https://doi.org/10.1021/acsami.7b08368, http://pubs.acs.org/journal/aamick.

Watson, G. S., Green, D. W., Schwarzkopf, L., Li, X., Cribb, B. W., Myhra, S., & Watson, J. A. (2015). A gecko skin micro/nano structure – A low adhesion, superhydrophobic, anti-wetting, self-cleaning, biocompatible, antibacterial surface. *Acta Biomaterialia*, *21*, 109–122. Available from https://doi.org/10.1016/j.actbio.2015.03.007, http://www.journals.elsevier.com/acta-biomaterialia.

Wen, L., Weaver, J. C., & Lauder, G. V. (2014). Biomimetic shark skin: Design, fabrication and hydrodynamic function. *Journal of Experimental Biology*, *217*(10), 1656–1666. Available from https://doi.org/10.1242/jeb.097097, http://jeb.biologists.org/content/217/10/1656.full.pdf + html.

Xiao, Yu, Wang, Wenxuan, Tian, Xiaohua, Tan, Xing, Yang, Tong, Gao, Peng, Xiong, Kaiqing, Tu, Qiufen, Wang, Miao, Maitz, Manfred F., Huang, Nan, Pan, Guoqing, & Yang, Zhilu (2020). A versatile surface bioengineering strategy based on mussel-inspired and bioclickable peptide mimic. *Research; a Journal of Science and its Applications, 2020.* Available from https://doi.org/10.34133/2020/7236946.

Xie, Y. Y., Wang, X. Q., Sun, M. Y., Qin, X. T., Su, X. F., Ma, X. F., Liu, X. Z., Zhong, C., & Jia, S. R. (2022). Heterochiral peptide-based biocompatible and injectable supramolecular hydrogel with antibacterial activity. *Journal of Materials Science*, *57*(8), 5198–5209. Available from https://doi.org/10.1007/s10853-022-06982-7, http://www.springer.com/journal/10853.

Xiong, Xueqing, Huang, Yanyan, Lin, Changxu, Liu, Xiang Yang, & Lin, Youhui (2019). Recent advances in nanoparticulate biomimetic catalysts for combating bacteria and biofilms. *Nanoscale*, *11*(46), 22206–22215. Available from https://doi.org/10.1039/c9nr05054j.

Yamamoto, M., Nishikawa, N., Mayama, H., Nonomura, Y., Yokojima, S., Nakamura, S., & Uchida, K. (2015). Theoretical explanation of the lotus effect: Superhydrophobic property changes by removal of nanostructures from the surface of a lotus leaf. *Langmuir: the ACS Journal of Surfaces and Colloids*, *31*(26), 7355–7363. Available from https://doi.org/10.1021/acs.langmuir.5b00670, http://pubs.acs.org/journal/langd5.

Yang, Y., Liang, Y., Chen, J., Duan, X., & Guo, B. (2022). Mussel-inspired adhesive antioxidant antibacterial hemostatic composite hydrogel wound dressing via photopolymerization for infected skin wound healing. *Bioactive Materials*, *8*, 341–354. Available from https://doi.org/10.1016/j.bioactmat.2021.06.014, http://www.keaipublishing.com/en/journals/bioactive-materials/.

Yang, Xiao, Zhang, Wei, Qin, Xuezhi, Cui, Miaomiao, Guo, Yunting, Wang, Ting, Wang, Kaiqiang, Shi, Zhenqiang, Zhang, Chao, Li, Wanbo, & Wang, Zuankai (2022). Recent progress on bioinspired antibacterial surfaces for biomedical application. *Biomimetics*, 7(3), 88. Available from https://doi.org/10.3390/biomimetics7030088.

Yan, Y., Li, Y., Zhang, Z., Wang, X., Niu, Y., Zhang, S., Xu, W., & Ren, C. (2021). Advances of peptides for antibacterial applications. *Colloids and Surfaces B: Biointerfaces*, *202*, 18734367. Available from https://doi.org/10.1016/j.colsurfb.2021.111682, http://www.elsevier.com/locate/colsurfb.

Yebra, D. M., Kiil, S., & Dam-Johansen, K. (2004). Antifouling technology – Past, present and future steps towards efficient and environmentally friendly antifouling coatings. *Progress in Organic Coatings*, *50*(2), 75–104. Available from https://doi.org/10.1016/j.porgcoat.2003.06.001.

Ye, Q., Zhou, F., & Liu, W. (2011). Bioinspired catecholic chemistry for surface modification. *Chemical Society Reviews*, *40*(7), 4244–4258. Available from https://doi.org/10.1039/c1cs15026j.

Ye, Z., Zhu, X., Mutreja, I., Boda, S. K., Fischer, N. G., Zhang, A., Lui, C., Qi, Y., & Aparicio, C. (2021). Biomimetic mineralized hybrid scaffolds with antimicrobial peptides. *Bioactive Materials*, *6*(8), 2250–2260. Available from https://doi.org/10.1016/j.bioactmat.2020.12.029, http://www.keaipublishing.com/en/journals/bioactive-materials/.

Yildiz, T., Durdu, S., Ozcan, K., & Usta, M. (2023). Characterization and investigation of biological properties of silver nanoparticle-doped hydroxyapatite-based surfaces on zirconium. *Scientific Reports*, *13*(1). Available from https://doi.org/10.1038/s41598-023-33992-5, https://www.nature.com/srep/.

Yuan, J., Zhang, D., He, X., Ni, Y., Che, L., Wu, J., Wu, B., Wang, Y., Wang, S., Sha, D., Zheng, S. Y., & Yang, J. (2021). Cationic peptide-based salt-responsive antibacterial hydrogel dressings for wound healing. *International Journal of Biological*

Macromolecules, *190*, 754–762. Available from https://doi.org/10.1016/j.ijbiomac.2021.09.019, http://www.elsevier.com/locate/ijbiomac.

Yu, Kai, Alzahrani, Amal, Khoddami, Sara, Cheng, John T. J., Mei, Yan, Gill, Arshdeep, Luo, Haiming D., Haney, Evan F., Hilpert, Kai, Hancock, Robert E. W., Lange, Dirk, & Kizhakkedathu, Jayachandran N. (2021). Rapid assembly of infection-resistant coatings: screening and identification of antimicrobial peptides works in cooperation with an antifouling background. *ACS Applied Materials & Interfaces*, *13*(31), 36784–36799. Available from https://doi.org/10.1021/acsami.1c07515.

Zardus, J. D., Nedved, B. T., Huang, Y., Tran, C., & Hadfield, M. G. (2008). Microbial biofilms facilitate adhesion in biofouling invertebrates. *Biological Bulletin*, *214*(1), 91–98. Available from https://doi.org/10.2307/25066663, http://www.biolbull.org/.

Zhang, Xin, Bai, Rushui, Sun, Qiannan, Zhuang, Zimeng, Zhang, Yunfan, Chen, Si, & Han, Bing (2022). Bio-inspired special wettability in oral antibacterial applications. *Frontiers in Bioengineering and Biotechnology*, *10*. Available from https://doi.org/10.3389/fbioe.2022.1001616.

Zhang, Junping, & Seeger, Stefan (2013). Silica/silicone nanofilament hybrid coatings with almost perfect superhydrophobicity. *Chemphyschem: a European Journal of Chemical Physics and Physical Chemistry*, *14*(8), 1646–1651. Available from https://doi.org/10.1002/cphc.201200995.

Zhang, X., Wang, L., & Levänen, E. (2013). Superhydrophobic surfaces for the reduction of bacterial adhesion. *RSC Advances*, *3*(30), 12003–12020. Available from https://doi.org/10.1039/c3ra40497h, http://pubs.rsc.org/en/journals/journalissues.

Zhang, W., Wang, R., Sun, Z. M., Zhu, X., Zhao, Q., Zhang, T., Cholewinski, A., Yang, F., Zhao, B., Pinnaratip, R., Forooshani, P. K., & Lee, B. P. (2020). Catechol-functionalized hydrogels: Biomimetic design, adhesion mechanism, and biomedical applications. *Chemical Society Reviews*, *49*(2), 433–464. Available from https://doi.org/10.1039/c9cs00285e, http://pubs.rsc.org/en/journals/journal/cs.

Zhang, C., Wu, B., Zhou, Y., Zhou, F., Liu, W., & Wang, Z. (2020). Mussel-inspired hydrogels: From design principles to promising applications. *Chemical Society Reviews*, *49*(11), 3605–3637. Available from https://doi.org/10.1039/c9cs00849g, http://pubs.rsc.org/en/journals/journal/cs.

Zhao, Y., Guo, Q., Dai, X., Wei, X., Yu, Y., Chen, X., Li, C., Cao, Z., & Zhang, X. (2019). A biomimetic non-antibiotic approach to eradicate drug-resistant infections. *Advanced Materials*, *31*(7). Available from https://doi.org/10.1002/adma.201806024, http://onlinelibrary.wiley.com/journal/10.1002/(ISSN)1521-4095.

CHAPTER 12

Future of biomimicry in the field of smart coatings

Saman Zehra
Corrosion Research Laboratory, Department of Applied Chemistry, Faculty of Engineering and Technology, Aligarh Muslim University, Aligarh, Uttar Pradesh, India

12.1 Introduction

Biomimetic coatings area cutting-edge area at the nexus of materials science, biology, and engineering, a subset of biomimicry or bioinspired technology (Fadok, 2022). The profound insight that nature has evolved perfect solutions to a wide range of problems over millions of years is the origin of biomimetic coatings. The natural world provides a wealth of creative design ideas, from self-cleaning surfaces fashioned after lotus leaves to antireflective coatings modeled after moth eyes (Jiang & Feng, 2010).

The need for high-performance, sustainable, and efficient materials and technologies is what drives the development of biomimetic coatings. Researchers and enterprises have looked for alternatives that are more in tune with the fundamentals of nature because conventional manufacturing and engineering methods frequently result in environmental damage and resource depletion (Haapala et al., 2013). This is where biomimicry, which uses biological systems as a model to develop solutions to human problems, represents a paradigm shift.

Biomimetic coatings provide practical surface coatings with exceptional qualities by using the inherent brilliance of biological adaptations and processes (Pereira et al., 2015; Shimomura, 2010; Xia, 2016). These coatings are designed to closely resemble or directly imitate the structural and functional characteristics present in biological things. The objective is to comprehend the fundamental mechanisms, components, and processes that control natural systems rather than only superficially imitating nature. This knowledge is the basis for creating coatings with features such as self-healing, water resistance, antifouling, adhesion, and optical qualities.

A number of causes, such as the pressing need for sustainable solutions, the need for sophisticated materials across various sectors, and the ongoing

Smart Biomimetic Coatings
DOI: https://doi.org/10.1016/B978-0-443-21738-8.00012-6

breakthroughs in materials science and nanotechnology, are driving the growing interest in biomimetic coatings. To develop coatings that might transform industries as diverse as aerospace, healthcare, automotive, architecture, and renewable energy, researchers and engineers are investigating fresh biomimetic principles.

Additionally, biomimetic coatings show potential for tackling important global issues including climate change mitigation and environmental conservation. These coatings have the ability to reduce resource consumption, cut waste, and improve the general eco-friendliness of products and technology by embracing the biomimicry principles. The future of biomimetic coatings is extremely important on a number of levels, from sustainability and technical progress to economic growth and environmental preservation. Appreciating the revolutionary potential of biomimetic coatings in diverse industries and sectors requires an understanding of their relevance. The future of biomimetic antifouling coating is represented in Fig. 12.1.

In this chapter, we will look at how biomimetic coatings, which provide environment-friendly solutions influenced by nature, are positioned to change the face of materials science and technology in the years to come. We will examine prospective applications, difficulties, and future views of biomimetic coatings in the next sections of this chapter as we dive into the changing trends and outlooks in this field.

12.2 The impact of biomimetic coatings on sustainable practices

Because biomimetic coatings provide cutting-edge solutions that are compatible with environmental stewardship, resource conservation, and eco-friendly technology, their influence on sustainable practices is extensive and diverse. By encouraging resource efficiency, minimizing environmental harm, and assisting in the development of more responsible and environment-friendly technology, biomimetic coatings have a beneficial effect on sustainable practices. Contribution of these coatings to increasing sustainability is probably going to grow as they develop and find new uses. The following are a few ways that biomimetic coatings promote sustainability, and the outline is illustrated in Fig. 12.2 (Jatsch et al., 2023; Ilieva et al., 2022):

- Reduced environmental footprint: In comparison to conventional coatings, biomimetic coatings frequently need fewer resources and chemicals during manufacture. Using fewer resources and producing less trash results in a lower environmental imprint.

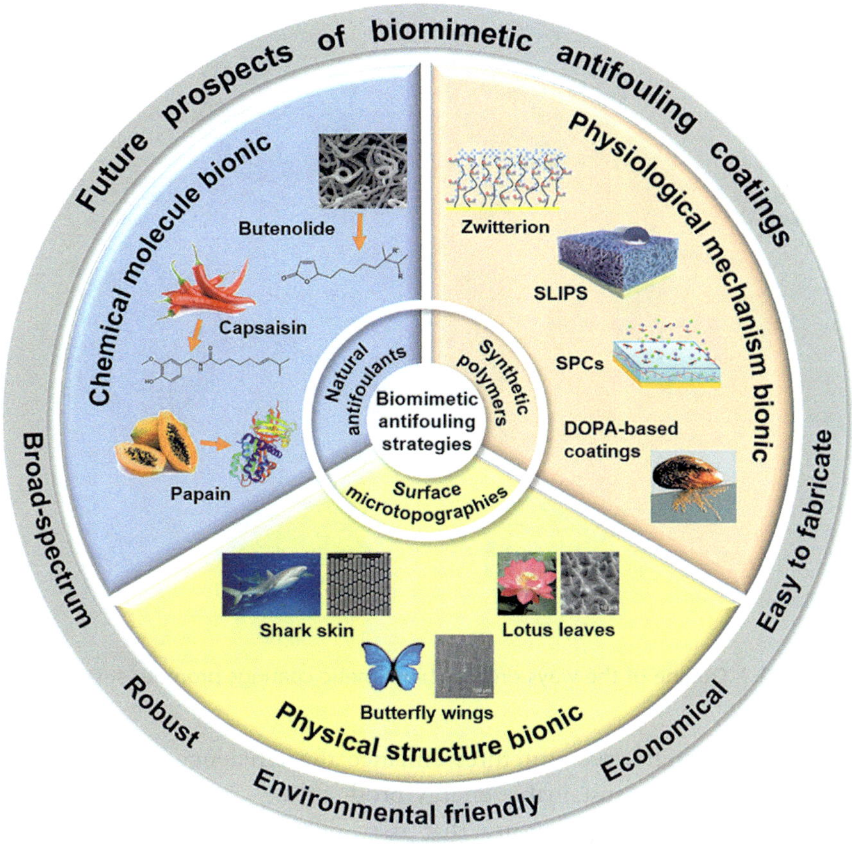

Figure 12.1 General illustration of the future prospect of biomimetic antifouling coatings. *From Chen, L., Duan, Y., Cui, M., Huang, R., Su, R., Qi, W. & He, Z. (2021). Science of the total environment, 766, 144469. https://doi.org/10.1016/j.scitotenv.2020.144469.*

- Longer product lifespan: Biomimetic coatings improve the robustness and endurance of goods and constructions. They aid in resource saving and waste reduction by lowering the frequency of replacements or maintenance.
- Reduced chemical usage: Many biomimetic coatings are designed to be self-cleaning or antifouling, reducing the need for harsh chemical cleaning agents. This minimizes chemical pollution and potential harm to ecosystems.
- Energy efficiency: Biomimetic coatings can improve the energy efficiency of various applications. For example, coatings inspired by

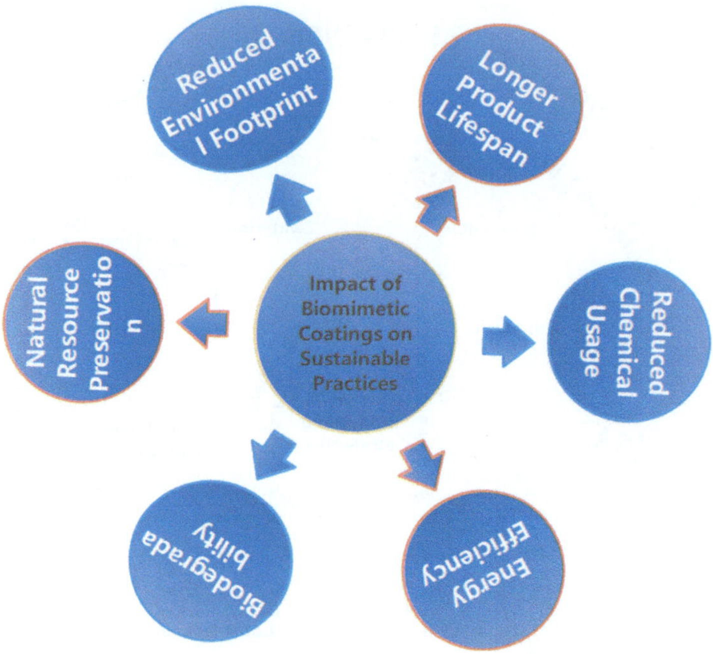

Figure 12.2 Outline of the ways on how biomimetic coatings promote sustainability.

natural antireflective structures enhance the efficiency of solar panels, leading to more sustainable energy production.

- Biodegradability: To ensure that they decompose organically at the end of their life cycle and lessen the load of persistent pollutants, certain biomimetic coatings are made from biodegradable materials.
- Natural resource preservation: Biomimetic coatings can reduce the wear and tear on machinery and equipment, preserving natural resources by extending the life of these assets.

12.3 Expanding sectors for biomimetic coatings

With their distinctive qualities and adaptability, biomimetic coatings are finding use in various industries. The potential influence of these coatings might be seen across many industries as they develop, providing creative answers to challenging problems (Ganeshkumar et al., 2023). The following sections discusses on some of the developing industries where biomimetic coatings are prospering (Srishti et al., 2023).

12.3.1 Aerospace and aviation

Biomimetic coatings are utilized in the aircraft sector to lower drag and increase fuel economy. For instance, coatings modeled after shark skin can reduce turbulence and improve an aircraft's aerodynamics.

12.3.2 Healthcare and biomedical equipment

The creation of biocompatible materials for surgical implants, medication delivery systems, and tissue engineering depends heavily on biomimetic coatings. They can improve the durability and functionality of medical equipment.

12.3.3 Automotive industry

Biomimetic coatings are advantageous for the automobile industry as they increase vehicle safety and economy. These coatings can improve self-cleaning abilities, lessen wind resistance, and offer antifogging qualities for windshields and mirrors.

12.3.4 Architecture and construction

Biomimetic coatings aid in the creation of energy-efficient building plans in sustainable architecture. Temperature and humidity may be controlled via coatings modeled after termite mounds and plant surfaces, which eliminates the need for heating and cooling equipment.

12.3.5 Marine and shipping

In the maritime sector, biomimetic coatings are used to stop biofouling on ship hulls, lowering fuel consumption and maintenance costs. These coatings imitate antifouling techniques of marine species.

12.3.6 Electronics and optics

Antireflective surfaces, optical coatings, and self-cleaning screens for electrical gadgets are all made possible by biomimetic coatings. They increase the longevity and visibility of screens.

12.3.7 Environmental remediation

Environmental uses of biomimetic coatings, such as soil restoration and water filtration, are being investigated. They can imitate filtration and adsorption capabilities of natural systems.

12.3.8 Space exploration

Biomimetic coatings are being studied for their potential to reduce problems with space debris and radiation exposure in space travel.

12.3.9 Food packaging and preservation

By emulating natural barriers against moisture, gases, and pollutants, biomimetic coatings are employed in food packaging to extend the shelf life and safety of perishable goods.

12.3.10 Defense and security

Military camouflage systems can use biomimetic coatings to provide adaptable coloring and concealment that are modeled after animal adaptations. The extraordinary potential of nature-inspired solutions to solve a wide range of difficulties in the modern world is demonstrated by the likelihood that fresh uses for biomimetic coatings will be discovered in developing industries as they continue to evolve.

12.4 Key insights on the future of biomimetic coatings

Future innovations, trends, and opportunities in the field of biomimetic coatings will influence it in the years to come (Srishti et al., 2023). Here are some salient conclusions:

1. Sustainability will be a major concern for biomimetic coatings in the future. These coatings are anticipated to be crucial in helping all sectors to reduce resource use, waste, and environmental effect.
2. Biomimetic coatings will keep improving and eventually serve several functions in one application. More and more coatings will have properties such as self-healing, self-cleaning, and anticorrosion.
3. Coatings will be more effective, long-lasting, and efficient thanks to developments in materials science, such as the creation of brand-new biomimetic materials and nanotechnology.
4. To maximize the potential of biomimetic coatings, cooperation between several disciplines such as biology, materials science, engineering, and design will be even more important.
5. As the advantages of biomimetic coatings are more generally understood, they will permeate a wider range of industries, such as agriculture, renewable energy, and consumer goods.

Therefore sustainability, creativity, teamwork, and a widening spectrum of applications will characterize the future of biomimetic coatings. These coatings have the potential to transform technology, lessen environmental impact, and contribute to a more robust and sustainable future as they become more incorporated into numerous sectors.

12.5 Limitations in the field of biomimetic coatings

Although the science of biomimetic coatings has advanced significantly, there are still many restrictions and difficulties. To realize the full potential of biomimetic coatings, scientists and engineers are actively attempting to address these challenges. Biological systems frequently have elaborate structures and are quite complex (Wolkenhauer et al., 2011). It can be difficult to replicate this complexity in coatings. To address this issue, researchers are creating sophisticated modeling and simulation methods that will help them better comprehend and recreate complex biological systems (Kriete and Eils, 2013). Advanced materials and nanotechnology also make it possible to create complex biomimetic coatings (Zhou et al., 2020). The duration and robustness provide another difficulty. There are questions regarding the long-term performance and upkeep needs of some biomimetic coatings as they could not be as resilient as conventional coatings. More durable and long-lasting biomimetic coatings are being developed as a result of advances in materials science and nanotechnology to meet this issue. Concerns about durability are also being addressed by research on self-repairing and self-healing coatings.

Scalability and cost are further issues in the industry. Widespread adoption may be constrained by the cost-effectiveness of the materials and the scalability of biomimetic coating manufacture. However, it is crucial to keep looking into scalable production techniques and reasonably priced biomimetic materials (Nazir et al., 2023). It may be possible to narrow the gap between research and commercialization by working with industrial partners. Biologists, materials scientists, engineers, and designers all have skills that are needed for biomimetic coatings. It can be difficult to collaborate effectively. Knowledge sharing and cooperative innovation may be supported through supporting multidisciplinary research and collaborations between government, business, and academic organizations.

Continuous investigation, cooperation, and invention in the area of biomimetic coatings are necessary to overcome these constraints. Biomimetic coatings have the potential to transform several sectors and contribute to sustainable and environment-friendly technology when these difficulties are overcome.

12.6 Conclusion

The future of the biomimetic coatings will be determined by innovation, sustainability, and cross-disciplinary cooperation. Looking ahead, it is certain that biomimetic coatings will continue to revolutionize sectors and provide innovative solutions to global problems. These coatings, which draw their inspiration from nature's beauty, will be at the forefront of sustainable practices, minimizing environmental footprints and advancing eco-friendly technology. With their multifunctional and specialized solutions, they will be crucial in the aerospace, healthcare, energy, and numerous other industries.

The development of biomimetic coatings will be influenced by improvements in materials, cross-industry innovation, and ethical issues. Their responsible incorporation into numerous applications will be guided by regulatory bodies and international cooperation. Future generations will be encouraged through education and awareness to investigate biomimicry concepts, ensuring that nature remains an endless source of inspiration.

In a world that is always changing, biomimetic coatings will promote sustainability, improve resilience, and reduce climate change. In conclusion, biomimetic coatings have a promising future and hold the promise of a world where technology and nature coexist peacefully for the benefit of both people and the environment. As we begin this thrilling trip, we discover that we are at the nexus of innovation and conservation, where the infinite wisdom of nature inspires solutions only constrained by our imagination.

Acknowledgments

One of the authors gratefully acknowledges funding from the Department of Science and Technology (DST), New Delhi, India, for the funding under the Women Scientist (WOS-A) program [File number: SR-WOS-A-ET-54-2019].

References

Kriete, A., & Eils., R. (2013). *Computational systems biology: From molecular mechanisms to disease*. Academic press.

Fadok, R.A. (2022). Massachusetts Institute of Technology.

Ganeshkumar, S., Kumar, A., Maniraj, J., Suresh Babu, Y., Kumar Ansu, A., Goyal, A., Kareem Kadhim, I., Saxena, K. K., Prakash, C., Altuijri, R., Ijaz Khan, M., & Hassan, A. M. (2023). Exploring the potential of nano technology: A assessment of nano-scale multi-layered-composite coatings for cutting tool performance. *Arabian Journal of Chemistry*, *16*(10), 105173. Available from https://doi.org/10.1016/j.arabjc.2023.105173, https://www.sciencedirect.com/science/article/pii/S1878535223006354.

Haapala, K. R., Zhao, F., Camelio, J., Sutherland, J. W., Skerlos, S. J., Dornfeld, D. A., Jawahir, I., Clarens, A. F., & Rickli, J. L. (2013). *Journal of Manufacturing Science and Engineering, 135.*

Ilieva, L., Ursano, I., Traista, L., Hoffmann, B., & Dahy, H. (2022). Biomimicry as a sustainable design methodology—Introducing the 'Biomimicry for Sustainability' framework. *Biomimetics*, 7(2), 37. Available from https://doi.org/10.3390/biomimetics7020037.

Jatsch, A. S., Jacobs, S., Wommer, K., & Wanieck, K. (2023). Biomimetics for sustainable developments—A literature overview of trends. *Biomimetics*, *8*(3). Available from https://doi.org/10.3390/biomimetics8030304, http://www.mdpi.com/journal/biomimetics.

Jiang, L., & Feng, L. (2010). *Bioinspired intelligent nanostructured interfacial materials*. World Scientific.

Nazir, A., Gokcekaya, O., Md Masum Billah, K., Ertugrul, O., Jiang, J., Sun, J., & Hussain, S. (2023). Multi-material additive manufacturing: A systematic review of design, properties, applications, challenges, and 3D printing of materials and cellular metamaterials. *Materials & Design*, *226*111661. Available from https://doi.org/10.1016/j.matdes.2023.111661.

Pereira, P., Monteiro, G., Prazeres, D. (2015). Biotechnologies and biomimetics for civil engineering.

Shimomura, M. (2010). NISTEP Science & Technology Foresight Center.

Srishti, Kumar, A., Sinhamahapatra, A. (2023), Biomimetics in smart coatings. In *Antiviral and antimicrobial smart coatings: Fundamentals and applications* (pp. 263–285). Elsevier, India. Available from https://doi.org/10.1016/B978-0-323-99291-6.00013-X, https://www.sciencedirect.com/book/9780323992916.

Wolkenhauer, O., Muir, A., Hooker, C. (2011). The complexity of cell-biological systems. *Handbook of the Philosophy of Science*. 10. North-Holland, Amsterdam. Available from https://doi.org/10.1016/B978-0-444-52076-0.50013-4, https://www.sciencedirect.com/science/article/pii/B9780444520760500134.

Xia, Z. (2016). *Biomimetic principles and design of advanced engineering materials*. Wiley. Available from 10.1002/9781118926253.

Zhou, J., Kroll, A. V., Holay, M., Fang, R. H., & Zhang, L. (2020). Biomimetic nanotechnology toward personalized vaccines. *Advanced Materials*, *32*(13). Available from https://doi.org/10.1002/adma.201901255.

Index

Note: Page numbers followed by "*f*" and "*t*" refer to figures and tables, respectively.

C

9780443217388